Personal Stress Management

Personal Stress Management

From Surviving to Thriving

Dianne Hales
with Julia Hales

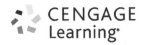
CENGAGE
Learning·

Australia • Brazil • Mexico • Singapore • United Kingdom • United States

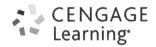

Personal Stress Management: From Surviving to Thriving
Dianne Hales, Julia Hales

Product Director: Dawn Giovanniello

Product Manager: Krista Mastroianni

Content Developer: Miriam Myers

Marketing Manager: Ana Albinson

Product Assistant: Marina Starkey

Senior Content Project Manager: Tanya Nigh

Digital Content Specialist: Jennifer Chinn

Intellectual Property Analyst:
Christine Myaskovsky

Intellectual Property Project Manager:
Erika Mugavin

Manufacturing Planner: Karen Hunt

Production Service and Compositor:
MPS Limited

Photo and Text Researcher:
Lumina Datamatics Limited

Art Director and Cover Designer:
Michael Cook

Text Designer: Liz Harasymczuk

Cover Image: Getty/Izf

For product information and technology assistance, contact us at
Cengage Learning Customer & Sales Support, 1-800-354-9706.

For permission to use material from this text or product,
submit all requests online at **www.cengage.com/permissions.**
Further permissions questions can be e-mailed to
permissionrequest@cengage.com.

Library of Congress Control Number: 2016933700

ISBN: 978-1-133-36431-3

Cengage Learning
20 Channel Center Street
Boston, MA 02210
USA

Cengage Learning is a leading provider of customized learning solutions with employees residing in nearly 40 different countries and sales in more than 125 countries around the world. Find your local representative at **www.cengage.com.**

Cengage Learning products are represented in Canada by
Nelson Education, Ltd.

To learn more about Cengage Learning Solutions, visit **www.cengage.com.**

Purchase any of our products at your local college store or at our preferred online store **www.cengagebrain.com.**

Printed in the United States of America
Print Number: 01   Print Year: 2016

Brief Contents

Preface **xi**

Part I Stress and Its Impact

CHAPTER 1   Understanding Stress   **1**

CHAPTER 2   Stress and Your Body   **20**

CHAPTER 3   Stress and Your Mind   **39**

Part II Stress on Campus

CHAPTER 4   Stress on Campus   **61**

CHAPTER 5   Your Personal Environment, Time, and Money   **79**

CHAPTER 6   Relationships, Social Health, and Stress   **101**

Part III Managing Stress

CHAPTER 7   Personal Change   **125**

CHAPTER 8   Psychological Approaches   **144**

CHAPTER 9   Stress-Resistant Health Habits   **166**

CHAPTER 10   Spirituality, Life Balance, and Resilience   **192**

CHAPTER 11   Occupational and Environmental Stress   **213**

Part IV Stress Reduction and Relaxation Techniques

CHAPTER 12   Breathing, Relaxation, and Guided Imagery   **232**

CHAPTER 13   Mindfulness, Meditation, and Self-hypnosis   **248**

CHAPTER 14   Physical Techniques   **264**

CHAPTER 15   Complementary, Alternative, and Creative Therapies   **282**

Glossary **296**

References **300**

Index **309**

Contents

Preface   **xi**

Part I Stress and Its Impact

CHAPTER 1
Understanding Stress   **1**

What Is Stress?   3

Stress: Good, Bad, and Neutral   4

Stress and the Dimensions of Health   5
  Physical Health   5
  Psychological Health   5
  Spiritual Health   5
  Social Health   5
  Intellectual Health   5
  Occupational Health   5
  Environmental Health   5

Stress in America   5

Types of Stressors   6
  Acute Stressors   6
  Episodic Acute Stressors   6
  Chronic Stressors   7

Common Stressors   7
  Daily Hassles   7
  Life Change Events   7
  Psychosocial Stressors   9
  Trauma   9

Inside Stress: The General Adaptation Syndrome   9

How the Body Responds to Stress   10
  Automatic Stress Responses   10
  Fight or Flight   10
  Freezing   10
  Submission   10
  Challenge Response Model   11
  Tend-and-Befriend Model   12
  Transactional or Cognitive-Reappraisal Model   12

How Much Stress Is Too Much?   13

Rethinking Stress   14
  The Stress Paradox   14
  Stress Mindsets   15
  From Surviving to Thriving   15

Chapter Summary   16

Stress Relievers   17

Your Personal Stress Management Toolkit   18

CHAPTER 2
Stress and Your Body   **20**

The Biology of Stress   22
  The Inside Story   22
  The Key Players   23
  Sounding the Stress Alarm   23

Stress and Susceptibility   24
  Biological Sex   24
  Race and Ethnicity   25
  Genes   25
  Family History   25

The Toll of Excess Stress   26

Stress and the Immune System   27

Stress and the Cardiovascular System   28

Stress and the Gastrointestinal System   29

Stress and the Muscles   30

Stress and the Skin   32

Stress and the Reproductive System   33

Stress and Cancer   33

Stress and Aging   34

Rx: Relax   35

Chapter Summary   35

Stress Relievers   36

Your Personal Stress Management Toolkit   37

CHAPTER 3
Stress and Your Mind   **39**

Psychological Health   41

Stress and the Brain   41

Perception-Based Theories of Stress   43
  Locus of Control   43
  Self-Efficacy   43
  Expectations   44
  Attributions   44

Taking Charge of Your Thoughts   45
  Thought Awareness   45
  Cognitive Restructuring/Reframing   46
  Rational Emotive Behavior Therapy   46
  Thinking Traps   47
  Why Worry?   48

Talking Back to Stress   48
  Self-Talk   49
  Negate the Negatives   49
  Affirm Yourself   50

Stress and Mental Health   50
  Anxiety   51
  Depression   51

Stress-Related Mental Disorders   52
  Adjustment Disorder   52
  Acute Stress Disorder   52
  Post-Traumatic Stress Disorder (PTSD)   53

Suicide   54

Harnessing the Powers of Your Mind   55

Chapter Summary   56

Stress Relievers   57

Your Personal Stress Management Toolkit   59

Part II Stress on Campus

CHAPTER 4
Stress on Campus   **61**

Students under Stress   63
  Gender Differences   64
  Students under Age 25   65
  Nontraditional-Age Students   65

Entering Freshmen and First-Generation College
    Students 66
Minority Students 66
Academic Stress 68
Inside Academic Stress 69
Your Study Style 69
Test Stress 71
Common Campus Stressors 73
Risky Behaviors 74
Illness and Disability 74
Violence and Crime 75
Coping with Campus Stress 76
Chapter Summary 76
Stress Relievers 77
Your Personal Stress Management Toolkit 78

CHAPTER 5
Your Personal Environment, Time,
and Money 79

Managing Your Personal Environment 82
Rules of Order 82
Your Study Space 82
Establishing Order 83
Managing Your Time 84
Day Planning 84
Visualize Your Time 84
Take Time for Yourself 85
Pre-empting Procrastination 86
Live in Real Time 86
The Myth of Multitasking 87
The Now Imperative 88
Time Management for Commuting and Working
    Students 88
Managing Your Money 89
Financial Homeostasis 90
Frugal Living 92
Personal Finances 101 93
Your Credit Score 93
Banking Basics 93
Avoid Debit and Credit Card Stress 94
Digital Financial Management 95
Debt Relief 95
Protect Your Private Information 96
Taking Control 96
Chapter Summary 97
Stress Relievers 98
Your Personal Stress Management Toolkit 99

CHAPTER 6
Relationships, Social Health,
and Stress 101

Social Health and Support 103
Getting Along with Others 104
Communicating 101 104
How Men and Women Communicate 106
Agreeable but Assertive 106
Forming Relationships 107
Family Ties 107
Friendship 107
Loneliness 108

Shyness 108
Social Anxiety 108
Living in a Wired World 109
Social Media on Campus 109
Online Eustress 109
Digital Distress 110
Sexual and Romantic Relationships 110
Gender Identity 111
Intimate Relationships 114
Cohabitation 114
Marriage 114
Marriage and Health 115
Resolving Conflict 115
Dysfunctional Relationships 116
Emotional and Verbal Abuse 116
Codependency and Enabling 117
Intimate Partner Violence 118
Sexual Victimization 118
When Love Ends 119
Breaking Up and Rejection 119
Divorce 119
Building Better Relationships 120
Chapter Summary 121
Stress Relievers 122
Your Personal Stress Management Toolkit 123

Part III Managing Stress

CHAPTER 7
Personal Change 125

Choosing Change 127
Why Change Seems Stressful 127
What You Need to Know about Change 127
What You Can and Can't Change 128
The Stages of Change 129
Precontemplation 129
Contemplation 130
Preparation 130
Action 131
Maintenance 131
Relapse 131
Is This the Best Time to Make
    a Change? 131
See the Steps of Change 132
Motivating Change: Go for Your Goals 133
Your Big Dream 133
Your Destination Goal 133
Setting Long-Term Goals 134
Your Short-Term Goals 134
The Language of Change 135
Loophole Language 135
Real Talk 135
Boosting Your Power to Change 136
Beyond Willpower 137
Making Personal Change Inevitable 137
Are You Getting in Your Own Way? 138
Changing for Good 139
Managing Your Behaviors 140
Chapter Summary 141
Stress Relievers 142
Your Personal Stress Management Toolkit 143

CHAPTER 8
Psychological Approaches 144

Psychological and Emotional Health 146
Emotional Intelligence 146
The Power of Positivity 148
  Emotional Spirals 148
  "Undoing" Stress 149
  Boost Self-Esteem 149
  Recognize Your Personality Traits 150
  Practice Self-Compassion 150
  Meet Your Needs 151
  Cultivate Gratitude 151
  Pursue Happiness 152
  Become Optimistic and Hopeful 153
Detoxifying Negative Feelings 154
  Fear 154
  Anger 155
  Mood Control 156
Taking Charge of Risky Behaviors 157
  Gambling 157
  Alcohol 157
  Drugs 159
  Tobacco 160
Strengthening Your Coping Muscles 161
Chapter Summary 162
Stress Relievers 163
Your Personal Stress Management Toolkit 164

CHAPTER 9
Stress-Resistant Health Habits 166

Physical Activity and Exercise 168
  The Stress of Sedentary Living 168
  Exercise, Stress, and the Brain 168
  Fitness Fundamentals 169
  Get F.I.T.T. 171
Sleep and Stress 171
  The Toll of Stress 171
  Student Night Life 173
  How Much Sleep Do You Need? 173
  Stress-induced Insomnia 174
  How to Get a Good Night's Sleep 174
  Napping 176
Healthy Eating 177
  Essential Nutrients 177
  Healthy Eating Guidelines 177
  Mindful Eating 178
  Nutrition and Mood 178
  Liquid Stress 178
Body Image and Stress 181
  "Fat Talk" 182
Weight and Stress 183
  Stress Fat 183
  Excess Weight 184
  Who's in Control of Your Weight? 184
  Beyond Diets 185
  Intuitive Eating 185
Stress and Disordered Eating 186
  Stress Eating 186
  Compulsive Overeating 186
  Binge Eating 186
  Eating Disorders 187
Creating a Stress-Resistant Lifestyle 187

  Physical Activity 187
  Better Sleep 187
  Healthier Eating 188
Chapter Summary 188
Stress Relievers 189
Your Personal Stress Management Toolkit 190

CHAPTER 10
Spirituality, Life Balance, and Resilience 192

Spirituality 194
  Spirituality and Health 194
  Spiritual Intelligence 194
  Enriching Your Spiritual Life 194
  The Power of Prayer 195
  Forgiveness 196
  Naikan 197
  Karma 197
Your Values 197
  Clarifying Your Values 198
  Compassion 198
  Altruism 199
A Life in Balance 200
Resilience 201
  Lessons from Resilient People 202
  Dealing with Setbacks 203
  Block Your Escape Routes 204
  No Failure to Fear 204
  The Power of Plan B—and C 204
  Relapse Rehearsals 205
Tools for Finding Meaning and Joy 205
  Expressive Writing and Journaling 205
  The Benefits of Expressive Writing and Journaling 206
  Types of Journaling 206
  Humor or Laughter Therapy 207
Coping with Life's Ups and Downs 209
Chapter Summary 209
Stress Relievers 210
Your Personal Stress Management Toolkit 212

CHAPTER 11
Occupational and Environmental Stress 213

Preparing for Your Future 215
  Balancing Work and School 215
  Building Your Resume While in College 215
  Choosing a Career 216
Finding a Job 216
  Networking 217
  Preparing for a Job Interview 217
  Handling Interview Stress 218
On the Job 218
  What Kind of Worker Are You? 218
  Time and Task Management 219
  Emotional Intelligence at Work 219
Occupational Stress 220
  Causes of Occupational Stress 220
  Coping with Occupational Stress 221
  Burnout 221
  Causes of Burnout 222
  The Stages of Burnout 222
  Job Loss and Unemployment 223

Environmental Stress 224
　Climate Change 225
　Pollution 225
　Noise 226
　Cell Phones 228
Chapter Summary 228
Stress Relievers 229
Your Personal Stress Management Toolbox 230

Part IV Stress Reduction and Relaxation Techniques

CHAPTER 12
Breathing, Relaxation, and Guided Imagery 232

Breathing 233
　Understanding Breathing 233
　The Benefits of Diaphragmatic Breathing 234
　What You Need to Know 235
　Introductory Breathing Exercise 235
Guided Imagery 238
　Understanding Guided Imagery 239
　The Benefits of Guided Imagery 239
　What You Need to Know 240
　Introductory Guided Imagery Exercise 240
Relaxation 241
　Understanding Relaxation 241
　The Benefits of Relaxation 241
　What You Need to Know 242
　ABC Relaxation 244
Chapter Summary 245
Stress Relievers 246
Your Personal Stress Management Toolkit 246

CHAPTER 13
Mindfulness, Meditation, and Self-hypnosis 248

Mindfulness 250
　Understanding Mindfulness 250
　The Benefits of Mindfulness 251
　What You Need to Know 251
　Mindfulness Skills 252
　Mindfulness-Based Stress Reduction (MBSR) 252
　Mindfulness Practices 253
Meditation 255
　Understanding Meditation 255
　The Benefits of Meditation 255
　What You Need to Know 256
　Meditation Practices 257
　Meditation Exercises 258
Self-Hypnosis 259
　Understanding Hypnosis 259
　The Benefits of Hypnosis 259
　What You Need to Know 260
　Self-Hypnosis Exercise 260
Chapter Summary 261

Stress Relievers 261
Your Personal Stress Management Toolkit 262

CHAPTER 14
Physical Techniques 264

Autogenics 265
　Understanding Autogenics 265
　The Benefits of Autogenics 266
　What You Need to Know 266
　The Stages of Autogenics 266
Biofeedback 267
　Understanding Biofeedback 267
　The Benefits of Biofeedback 267
　What You Need to Know 268
Yoga 268
　Understanding Yoga 269
　The Benefits of Yoga 276
　What You Need to Know 276
Tai Chi 276
　Understanding Tai Chi 277
　The Benefits of Tai Chi 277
　What You Need to Know 277
Pilates 278
　Understanding Pilates 278
　The Benefits of Pilates 278
　What You Need to Know 278
Dance or Movement Therapy 278
Chapter Summary 279
Stress Relievers 280
Your Personal Stress Management Toolkit 280

CHAPTER 15
Complementary, Alternative, and Creative Therapies 282

Complementary and Alternative Medicine (CAM) 283
　Understanding CAM 283
CAM for Stress Management 284
　Alternative Medical Systems 284
　Mind–Body Medicine 285
　Manipulative and Body-based Methods 285
　Biologically-based Therapies 287
　Energy Therapies 288
　Other Complementary and Alternative Techniques 288
Creative or Expressive Therapies 289
　Art Therapy 290
　Music Therapy 291
Chapter Summary 293
Stress Relievers 293
Your Personal Stress Management Toolkit 294

Glossary 296

References 300

Index 309

Key Features

Pre-Chapter Check-in

Every chapter begins with a self-assessment that focuses on a specific aspect of stress related to a student's life:

Your Stress Signals   2
Where Do You Feel Stress?   21
Are You in Balance?   40
Student Stress Scale   62
Where Does Your Time Go?   80
Is Your Relationship Healthy?   102
What Would You Change?   126
How Are You Doing?   145
Healthy Habits Inventory   167
How Satisfied Are You with Your Life So Far?   193
Rate Your Job Stress   214
How Do You Normally Breathe?   233
How Mindful Are You?   249
Which Mind-Body Practice Is Best for You?   265
Have You Tried Complementary, Alternative, or Creative Therapies?   283

Check-ins

These are quick in-text self-assessments that ask students direct, personal questions that they can relate and response to or that present an intriguing concept or research finding.

Stress Relievers

These are quick, practical steps that students can take immediately or in the near future to reduce stress. The Stress Relievers appear in the text and are summarized at the end of every chapter.

Your Personal Stress Management Toolkit

Because students are all different, with different backgrounds, personalities, life circumstances, and stressors, there is no one-size-fits-all stress management technique for them to use for every stressor they encounter in life. As they progress through your course, students can use this unique interactive feature to assemble a collection of coping strategies—a toolkit for personal stress management—that they can tailor to specific situations and stressors.

To build this toolkit, each chapter includes:

Reflection (a self-assessment designed to deepen students' self-understanding)

Getting to Know Your Personal Stress   18
How Relaxed Are You?   37
Are You Internal or External?   59
Are You Showing Signs of Campus Stress?   78
Do You Have a Procrastination Problem?   99
Building Blocks of a Good Relationship   123
Dream Big   143
How Grateful Are You?   164
Stress Eating   190
A Day in Your Life   212
How Green Is Your Lifestyle?   230
What Are Your Tension Targets?   246
Are You Present?   262
Why Try a Mind-Body Technique?   280
Should You Try a Complementary, Alternative, or Creative Therapy?   294

Technique (a practical stress-reducing technique for students to put to immediate use and continue indefinitely in the future)

Introductory Breathing Exercise   18
Tense and Relax Exercise   37
Mindfulness Meditation   59
Mindful Studying   78
Complete the Incompletes   100
Listen Up!   123
Create a Timeline   143
Taming a Toxic Temper   165
Get a Grip on Stress Eating   191
Pie Chart   212
Instant Stress Relievers to Go   230
Breathing for Tension Relief   247
Sitting Meditation   262
Introductory Autogenics Exercise   281
Express Your Stress   295

Preface

To the Student

However old you are, wherever you came from, whatever your goals, the only sure thing in your life is stress. Don't assume that's all bad. Although you may have thought of it as an enemy to avoid whenever possible, stress isn't innately and invariably dangerous. In fact, it is an unavoidable part of life.

There is no magic, no hidden secret to dealing with stress. There are, however, techniques and tools that can empower you to approach stress as a challenge rather than a threat. You will discover and master them in *Personal Stress Management*. You will see how stress can serve as a catalyst for developing greater strength and even greater wisdom. You will discover that stress, rather than breeding anxiety or aggression, can foster caring and compassion. You will learn how stress can lead to greater meaning and sense of purpose and strengthen human connections. Although you can never avoid or eliminate difficulties and disappointments, you can change the way you think about them. This is the key to changing the way you respond to stress—physically, mentally, and emotionally.

A key premise of this book is that stress is always personal. The very same experience—whether it be auditioning for a dance video, zip-lining, or studying abroad—might seem thrilling to one person and terrifying to another. No one has your unique mix of values and vulnerabilities, genetic predispositions and childhood experiences, social support and individual aptitudes. That's why learning about stress begins with learning about yourself. You—and only you—can transform your thinking, which in turn can transform your feelings, your behaviors, and your responses to stress.

Personal Stress Management, based on decades of scientific research and clinical practice, presents a positive, proactive, research-based view of stress—not as an ordeal to survive, but as an opportunity to thrive. As you will discover, this book—like this class—is different in one critical way: Your other courses prepare you for further academic pursuits and a future career; *Personal Stress Management* prepares you for life.

To the Instructor

Your students know about stress. They live with it every day, whether they're cramming for a final, figuring out how to live on a budget, juggling a part-time job, or dealing with a difficult roommate. Today's undergraduates report greater stress and more sources of stress than students did twenty years ago, and higher percentages say they frequently feel overwhelmed.

As the author of *An Invitation to Health*, the leading college health textbook, I have always considered the ability to cope with stress a key determinant of student health. Managing stress, like maintaining good health, is one of the most important lessons students can learn in college. This is the reason I wanted to write a textbook on stress management.

I collaborated on this project with my daughter, Julia Hales, who has a graduate degree in psychology and extensive experience in counseling clients of all ages. She adapted therapy-based techniques into practical strategies and skills that students can apply immediately in their daily lives.

Personal Stress Management presents a positive, proactive, evidence-based approach. Although we discuss the negative effects of excess stress, we take a new perspective. As we see it, stress can be an opportunity for learning and growth that enables individuals to thrive—that is, to function at a higher level both psychologically and physically, build mental toughness, clarify values, enrich relationships, and deepen appreciation for life.

Among the features that set *Personal Stress Management* apart from existing texts are:

- **Student Focus.** An entire section examines students under stress in their classrooms and in their roles as friends, roommates, partners, parents, employees, and members of larger communities. Three chapters address concerns such as academic and test stress; first-year, first-generation, and community college challenges; time management; financial issues; social networking; sex on campus; and relationships (virtual and actual).

- **Diversity and Stress.** Gender, race, ethnicity, and culture have an enormous impact on stress and its effects on individuals and families. An Asian-American, a Hispanic, a Caucasian, and an African-American student may experience a similar situation as extremely to slightly to not at all stressful. Understanding such differences, we believe, can provide students with insight into themselves and their classmates.

- **Stress and Health.** *Personal Stress Management* reports on the most recent stress-related findings from psychoneuroimmunology, neuroscience, exercise physiology, nutrition, and medicine. While other texts emphasize stress and disease, we provide substantive coverage of how healthy habits, such as regular exercise, better sleep habits, and good nutrition, defend against stress and prevent burnout.

- **The Psychology of Stress.** We explore the relationship of stress to anxiety, depression, unhealthy risk-taking, and traumatic experiences (reported by the majority of undergraduates). We also highlight the contributions of positive psychology, including insights on the "stress paradox" (the observation that a certain degree of stress, rather than low or no stress, is linked to greater life satisfaction) and the impact of a "stress-is-enhancing" versus a "stress-is-debilitating' mindset. As part of our integrated mind-body-spirit approach, we report on the role of spirituality and related practices as well as the contributions of happiness, gratitude, and resilience.

- **Personal Change.** The most constant stressor in life is change, yet other texts provide minimal, if any, coverage of scientific research on the subject. *Personal Stress Management* devotes a chapter to the ground-breaking transtheoretical model of change and the stages of behavioral change. In addition, within each chapter, we translate theory and research into practical stress management "tools" that students can implement and evaluate. By choosing those they find most useful, they can assemble their own customized "Personal Stress Management Toolkit" by the end of the term.

A class in stress management can and should be transformational. Unlike instruction that presents only factual information, teaching students about stress provides a unique opportunity to share knowledge in ways that promote both learning and personal growth. We created *Personal Stress Management* as a tool for you to use to equip students with the insights and skills that will help them now and in the years to come.

We are excited by the opportunity to work with you to engage students in a dynamic new approach to managing stress. We welcome your comments and look forward to hearing from you.

Supplemental Resources

Health MindTap for *Personal Stress Management: From Surviving to Thriving*

A new approach to highly personalized online learning. Beyond an eBook, homework solution, digital supplement, or premium website, MindTap is a digital learning platform that works alongside your campus LMS to deliver course curriculum across the range of electronic devices in your life. MindTap is built on an "app" model, allowing enhanced digital collaboration and delivery of engaging content across a spectrum of Cengage and non-Cengage resources.

Diet & Wellness Plus

Diet & Wellness Plus helps you understand how nutrition relates to your personal health goals. Track your diet and activity, generate reports, and analyze the nutritional value of the food you eat. Diet & Wellness Plus includes over 75,000 foods, as well as custom food and recipe features. The Behavior Change Planner helps you identify risks in your life and guides you through the key steps to make positive changes.

Instructor Companion Site

Everything you need for your course in one place! This collection of book-specific lecture and class tools is available online via www.cengage.com/login. Access and download PowerPoint presentations, images, instructor's manual, videos, and more.

Global Health Watch

Bring currency to the classroom with Global Health Watch from Cengage Learning. This user-friendly website provides convenient access to thousands of trusted sources, including academic journals, newspapers, videos, and podcasts, for you to use for research projects or classroom discussion. Global Health Watch is updated daily to offer the most current news about topics related to nutrition.

Cengage Learning Testing Powered by Cognero

This flexible online system allows the instructor to author, edit, and manage test bank content from multiple Cengage Learning solutions; create multiple test versions in an instant; and deliver tests from an LMS, a classroom, or wherever the instructor wants.

Acknowledgments

Many people contributed to the creation of *Personal Stress Management* over the last several years. I will always be grateful for the support and friendship of my original editorial team at Cengage—Sean Wakely, Aileen Berg, Yolanda Cossio, and Nedah Rose. I applaud and appreciate Krista Mastroianni, product manager, who enthusiastically adopted this project, and Miriam Myers, senior content developer, who expertly took up the reins and shepherded *Personal Stress Management* through completion.

I thank Michael Cook, senior designer, and his design team; Marina Starkey for her invaluable aid as our product assistant; Tanya Nigh, senior content project manager; Lynn Lustberg of MPS Limited; Gopala Krishnan Sankar, our photo researcher; Christine Myaskovsky, who managed the overall permissions; and to Kellie Petruzzelli, who supervised the ancillaries.

Finally, I would like to thank the reviewers whose input has been invaluable in sharpening our vision and creating this book.

Chalyce Carlsen, Utah State University
Paul Bondurant, MS. Macomb Community College
Robert Hess, MS, LAT, ATC, Community College
    of Baltimore County
Leigh Hilger, Western Carolina University
Dr. Jerome Kotecki, Boston State University
Melissa Lee, MS, MBA, Florida Atlantic University
Allison B. Oberne, MA, MPH, CPH, College of Public Health
Desiree D. Reynolds, Indiana University Bloomington
Dr. Margaret M. Shields, University of Alabama
Stephen P. Sowulewski (Associate Professor of Health),
    Reynolds Community College
Deborah Wuest, Ithaca College

About the Authors

Dianne Hales is the author of *An Invitation to Health*, *An Invitation to Wellness*, and *An Invitation to Personal Change*. Her trade books include *Mona Lisa: A Life Discovered*, *La Bella Lingua*, *Just Like a Woman*, and *Caring for the Mind*, with translations into Chinese, Japanese, Italian, French, Spanish, Portuguese, German, Dutch, Swedish, Danish, Polish, and Korean. A graduate of Columbia University Journalism School, Dianne served as a contributing editor for *Parade*, *Ladies' Home Journal*, *Working Mother*, and *American Health* and has written more than 1,000 articles for national publications. Her writing awards include honors from the American Psychiatric Association. The American Psychological Association, and the Council for the Advancement of Scientific Education. The government of Italy bestowed its highest honor—knighthood, with the title *Cavaliere dell' Ordine della Stella della Solidarietà Italiana* (Knight of the Order of the Star of Italian Solidarity)—in recognition of her book *La Bella Lingua* as "an invaluable tool for promoting the Italian language."

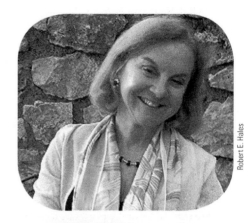

Julia Hales, who earned a baccalaureate in psychology and sociology from the University of California, Davis and a master's in counseling psychology with an emphasis in marital and family therapy from the University of San Francisco, has worked as a therapist and researcher in schools, treatment centers, hospitals, and universities. Her clinical experience includes individual and group therapy for children, adolescents, and adults with developmental and mental disorders, crisis intervention, psychological assessment, and social skills training. Drawing on her professional expertise, Julia developed and adapted psychoeducational materials, including cognitive behavioral therapy (CBT), solution-focused therapy, self-assessments, and mindfulness-based exercises, for *Personal Stress Management*.

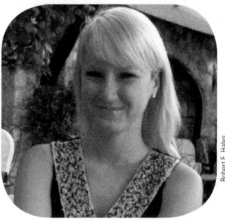

Personal Stress Management

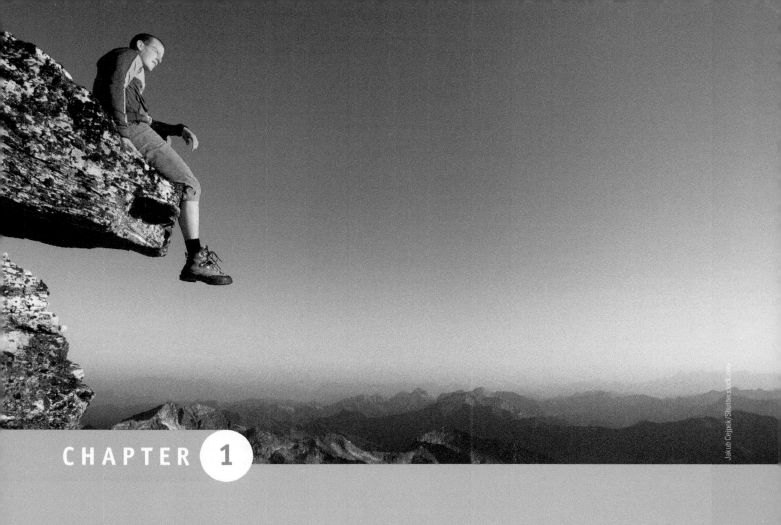

Jakub Cejpek/Shutterstock.com

CHAPTER 1

Understanding Stress

After reading this chapter, you should be able to:

1.1 Describe the concept of stress.

1.2 Differentiate among eustress, distress, and neustress.

1.3 Assess the effects of common stressors on the overall well-being of individuals.

1.4 Analyze the experience of stress in America.

1.5 Classify the most common types of stressors.

1.6 Identify common causes of stress.

1.7 Describe how different proposed models explain the "fight-or-flight" physiological stress response of the body.

1.8 Discuss theories and models that describe responses to stress.

1.9 Explain the Yerkes-Dodson law.

1.10 Summarize the positive and negative aspects of stress (stress paradox).

How can you tell when you're stressed? Does your heart race? Do your shoulders feel tight? Do you bite your nails, grind your teeth, scratch at a cut or bug bite? Does your stomach churn or your head ache? Do you eat more or less than usual? Do you have problems falling or staying asleep?

As you tune into your body and observe your behavior, you can hone your ability to spot stress signals before you feel overwhelmed. Read through the list of warning signs below, and check any that apply to you.

_____ Physical symptoms, including chronic fatigue, headaches, indigestion, and diarrhea.
_____ Sleep problems.
_____ Frequent illnesses or worrying about getting sick.
_____ Self-medicating, including use of alcohol and drugs (legal and otherwise).
_____ Problems concentrating on studies or work.

_____ Feeling irritable, anxious, angry, or apathetic.
_____ Working or studying longer and harder than usual.
_____ Exaggerating, to yourself and others, the importance of what you do.
_____ Becoming accident-prone.
_____ Breaking rules, whether it's a curfew at the dorm or a speed limit on the highway.
_____ Going to extremes, such as drinking too much, overspending, or gambling.

If you checked one or more of these red flags, pay closer attention to both the number and the intensity of stressors in your life.

Start tracking symptoms as they develop, and look for patterns that may help you recognize, avoid, or cope better with your stress triggers.

Y ou know about stress. You live with it every day—whether you're a full- or a part-time student, enrolled in a community college or a private university. You may lose your cell phone, blow your budget, or fail a test. You may be juggling school and a job, missing your family, uncertain about a major, or worried about your job prospects. If—like more undergraduates than ever—you're older than the traditional college student, you may be breathlessly keeping up with children, rent, housework, and homework. Your life can be confusing, engaging, exhausting, thrilling, terrifying—sometimes all in the course of a single day.

You aren't alone. According to the American College Health Association (ACHA) national surveys, stress ranks as the number-one barrier to academic achievement in college.[1] First-year, female, minority, and first-generation students register the most stress, but no one is immune.[2] What you may *not* know about stress is that you have more control over it than anyone or anything else—even if at times you may not feel this way.

Stress is an unavoidable part of living, loving, learning, growing, relating, trying, failing, stretching, and achieving. But simply by being human, you are magnificently equipped to manage it. Our species would have died out eons ago if we were not in possession of remarkable skills for adapting to new challenges and circumstances. You, as a descendant of resourceful, resilient ancestors, are hardwired to cope.

Although you may have thought of it as an enemy to avoid whenever possible, stress isn't innately and invariably dangerous. When viewed as a challenge rather than a threat, stress serves as a catalyst for developing greater strength and even greater wisdom.[3] Rather than breeding anxiety or aggression, stress can foster caring and compassion; rather than increasing anxiety and depression, it can lead to greater meaning and sense of purpose; rather than isolating you from others, it can strengthen human connections. When understood and accepted, stress can be beneficial and even essential for health and growth.

As you progress through college, you will not be able to anticipate every challenge or prepare for every contingency. But you can take steps that will help you avoid some stressors, reduce the negative impact of others, and learn and grow from stressful experiences. By assessing your life situation realistically, without exaggerating or downplaying problems and obstacles, you can determine where you are and what you need to make the most of your circumstances. Although you can never avoid or eliminate difficulties and disappointments, you can change the way you think about them. This is the key to changing the way you respond to stress—physically, mentally, and emotionally.

Personal Stress Management, based on decades of scientific research and clinical practice, presents a positive, proactive, research-based way of thinking about stress—not as an ordeal to survive, but as an opportunity to thrive. It will help you learn to anticipate stressful events, overcome obstacles, reduce unnecessary stress, prevent stress overload, and find alternatives to an endless cycle of alarm, panic, and exhaustion.

A key premise of this book is that stress is always personal. The very same experience—auditioning for a dance video, zip-lining, studying abroad—might seem thrilling to one person and terrifying to another. No one views something unknown or potentially upsetting exactly the way you do. No one has your unique mix of values and vulnerabilities, genetic predispositions and childhood experiences, social support and individual aptitudes. That's why learning about stress begins with learning about yourself. You—and only you—can transform your thinking, which in turn can transform your feelings, your behaviors, and your responses to stress.

As you will discover, this class is different in one critical way: Your other courses prepare you for further academic pursuits and a future career; *Personal Stress Management* prepares you for life.

What Is Stress?

In everyday life, stress has become a catch-all phrase for everything that goes wrong. We use "**stress**" to describe what's going on inside us—thoughts, feelings, physical symptoms—and what's happening around us. The word itself comes from the Latin *stringere,* which means "to draw tight." In physics, stress means strain, pressure, or force on a system. In psychology, the word can refer to an external force that causes someone to become tense or upset, and/or to an internal state of arousal, and/or the physical response of the body when it must adapt or adjust to a challenge.

Dr. Hans Selye, the father of scientific research into stress, defined it as "the non-specific response of the body to any demand made upon it." As he demonstrated, laboratory animals and people respond in the same way to a **stressor** (anything that triggers a state of arousal), regardless of whether it is positive or negative: by mobilizing internal resources and tensing for action.

Unlike the physical threats that endangered our early ancestors, most contemporary stressors do not pose an immediate threat to our lives, and a physical response cannot resolve conflict or ease fear, worry, and anger. For higher primates like humans, **perception** (one's way of evaluating, understanding, and interpreting a situation) has emerged as a critical factor because it influences how you evaluate and react to stress. The American Institute of Stress, created by Selye as a nonprofit clearinghouse of

stress The nonspecific response of the body to any demands made upon it; may be characterized by muscle tension and acute anxiety, or may be a positive force for action.

stressor An event or situation that an individual perceives as a threat; precipitates either adaptation or the stress response.

perception A person's cognitive (mental) interpretation of events.

A wedding brings the joy of eustress, while a car crash triggers distress. Watching televised coverage of a terrorist attack or natural disaster can cause neustress, even though it doesn't affect you directly.

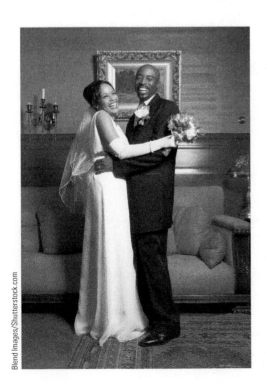

Blend Images/Shutterstock.com

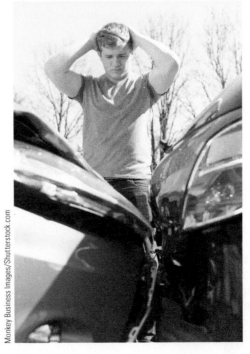

Monkey Business Images/Shutterstock.com

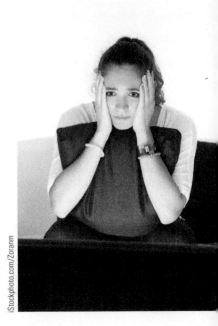

iStockphoto.com/Zoranm

stress-related information, incorporates perception into its most recent definition by describing stress as "a condition or feeling experienced when a person perceives that demands exceed the personal and social resources the individual is able to mobilize."[4] Your perception of whether or not you can handle a challenge—not the situation itself—determines whether or not you experience stress.

Stress: Good, Bad, and Neutral

"Stress is not necessarily something bad," noted Hans Selye, who coined the word "**eustress**" (the Greek prefix *eu* means "good") for the positive, energizing stress that challenges us to grow, adapt, and find creative solutions. When you're gaming with friends, stress strengthens your concentration; when you're taking a tough exam, it sharpens your thinking; when you're walking on a deserted street at night, it alerts you to potential dangers. However, too much eustress can also be problematic. A wedding, for instance, is a joyful event, but planning and organizing can create anxiety and take up so much time that they interfere with other commitments.

Certain forms of eustress are so thrilling that you've probably paid money to experience them—by riding a roller-coaster, for instance, or going to a scary movie. Such experiences, which we think of as stimulating rather than stressful, involve only moderate amounts of stress, and are time-limited. Anxiety makes us uncomfortable; stress helps us to rise to the occasion by speeding thought processes and making the most of internal resources.

Although stress can be helpful in keeping you alert for a limited time, intense or prolonged stress can strain body and brain. "**Distress**," the negative stress caused by trauma, loss, and other upsetting occurrences, depletes or even destroys life energy. Rather than mobilizing our internal resources, distress undermines well-being, targets vulnerable organs, and gets in the way of our ability to reach our fullest potential. Distress breeds overreaction, confusion, poor concentration, and performance anxiety. We cannot function at our best; we feel off, distracted, or edgy. As discussed in Chapter 2, we're more likely to develop physical symptoms and ailments.

Some experts have introduced another category: "**neustress**," or neutral stressors caused by an upsetting event that does not affect us immediately or directly but that may trigger anxiety, sadness, fear, and other stressful feelings. For example, an airplane crash or a mass shooting

reported in the media may deeply upset you. You experience emotions commonly related to stress, but your response is briefer and less severe than if you or a loved one had been in danger.

....

✔ **Check-in:** Stress in your life

Give an example of eustress that you experienced recently. What were the circumstances? How did you feel during and after the experience?

Give an example of distress in your life. Describe the circumstances and how you felt during and after the experience.

Give an example of neustress that may have affected you and how you felt as a result.

TABLE 1.1 Types of Stressors

Eustress—Sources of Stress in Daily Life with Positive Connotations:
Committed relationship
Marriage
Promotion
Having a Baby
Winning Money
New Friends
Graduation
Distress — Sources of Stress in Daily Life with Negative Connotations:
Breaking up
Divorce
Punishment
Injury
Rejection, anger, and other negative feelings
Financial Problems
Work Difficulties
Neustress—Stress with Neither Negative nor Positive Connotations:
An explosion, mass shooting, plane crash, or terrorist attack that does not affect you or your loved ones
A natural disaster, such as a tornado or flood, that does not affect you or your loved ones
A public health threat, such as an Ebola outbreak
An environmental threat, such as global warming

eustress Positive stress, which stimulates a person to function properly.

distress A negative stress that may result in illness.

neustress Neutral stressors that do not affect us immediately or directly but that may trigger anxiety, sadness, fear, and other stressful feelings.

Stress and the Dimensions of Health

✔ **Check-in:** The dimensions of health

As you read the following section, ask yourself which dimensions of your health are most affected by stress. How so?

More than the absence of disease or infirmity, **health** is the process of discovering, using, and protecting all the resources within your body, mind, spirit, family, community, and environment. From a **holistic** perspective, which looks at health and the individual as a whole rather than part by part, stress can have an impact on every dimension of well-being:

Physical Health

Stress triggers molecular changes within your body that affect your heart, muscles, immune system, bones, blood vessels, skin, lungs, gastrointestinal (digestive) tract, and reproductive organs. As explained in Chapter 2, these physiological changes, although useful in the short term, can make us more susceptible to many illnesses, worsen existing health conditions, and speed up the aging process.

Psychological Health

Chronic stress affects both thoughts and feelings, impairing your ability to learn and remember and contributing to anxiety and depression. Negative emotions linked with excess stress, such as anger and fear (see Chapter 8), can be harmful to both mind and body. Positive emotions and attitudes, such as compassion and gratitude, can buffer the ill effects of stress and enhance satisfaction and genuine happiness.

Spiritual Health

Stress can undermine your ability to identify your basic purpose in life and to achieve your full potential). When nurtured, your spirit can imbue your life with meaning and help you both resist and recover from stress (see Chapter 10).

Social Health

Your relationships with your family, friends, co-workers, and loved ones—whether comforting or complicated, frustrating or fulfilling— affect and are affected by the stress in your life. Skills such as communicating clearly and resolving conflicts, discussed in Chapter 5, can both strengthen your ties to others and reduce your stress level.

Intellectual Health

Intellectual health encompasses your ability to learn from life experience, your openness to new ideas, and your capacity to question and evaluate information. Even mild stressors can interfere with your brain's functioning by impairing sleep, dampening creativity, disrupting concentration and memory, and undermining your ability to make good choices and decisions.

Occupational Health

Most undergraduates—about 60 to 70 percent— are employed, with 20 percent working full-time year-round. They are more likely to feel overwhelmed and report greater anxiety and stress than students without jobs. Many factors contribute to job stress; these can range from the workplace environment to office politics to sexual harassment (see Chapter 11). Employees in dead-end jobs with little or no control or status are especially vulnerable to stress-related problems such as hypertension.

Environmental Health

External forces such as pollution, noise, natural disasters, exposure to toxic chemicals, and threats to your safety can cause or intensify stress. These days you also have to cope with a byproduct of our 24/7, nonstop digital world: **technostress**, created by an unending barrage of texts, tweets, e-mails, notifications, blogs, alerts, Instagrams, pins, pokes, streaming videos, and other digital distractions. Although you can't control every aspect of your environment, you can create a buffer zone that protects you from constant intrusions (see Chapter 11).

Stress in America

Every year the American Psychological Association asks men and women across the country to rank their stress level on a scale of 1 (little or no stress) to 10 (a great deal of stress). In its most recent *Stress in America* survey, the average stress level was 5.1, significantly higher than the 3.8 Americans see as a healthy stress rating.

Here are some other key findings: [1]

- About a third of adults report that their stress has increased over the past year; about a quarter say they experienced "extreme" stress (a rating of 8, 9, or 10).

- Adults reporting extreme stress are twice as likely to describe their health as "fair" or "poor," compared to those with low stress levels, who are more likely to say their health is "very good" or "excellent."

health A state of complete well-being, including physical, psychological, spiritual, social, intellectual, and environmental dimensions.

holistic A view of health and the individual as a whole rather than part by part.

physical health The functioning of the cells, tissues, organs, and systems that make up the body.

psychological health Psychological health encompasses both our emotional and mental states—that is, our feelings and our thoughts—and involves the ability to recognize and express emotions, to function independently, and to cope with the challenges of stress.

spiritual health The principles and values that guide a person and give meaning, direction, and purpose to life.

social health The ability to interact effectively with other people and the social environment to develop satisfying relationships and fulfill social roles.

intellectual health Ability to learn from life experience, accept new ideas, and question and evaluate information.

occupational health The ability to work productively, to meet job requirements, and to gain satisfaction from completion of assigned responsibilities.

- Across the nation younger respondents experience higher stress levels. Millennials (born in the 1980s and 1990s) report an average stress level of 6.0 and Gen-Xers (born between 1965 and 1980) of 5.8, compared to 4.3 for Baby Boomers.

- Women report higher stress levels than men (5.3 versus 4.9 on a 10-point scale).

- Almost one-third of adults report that stress has a very strong or strong impact on their body/physical health and mental health.

- The most common sources of stress nationwide are money, work, and family responsibilities, followed by personal health concerns, health issues affecting family members, and the economy.

- Adults in urban areas report a significantly higher stress level (5.6) than those in suburban (5.0) and rural (4.7) settings

- Nearly seven in ten adults report that they have experienced discrimination, including being harassed, threatened, or treated with less respect, on the basis of age, race or ethnicity, disability, sexual orientation, gender, or gender identity. Six in ten of these individuals encountered some form of discrimination on a daily basis.

- Regardless of its cause, individuals experiencing discrimination report greater stress and poorer health. Hispanics reporting discrimination had higher levels than those who did not (6.1 compared to 5.1); the stress level of Blacks reporting discrimination averaged 5.5, compared with 3.8 for African-Americans who did not experience it.[5]

Types of Stressors

Stressors—internal or external demands that upset balance and affect physical and psychological well-being—come in all varieties: big, small, brief, long, intense, mild, trivial, terrible. To evaluate the impact of a stressor, consider three crucial factors:

- Frequency: How often does it occur?

- Intensity: How intense is your response?

- Time: For how long does your stress response continue?

During your first days on campus, you may have felt nonstop stress as you struggled to get your bearings, find your classes, buy books, start assignments, meet people, and complete time-consuming paperwork. As you settled into a routine, you may have felt that you could at least come up for air occasionally.

Some stressors don't occur very often, but when they do, they're intense. You may be cruising along the highway and spot a state trooper's car, siren roaring and lights flashing, behind you; or your plane may hit a sudden batch of turbulence and bounce violently. In seconds, your stress levels spike. When the trooper passes you by or the plane stabilizes, your body calms itself and returns to a state of balance.

What matters most to your health is the duration of stress—how long your body and brain remain in a state of arousal. If prolonged or repeated, even subtle forms of stress, such as worry about finding a job, can undermine your physical and psychological well-being.

Acute Stressors

An **acute stressor** is time-limited. You reach for your wallet and it's not where you thought you left it. As you search frantically through pockets, peer under seat cushions, and try to recall the last time you used it, your heart pounds; beads of sweat may form on the back of your neck. After what feels like an eternity, you remember that you wore your roommate's jacket the evening before, and sure enough, your wallet is still in the pocket. The crisis is over; you take a deep breath; your body calms itself, and your distress quickly dissolves.

> **Stress Reliever:** Refocus
>
> Upload a photo of a favorite person, place, or pet to your cell phone or computer.
>
> As soon as you start feeling stressed, click on it. Block all other thoughts, and focus completely on the happiness you associate with this image. Breathe slowly and deeply.

Episodic Acute Stressors

Some situations, events, or encounters, such as a challenging semester-long internship or a slow recovery from a serious injury, where exposure to one or more acute stressors can be frequent and repeated, can be called **episodic acute stressors**. As distress mounts, you may find yourself misplacing things, forgetting deadlines, losing forms, or not charging your phone. Something always seems to be going wrong, and you feel increasingly tense and irritable. In addition to frayed nerves, episodic acute stress can cause headaches, stomachaches, and other stress-linked symptoms described in Chapter 2.

environmental health The impact the world around you has on well-being and the impact you can have by protecting and preserving the environment.

technostress Tension and anxiety associated with technology and the nonstop barrage of digital media.

acute stressor A short-term event or situation that an individual perceives as a threat.

episodic acute stressor Frequent and repeated experience of an acute stressor.

Chronic Stressors

Chronic stressors, or long-term stressors, are ongoing problems that grind on and on relentlessly. You may be living with the world's messiest roommate; your boss may be micromanaging everything you do; your brother may have gambled away the money you loaned him. While your body returns to its normal resting state shortly after an acute or time-limited stress, chronic stressors—either repeated or prolonged—reactivate the stress response time and again, affecting every aspect of your life. You may develop chronic health problems or feel so worn out that you lose hope and become depressed.

Common Stressors

Whether trivial or traumatic, the entire range of events that fill our days can spike our stress levels. The following sections explain why.

Daily Hassles

Your phone battery dies; the ATM eats your debit card; you can't find an overdue library book; you lose $20 playing fantasy football. "No big deal," you may tell yourself—and you're right; yet string several such upsets together, and you find yourself in the middle of a miserable, no good, very bad day. Over time, irritations that seem like "small stuff" can have big consequences for your health, particularly if combined with chronic stress.[7]

What matters more than how many hassles you encounter is how you view and respond to them. In national surveys, the most commonly named sources of everyday stress involve scheduling, errands, commuting, social media, and routine chores.[8] These normal and expected parts of everyone's life are neither life-threatening nor even physically challenging; they become stressful when we view them as unwanted impositions that interfere with what we would rather be doing.

✔ **Check-in:** What's hassling you?

List your top three hassles. On a scale of 1 (totally trivial) to 10 (life-shattering), how would you rate each of them? Can you identify a simple step that might make at least one of them less stressful?

Life Change Events

In the course of twelve months, you may start a new school, move, change jobs, sprain your ankle, and fall in love. The good, the bad, and the mundane may merge together in the whirl of day-to-day experience, but "life change events" (defined as occurrences that require some sort of psychological or social adjustment) can have a cumulative effect. A series of too-intense pressures or too-rapid changes can push anyone closer and closer to exhaustion—and illness.

Stress experts Drs. Thomas Holmes and Richard Rahe first documented an association between stressful life events and the onset of a disease. Their Schedule of Recent Experiences (SRE) evaluates individual levels of stress and potential for coping on the basis of life change units, determined by the degree of readjustment necessary to adapt successfully to an event. The death of a partner or parent ranks high on the list, but even positive events, such as a vacation trip, involve some degree of stress. Each individual responds to changes differently, and the consequences vary from person to person.

Take the quiz on page 8 to assess how much your life has changed in the last year.

✔ **Check-in:** Holmes-Rahe stress inventory

If you score high, think about the reasons why there has been so much turmoil in your life. Some events, such as a sister's accident or a devastating hurricane, are beyond your control. But even so, you can respond in ways that may lower stress and protect you from disease.

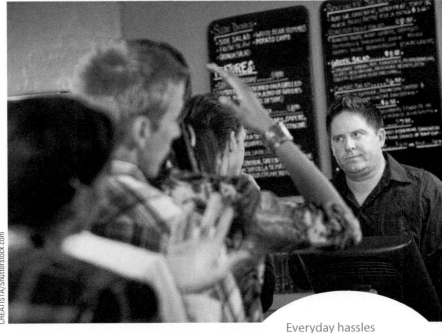

Everyday hassles like waiting in long lines are a common stressor.

chronic stressor Unrelenting demands and pressures that go on for an extended time.

TABLE 1.2 Holmes-Rahe Stress Inventory

The Social Readjustment Rating Scale

INSTRUCTIONS: Mark down the point value of each of these life events that has happened to you during the previous year. Total these associated points.

Life Event	Mean Value
1. Death of spouse	100
2. Divorce	73
3. Marital separation from mate	65
4. Detention in jail or other institution	63
5. Death of a close family member	63
6. Major personal injury or illness	53
7. Marriage	50
8. Being fired at work	47
9. Marital reconciliation with mate	45
10. Retirement from work	45
11. Major change in the health or behavior of a family member	44
12. Pregnancy	40
13. Sexual difficulties	39
14. Gaining a new family member (i.e. birth, adoption, older adult moving in, etc.)	39
15. Major business readjustment	39
16. Major change in financial state (i.e. a lot worse or better off than usual)	38
17. Death of a close friend	37
18. Changing to a different line of work	36
19. Major change in the number of arguments w/spouse (i.e. either a lot more or a lot less than usual regarding child rearing, personal habits, etc.)	35
20. Taking on a mortgage (for home, business, etc.)	31
21. Foreclosure on a mortgage or loan	30
22. Major change in responsibilities at work (i.e. promotion, demotion, etc.)	29
23. Son or daughter leaving home (marriage, attending college, joined mil.)	29
24. In-law troubles	29
25. Outstanding personal achievement	28
26. Spouse beginning or ceasing work outside the home	26
27. Beginning or ceasing formal schooling	26
28. Major change in living condition (new home, remodeling, deterioration of neighborhood or home etc.)	25
29. Revision of personal habits (dress manners, associations, quitting smoking)	24
30. Troubles with the boss	23
31. Major changes in working hours or conditions	20
32. Changes in residence	20
33. Changing to a new school	20
34. Major change in usual type and/or amount of recreation	19
35. Major change in church activity (i.e. a lot more or less than usual)	19
36. Major change in social activities (clubs, movies, visiting, etc.)	18
37. Taking on a loan (car, tv, freezer, etc.)	17
38. Major change in sleeping habits (a lot more or a lot less than usual)	16
39. Major change in number of family get-togethers (" ")	15
40. Major change in eating habits (a lot more or less food intake, or very different meal hours or surroundings)	15
41. Vacation	13
42. Major holidays	12
43. Minor violations of the law (traffic tickets, jaywalking, disturbing the peace, etc.)	11

Now, add up all the points you have to find your score.

150 pts or less means a relatively low amount of life change and a low susceptibility to stress-induced health breakdown.

150 to 300 pts implies about a 50% chance of a major health breakdown in the next 2 years.

300 pts or more raises the odds to about 80%, according to the Holmes-Rahe statistical prediction model.

Source: http://www.stress.org/holmes-rahe-stress-inventory

Psychosocial Stressors

Psychosocial stressors don't pose an immediate threat to survival. No one pulls a gun; no fire breaks out; no railing gives way as you lean on it. But "nonevents," such as conflict with a friend or relative, can have painful, long-lasting repercussions that affect your sense of self and self-worth and alter immune responses for months.[9] Those involving rejection, not belonging, and isolation can trap individuals in self-blame and other negative thinking patterns. Some psychosocial stressors, such as a parent's illness or a cancelled scholarship, may trigger specific physiological responses as well as emotional ones. The strongest antidote, as researchers have documented, is **social support**—the comfort, caring, and compassion you receive from family, friends, and others.[10] (See Chapter 5 on relationships and stress.)

Socioeconomic status has an inverse relationship with stress: the lower income falls, the greater the stress—and the higher the levels of stress hormones such as cortisol.[11] Poverty makes every aspect of daily life more stressful—from having to live in crowded, low-quality housing in dangerous neighborhoods to lacking resources for health care. It also can foster unhealthy behaviors, such as poor sleep, substance abuse, smoking, violence, and aggression.[12] Individuals in the lowest socioeconomic levels are more than three times as likely to suffer from depression, heart disease, and diabetes, and to die prematurely, as those earning the highest incomes.[13]

Although money can buffer the ill effects of financial stress, it cannot buy happiness or eliminate stress. If you are financially secure, you are able to meet your basic needs for safety, survival, and shelter. Beyond this level, more money does not bring greater fulfillment or protection from stress.

Earning money presents challenges of its own. As discussed in Chapter 11, occupational stressors can take many forms—from a noisy, open-office environment to sexual harassment to anxiety over potential layoffs. Workers who lose their jobs must deal with the stress of multiple losses: the loss of a paid position, a daily routine, and the camaraderie of coworkers, as well as the possible loss of the ability to support themselves and their families. Even if you're not working while in school, you may worry about your parents' job security or about your own employment prospects in the future.

Trauma

Cars crash; floods wipe out entire neighborhoods; shooters open fire on peaceful campuses. **Trauma** (an event that is extremely upsetting, frightening, or disturbing to those experiencing or witnessing it)

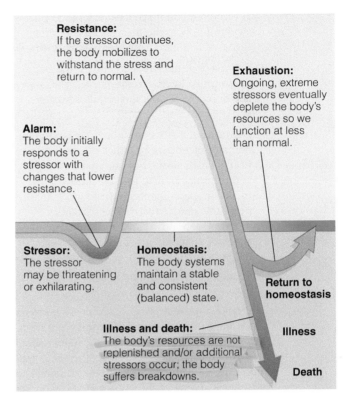

Resistance:
If the stressor continues, the body mobilizes to withstand the stress and return to normal.

Exhaustion:
Ongoing, extreme stressors eventually deplete the body's resources so we function at less than normal.

Alarm:
The body initially responds to a stressor with changes that lower resistance.

Stressor:
The stressor may be threatening or exhilarating.

Homeostasis:
The body systems maintain a stable and consistent (balanced) state.

Return to homeostasis

Illness and death:
The body's resources are not replenished and/or additional stressors occur; the body suffers breakdowns.

Illness

Death

FIGURE 1.1 General Adaptation Syndrome (GAS): The three stages of Selye's GAS are alarm, resistance, and exhaustion.

occurs so often that half of all Americans—about 60 percent of men and 50 percent of women—report at least one potentially traumatizing event during the course of their lives.[14] Certain groups, including veterans who have served in combat zones, are even more likely to experience trauma and its consequences. (See Chapter 3 for a discussion of trauma-related mental disorders.) Severe trauma-related conditions can cause disabling symptoms that persist for years or decades. However, with appropriate support and the passage of time, most people manage to move forward with their lives in an adaptive manner.

Inside Stress: The General Adaptation Syndrome

Our bodies, Hans Selye postulated, continually strive to maintain a stable and consistent physiological state, called **homeostasis**. When a stressor—physical, psychological, emotional, environmental—disrupts this state, it triggers a nonspecific physiological response, consisting of three distinct stages:

1. *Alarm.* As it becomes aware of a stressor, the body mobilizes various systems for action.

social support An individual's knowledge or belief that he or she is cared for and loved, belongs to a network or community, and has a mental obligation with others in the network.

trauma An intensely upsetting, scary, or disturbing event.

homeostasis The body's natural state of balance or stability.

Levels of certain hormones rise; blood pressure and flow to the muscles increase; the digestive and immune systems slow down.

2. *Resistance.* If the stress continues, the body draws on its internal resources to try to sustain homeostasis, but this requires greater and greater effort.

3. *Exhaustion.* If stress continues long enough, normal functioning becomes impossible. Even a small amount of additional stress at this point can lead to a breakdown. In animal experiments, Selye found that persistent stress caused illnesses similar to those seen in humans, such as heart attacks, stroke, kidney disease, and rheumatoid arthritis.

Selye's theory has been criticized as being too abstract and failing to take into account variations among individuals and differences between minor and major stressors and positive and negative stress. However, although the GAS model fails to take these variations and differences into account, it nonetheless remains fundamental to our understanding of the impact of stress on the body.

How the Body Responds to Stress

Over more than a century of scientific study, researchers have formulated models to describe how our bodies and brains react under stress. They include:

Automatic Stress Responses

Prehistoric humans faced constant life-or-death dangers. Without warning, a saber-toothed tiger might pounce, or an enemy tribe might attack. Our ancestors evolved quick reactions that required no conscious thought but mobilized their bodies in ways that helped ensure the survival of our species.

Fight or Flight

Physiologist Walter Cannon, another pioneer in stress research, dubbed the complex, near-instantaneous sequence of internal changes that kicks in when you confront any potential danger the **"fight or flight" response.** When your brain perceives a threat, it sounds the body's alarm and sends signals for production of natural stimulants that speed up thinking, heart rate, breathing, immunity, metabolism, and blood flow.

Your heart beats harder to pump blood to your large muscles; you breathe more rapidly to take in more oxygen.

Your body mobilizes energy and delivers it to the brain, heart, and lungs; shuts off nonessential functions like digestion and the sex drive, and ramps up the immune system to prepare for quick healing in case of injury. This classic threat response primes you to run for your life or go on the offense and fight back.

In interpersonal situations in contemporary life, individuals "fight" by arguing, opposing, demanding, criticizing, accusing, insisting, or refusing. Alternatively, they may take flight—by physically removing themselves or by withdrawing, not talking, dissociating, changing the topic, or otherwise "checking out."

Freezing

Scientists have identified an acute stress response that may precede fight or flight: **freezing**, a survival mechanism that stems from some of the oldest circuits within the brain.[15] Animals, like deer suddenly caught in the headlights of a car, often stop as soon as they become aware of a danger. In the wild, freezing makes them less likely to be detected by a bear or coyote that has not yet caught their scent and may delay an attack if the predator is nearby.

Freezing may last for seconds or minutes—although it may feel longer. As evolutionary scientists explain, early humans also may have frozen in place at the sight or sound of a potential hazard, using this time to stop, look, listen, assess what was happening, and mobilize for action. If, for instance, they spotted a lion at some distance, they would turn and flee. If the beast was already charging at them, they braced for a fight.

Submission

If unable to flee from or fight off a predator, animals may become immobile in the hope that their attacker will lose interest. In humans, this sort of reaction is called dissociation. Their minds go blank. Too overwhelmed to say a word or move a muscle, they submit, forfeit, yield, give up or give in, lower their expectations, settle, agree with others, or surrender their aspirations.[16]

Submission occurs when no other option seems possible. Hostages held by armed gunmen, for instance, comply with their orders because they fear for their lives. In a less dramatic situation, you might discover that a friend's romantic partner is cheating, but you may not say anything because you fear that the emotional fallout would be devastating for everyone.

fight or flight response The body's automatic physiological response that prepares the individual to take action upon facing a perceived threat or danger.

freezing A survival mechanism that stems from some of the oldest circuits within the brain; freezing gives a person time to stop, look, listen, and assess what is happening in the face of a stressor.

submission If unable to flee from or "fight off" a stressor, a person may give up or give in, agree with others, or surrender his or her aspirations.

✔ **Check-in:** Your stress selfie

Think back to a recent stressful experience. Did you react by fighting, taking flight, freezing, or submitting?

Imagine what you looked like in that situation. What thoughts were running through your mind? Describe or draw this image.

What steps could you have taken to respond differently? Write them down as a reminder of what to do in the future.

Challenge Response Model

Imagine that you are an athlete preparing for an Olympic final or a paramedic racing to an accident scene. Just as in the fight-or-flight response, your body mobilizes—not to save your life, but to perform at your peak. Your heart pumps more blood through your body; you breathe more deeply to take in more oxygen; your pupils dilate to take in more light; your hearing sharpens; your brain focuses. You are ready to give your all.

Unlike a threat response, which rewires the brain to heighten a sense of danger, a **challenge response** strengthens connections between the parts of the brain that suppress fear and enhance learning and positive motivation.[17] In studies of people in high-stakes situations, the challenge response consistently predicted better performance under pressure than either the fight-or-flight reaction or the absence of any stress response. Students scored higher on exams; athletes ran faster, jumped higher, or scored more points for their team.

What determines if you react with a threat response or a challenge response? The most important factor is how you perceive your ability to handle it. As you size up a stressor, you consciously or unconsciously ask yourself: How tough is this going to be? Do I have the skills or resources I need to handle it? Where can I turn for help? Just as in the cognitive reappraisal model of stress (see page 12), you respond differently if you believe that the challenge exceeds your resources or if you believe you can cope with it successfully.

Individuals who consistently respond to stress as if it were a challenge rather than a threat are more likely to:

- Focus on their resources
- Acknowledge their personal strengths

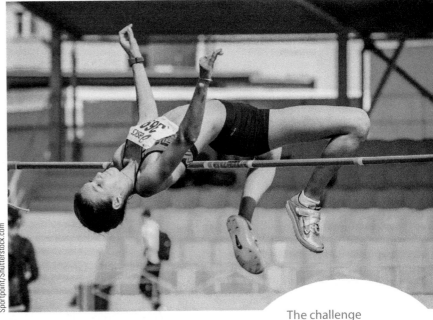

Sportpoint/Shutterstock.com

- Think about how they prepared for a particular challenge in the past
- Remember how they overcame previous challenges
- Imagine the support of their loved ones
- Pray or know that others are praying for them[18]

The challenge response mobilizes energy and concentration so athletes can perform at their peak.

🌀 **Stress Reliever:** Turn a Threat into a Challenge

As soon as you notice early stress signals, think of how they are preparing you to meet a challenge.

Pounding heart? Tell yourself that you are getting more energizing blood throughout your body.

Sweaty palms? They signal anticipation and excitement.

Butterflies in your stomach? The nerve cells in your digestive tract are telling you that something significant is happening.

Take a deep breath to sense your inner energy.

Ask yourself: What step should I take now to make the most of this moment?

challenge response A physiological response that strengthens connections between the parts of the brain that suppress fear and enhance learning and positive motivation so as to prepare and enable a person to face a stressor directly.

Tend-and-Befriend Model

The classic threat response that prepares us for fight or flight can make people angry, defensive, aggressive, or withdrawn. But some individuals respond differently under pressure and become more caring, compassionate, and cooperative. The reason, according to the **tend-and-befriend** model, is that an urge to forge social connections under stress may be, like fight-or-flight, an essential survival instinct, especially for the females of a species.

Rather than the "stand and defend" reaction of the men in a prehistoric tribe or clan, the women may have responded by "tending" to offspring in harm's way and "befriending" those who would threaten them.[19] Women may not be as innately driven as men to opt for fight or flight because estrogen and other female hormones may moderate the effects of the powerful stress hormones.[20] However, in times of crisis, persons of both sexes may become more trusting, generous, and willing to risk their own well-being to protect others.[21]

The tend-and-befriend response creates what some call the "biology of courage[22]," a physiological state that reduces fear and induces hope. The very acts of connecting and caring for others enable individuals to overcome feelings of powerlessness and hopelessness by inducing increases in several key brain chemicals, including:

- Oxytocin, which regulates the social caregiving system so you feel less fear and more empathy, connection, and trust.

- Dopamine, which boosts optimism about ability to cope and primes the brain for action so you don't freeze under pressure.

- Serotonin, which enhances your perception, intuition, and self-control so you can understand what is needed and take the most effective action.

Although the tend-and-befriend response may have evolved to protect children, it can emerge in response to any challenge you face. This is why nothing may help you more than helping others when you're feeling overwhelmed. When you reach out to tend and befriend someone in need, you benefit as well.[23] (See Chapter 10 for more on the benefits of altruism.)

Transactional or Cognitive-Reappraisal Model

The **Transactional or Cognitive-Reappraisal Model**, developed by psychologist Richard Lazarus, is a framework for evaluating the processes of coping with stressful events. In his view, stress is "neither an environmental stimulus, a characteristic of the person, nor a response but a relationship between demands and the power to deal with them without unreasonable or destructive costs."[24] The level of stress you experience depends on your appraisal of a stressor and on the social and cultural resources available to deal with it.

According to this model, stress stems from an interaction or "transaction" between a person and a stress-inducing trigger. When individuals confront a stressor—whether it's a painful injury or an argument with a partner—they make immediate judgments about whether it poses a threat and whether they will be able to respond to it. Lazarus identified four stages in this process:

- The *primary appraisal* is the evaluation of the significance of the stressor or threatening event. You judge its severity based on previous experience, self-knowledge, and available information about the challenge. You determine whether or not it is threatening or thrilling, positive or negative, controllable or overwhelming, major or minor. If you do not perceive any danger, you do not experience a stress response because your well-being is not at stake.

- If you perceive the situation as threatening, you proceed to the *secondary appraisal* and assess whether you have the power and social, cultural, financial, and other resources to act. In essence, you ask yourself: What can I do about this? Can I control it? If you perceive that you can cope with the stressor, you experience positive stress. If you conclude that you may not be able to handle the stressor, you experience negative stress.

tend-and-befriend A behavioral response to stress characterized by increased feelings of trust and compassion and an urge to force social connections.

Transactional or Cognitive Reappraisal Model A framework for evaluating the process of coping with a stressful event in four stages (primary appraisal, secondary appraisal, coping, and reevaluation); based on the theory that the level of stress that people experience depends on their assessment of a stressor and on the social and cultural resources available to deal with it.

When dealing with stress, women often "tend-and-befriend" by forging supportive social connections.

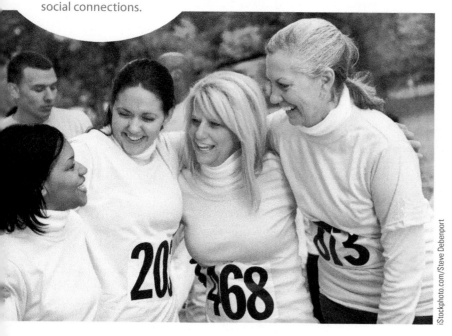

iStockphoto.com/Steve Debenport

- In the *coping* stage, you may try a variety of efforts and processes with different outcomes. These include:
  - problem-based coping, used when you feel you have control of the situation. For instance, you might deal with the stress of a failing grade by setting up a study schedule for upcoming exams.
  - emotion-based coping, used when you feel you have little control of the situation. You might try avoidance (cutting class so you don't have to see the instructor), distancing yourself (telling yourself the bad grade doesn't really matter), venting your frustration in an argument with a friend, or numbing yourself with alcohol or a drug.
- In the fourth stage of *reappraisal*, you evaluate the outcome in terms of your emotional well-being, ability to function, and health behaviors. Depending on whether or not the original stressor has been eliminated, you may need to try again or use a different approach.[25] If, for example, you realize you can't keep skipping class after blowing the midterm, you make up any late assignments, ask the instructor for extra-credit assignments, and focus on studying for future exams.

✔ **Check-in:** Appraise your stress.

When stressed, ask yourself:

What is happening?

Is it in any way a threat to my safety?

What can I do about it?

Is this strategy working?

If not, what else can I do?

How Much Stress Is Too Much?

Stress is essential for a productive life. With too little stress, we might not be motivated enough to work toward our goals. Stress energizes and stimulates us to get up, keep moving, reach out, accomplish something—up to a point. With too much stress, however, you can't function at your best. But when your stress level is neither too high nor too low, but just right, you become energized, effective, and efficient.

Psychology explains this phenomenon in terms of the **Yerkes-Dodson Principle** (named for the psychologists who first described it in 1908). In laboratory experiments, these researchers found that mild electrical shocks motivated rats to complete a maze, but when the shocks became too strong, the rats scurried around in random directions to escape. Their conclusion: increasing stress can boost performance—but only up to a certain point.

Your optimal level of stress or arousal differs from everyone else's and varies for different tasks. If you are synching your laptop and cell phone, you need to be just attentive enough to avoid mistakes. If you're engaged in a more complex task, such as composing an essay, you might require a greater sense of arousal to concentrate

Yerkes-Dodson Principle The theory that increased stress or arousal can help improve performance, but only up to a certain point, and that excess stress diminishes performance and can undermine health.

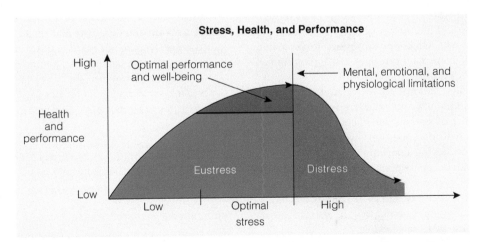

FIGURE 1.2 Stress, Health, and Performance. Stress can energize you to perform at your best—but only to a certain extent. Excess stress drains energy and impairs performance.

and organize your thoughts. But if writing is especially stressful, perhaps because English is your second language, you might become so anxious that you can't think through what you want to say.

Rethinking Stress

Many people view stress as a health menace—with reason. Although it rarely causes disease, stress can trigger molecular changes that make individuals more susceptible to many illnesses. Its impact on psychological well-being is no less significant. Excess stress can undermine the ability to learn, sleep, perform at your best, and cope with day-to-day hassles. As discussed in Chapter 3, it also can worsen depression, anxiety, and other mental disorders.

So would you be better off if you could avoid or eliminate stress? Read through the following section before you answer.

The Stress Paradox

When swamped by deadlines and demands, you might wish that life's difficulties could magically disappear or that you could find a way to dodge difficult experiences or numb the discomfort they cause. But what might a stress-free life look like? Would you drop out of school? Cut ties with your family? Quit your job? Break up with your partner? Stop saving money for the hiking adventure you've been planning for years? And if you did, would you feel happier? Probably not.

As researchers have meticulously documented, happy lives are not stress-free, nor does a stress-free life guarantee happiness. In countries around the globe, higher levels of stress are associated with greater well-being. Even though people would like to worry less, stress seems to go along with what we want most: love, health, and satisfaction with our lives. Psychologists call this the "**stress paradox.**"

In a large national survey of American adults ages 18 through 78, individuals reporting the highest number of stressful life events were the ones most likely to describe their lives as meaningful. Stress may be the consequence of engaging in roles, taking on responsibilities, and pursuing goals that fuel our sense of purpose. The most common sources of stress—relationships, jobs, health, parenting, caregiving—are also the greatest sources of life satisfaction.

"Stress is what happens when something you care about is at stake," says psychologist Kelly McGonigal, author of *The Upside of Stress,* "Rather than being a sign that something is wrong with your life, feeling stressed can be a barometer for how engaged you are in activities and relationships that are personally meaningful."[26] (See Chapter 10 for more on finding meaning in life).

Trying to avoid stress often backfires because of a vicious cycle called stress generation. As psychological research has shown, individuals who try to steer clear of difficulties end up creating more distress because they often turn to self-destructive distractions, substances, and other escapes. If you adopt a stress-avoidant perspective, anything in life that causes stress looks like a problem: If you feel stressed at school, you blame the instructors. If you experience stress in a relationship, you think there's something wrong with your partner. If trying to make a healthful change in your diet is stressful, you give up and go back to eating junk food. If you believe that life should be less stressful, you may begin to feel inadequate. If you were only strong, smart, or good enough, you wouldn't be stressed. You see stress as a personal failure, and you're more likely to feel hopeless and to become depressed.

What does lead to greater optimism, energy, and fulfillment? Although it may seem like another paradox, the answer is embracing stress. When you accept challenge and change as part of life's rich blend of experiences, you move beyond fear to acceptance and anticipation. You build your coping muscles, connect with your innermost values, and join forces with others. You face challenges head on and, win or lose, you learn from them. Because of—not despite—stress, you grow into your best and fullest self.

✔ **Check-in:** What would you subtract?

Reflect back on the last year and recall the days you considered very stressful. Think about everything that happened on those days.

If you could subtract them from your life experience, what would you be taking away? Challenges that you are now proud you've met? Relationships that you hold dear? Experiences that helped you grow?

You might have spared yourself some discomfort, but you also could have missed out on invaluable experiences.

stress paradox The observation that the most stressful aspects of life also bring the greatest satisfaction and joy.

Stress Mindsets

Is stress beneficial or harmful, enhancing or debilitating? Your answer may be more important than you might guess. The reason: the power of "**mindset**," the mental frame or lens that selectively organizes information, thereby orienting individuals toward a unique way of understanding experiences that shapes their choices and behaviors.[27]

Mindsets are beliefs that bias how you think, feel, and act and thereby shape your reality. Rather than preferences or opinions, mindsets reflect your philosophy of how life works. If you believe that the world is a dangerous place, you may see a potential threat everywhere you look. If you believe that money is the key to happiness, you may base key decisions, like choosing a major or career, solely on the financial bottom line.

People who believe that stress improves performance, productivity, learning, well-being, and personal growth have a "stress-is-enhancing" mindset; those who think that it impairs these functions, a "stress-is-debilitating" mindset.[28] Your stress mindset may influence the impact of stress as much as other variables such as the severity of a stressor or your capacity to cope.

In an eighteen-year study—the first to examine the association between perception of stress and cardiovascular health in a large population—researchers followed 7,268 men and women who were asked to rate the extent that stress had affected their health on a range from "not at all" to "extremely." When other variables such as age and overall well-being were accounted for, those who said that stress had affected their health "a lot" or "extremely" were 49 percent more likely than other participants to have a heart attack or die of heart disease. Only participants who reported that stress had affected their health "a lot" or "extremely" (8 percent) had an increased risk of coronary heart disease.[29]

Stress about stress, this suggests, may increase cortisol and promote inflammation as well as elevating blood pressure and heart rate. People who believe that stress is making them sick, who anticipate a decline in health as a result of stress, and who feel they can do little or nothing to control their stress or their fate also may engage in more unhealthy behaviors, such as smoking, drinking, and physical inactivity.[30]

Mindsets, however powerful, can be changed. In various anxiety-inducing experiments, volunteers who faced tasks such as solving math problems in their heads or speaking in public were given different messages. Some were told that their bodies were preparing them to perform at their best and encouraged to say "I am excited" when they felt their muscles tense or their hearts race. These participants consistently performed much better and appeared more relaxed than those who were told that they should simply stay calm. Viewing the challenge as an opportunity rather than a threat and interpreting the physiological arousal as excitement rather than anxiety changed their mindsets.[31]

....

✔ **Check-in:** To what extent do you feel that the stress in your life has affected your health?

....

____Not at all;

____Slightly:

____Moderately;

____A lot;

____Extremely

Why? What do you think are the implications of your answer?

....

From Surviving to Thriving

As psychologists define it, **thriving**—also dubbed hardiness, grit, resilience, or posttraumatic growth—refers to "enhanced psychological and physical functioning after successful adaptation."[32] You thrive when you respond to

mindset The mental frame or lens that selectively organizes information, thereby orienting individuals toward a unique way of understanding experiences that shapes their choices and behaviors.

thriving Enhanced psychological and physical functioning after successful adaptation to stressors and change. It is also known as hardiness, grit, resilience, or posttraumatic growth.

Learning to meet challenges and manage stress are among the most valuable lessons college can provide.

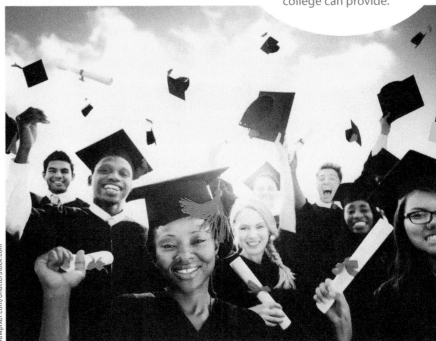
Rawpixel.com/Shutterstock.com

stress creatively and acquire even more potent skills to use in the future. You become stronger, smarter, more confident, committed, engaged, and fulfilled than ever would be possible if you shirked responsibility and coasted through life.

Stressful experiences can fundamentally change individuals for the better, yielding benefits such as mental toughness, heightened awareness, new perspectives, a sense of mastery, clearer priorities, deeper relationships, and greater appreciation for life.[33] When you look at stress this way, life doesn't become less stressful, but it does become more meaningful. You progress through an "upward spiral of flourishing," in which psychological approaches such as those discussed in Chapters 3 and 8 generate positive emotions, such as optimism and gratitude, and lead to a positive reappraisal of stress.[34]

Although at times undeniably unpleasant, tough, and even heart-breaking, stress provides lessons greater than those taught in classrooms. Without the contrast of stress, you would not appreciate pleasures in quite the same way. More than that, you might not explore all your possibilities, develop all your talents and strengths,

and savor the sense of mastery that comes when you face stress head on, learn from it, and move forward. This is the difference between distress and challenge, between surviving and thriving.

diaphragmatic or abdominal breathing Inhaling in a way that causes the diaphragm to contract and move down, drawing air deep into the lungs.

 Stress Reliever: Make the Most of Stress

Choose to remember your most important values so you find meaning in everyday stress.

Have open and honest conversations with trusted friends about your struggles so you feel less alone.

View your body's stress response as a resource to help you handle pressure and rise to a challenge.

Go out of your way to help someone so you can access the biology of courage and hope.

Chapter Summary

- In psychology, "stress" can refer to an external force that causes someone to become tense or upset, and/or to an internal state of arousal, and/or to the physical response of the body when it must adapt or adjust to a challenge. Dr. Hans Selye, a pioneer in studying physiological reactions to a challenge, defined stress as "the non-specific response of the body to any demand made upon it."

- Perception (one's way of evaluating, understanding, and interpreting a situation) is critical in how we respond to stress. Stress is experienced when we perceive that a demand exceeds the personal and social resources we are able to mobilize.

- The three major types of stress are "eustress," (the positive, energizing stress that challenges us to grow, adapt, and find creative solutions), "distress," (the negative stress caused by trauma, loss, and other upsetting occurrences), and "neustress," (a response to stressors that do not affect us directly but that may trigger stressful feelings).

- Stress can have an impact on every dimension of well-being: physical; psychological and emotional; spiritual; social; intellectual; occupational; and environmental.

- Stressors vary in frequency, intensity, and duration. Acute stress is time-limited and resolves fairly quickly. Episodic acute stress occurs periodically. Chronic or long-term stress poses the greatest danger to physical and psychological health.

- Stress experts Drs. Thomas Holmes and Richard Rahe documented an association between stressful life events and the onset of disease. Their Schedule of Recent Experiences (SRE) evaluates individual levels of stress and potential for coping on the basis of life change units and the degree of readjustment they require to adapt successfully.

- Trauma (an intensely upsetting, scary, or disturbing event) occurs so often that half of all Americans report at least one potentially traumatizing event during the course of their lives. Severe trauma-related conditions can cause disabling symptoms that persist for years or decades.

- The General Adaptation Syndrome (GAS), as defined by Hans Selye, consists of three distinct stages: *Alarm,* when the body mobilizes various systems for action; *Resistance,* as the body makes greater efforts to try to sustain the state of physiological balance called homeostasis; and *Exhaustion*, when normal functioning becomes impossible.

- Physiologist Walter Cannon described the survival mechanism with which humans react to stress as the "fight or flight" response, in which the brain signals for production of natural stimulants that speed up thinking, heart rate, breathing, immunity, metabolism, and blood flow to prime individuals to either fight or take flight.

- Other acute stress reactions are: 1) freezing in place when confronting a potential hazard; and 2) submission, in which a person simply yields because a stressful situation seems too overwhelming to do anything else.

- A challenge response to stress strengthens connections between the parts of the brain that suppress fear and enhance learning and motivation to boost performance under pressure. Some describe its effects as "the biology of hope."

- Another stress reaction is to "tend-and-befriend," or to respond to danger by caring for offspring and by reaching out to others for protection and support. Women may be more likely than men to act in this way because of the moderating effects of female hormones such as oxytocin and estrogen.

- Psychologist Richard Lazarus's Transactional or Cognitive-Reappraisal Model defines stress as "a relationship between demands and the power to deal with them without unreasonable or destructive costs." The level of stress depends on an interaction or "transaction" between a person and a stress-inducing trigger.

- According to the Yerkes-Dodson principle (named for the psychologists who first described it), increasing stress can boost performance—but only up to a certain point. The optimal level of stress or arousal differs for different individuals and for different tasks.

- The stress paradox refers to the observation that higher, not lower, levels of stress are linked to greater life satisfaction. The reason is that many of the challenges that can provoke stress also are the source of meaningful experiences.

- A "stress-is-enhancing" or "stress-is-debilitating" mindset can shape your beliefs about the impact of stress on well-being. Individuals who view stress as hazardous are more likely to develop serious stress-related health problems.

- Although often seen as a danger or threat, stress can also be viewed as an opportunity for learning and growth that enables individuals to thrive—that is, to function at a higher level both psychologically and physically. The potential positive benefits of stressful experiences include mental toughness, heightened awareness, new perspectives, a sense of mastery, clearer priorities, deeper relationships, greater appreciation for life, and an increased sense of meaningfulness.

STRESS RELIEVERS

Refocus

Upload a photo of a favorite person, place, or pet to your cell phone or computer. As soon as you start feeling stressed, click on it. Block all other thoughts, and focus completely on the happiness you associate with this image. Breathe slowly and deeply.

Turn a Threat into a Challenge

As soon as you notice early stress signals, think of how they are preparing you to meet a challenge.

- Pounding heart? Tell yourself that you are getting more energizing blood throughout your body.

- Sweaty palms? They signal anticipation and excitement.

- Butterflies in your stomach? The nerve cells in your digestive tract are telling you that something significant is happening.

- Take a deep breath to sense your inner energy. Ask yourself: What step should I take now to make the most of this moment?

Make the Most of Stress

- Choose to remember your most important values so you find meaning in everyday stress.

- Have open and honest conversations with trusted friends about your struggles so you feel less alone. View your body's stress response as a resource to help you handle pressure and rise to a challenge. Go out of your way to help someone so you can access the biology of courage and hope.

Because we are all different, with different backgrounds, personalities, life circumstances, and stressors, there is no one-size-fits-all stress management technique—nor even one magic weapon—for you to use for every stressor you encounter in life. As you progress through this course, your goal is to assemble a broad repertoire of coping strategies—a toolkit for personal stress management—that you can tailor to specific situations and stressors.

There is no magic or hidden secret to this process. Stress management consists of tested techniques and skills that you can master in the same way that you learned to ride a bike, drive a car, speak a new language, or write HTML code—step by step, lesson by lesson, day by day. The tools and techniques in this book are designed to reinforce what you're learning about stress management.

REFLECTION: Getting to Know Your Personal Stress

This exercise can help you get in touch with what defines your personal stress so you are more aware of what's happening. Below are words that are often used to explain stress in terms of feelings, physical sensations, and behaviors. Check the words that reflect your personal stress. Add any other terms that may come to mind.

Feelings: How do you feel when under stress?
_____ Anxious
_____ Scared
_____ Nervous
_____ Excited
_____ Overwhelmed
_____ On edge
_____ Apprehensive
_____ Sad
_____ Frustrated
_____ Lost
_____ Depressed
_____ Freaked out
_____ Uneasy
_____ Fretful
_____ Frightened
_____ Worried
_____ Overcommitted
_____ Exhausted
_____ Swamped
_____ Out of control
_____ Fragile
_____ Irritable

Physical Sensations: What happens in your body under stress?
_____ Tense (muscle tension)
_____ Restless
_____ Weak
_____ On high alert
_____ Achy
_____ Chest pains
_____ Stomachache
_____ Nausea
_____ Fidgety
_____ Trouble sleeping
_____ Lack of appetite
_____ Excessive appetite
_____ Dizzy
_____ Jittery
_____ Problems breathing
_____ Headache
_____ Weepy

Behavior: How do you act under stress?
_____ Avoiding tasks
_____ Not completing tasks
_____ Obsessive thinking
_____ Unable to concentrate
_____ Getting caught in negative thinking traps
_____ Not sleeping
_____ Oversleeping
_____ Not eating
_____ Overeating
_____ Changing your normal routine
_____ Excessive exercise
_____ Excessive TV watching, game playing, etc.
_____ Using substances (alcohol, tobacco, drugs) in excess
_____ Getting in arguments/taking stress out on others
_____ Avoiding social situations
_____ Pulling away from family or friends
_____ Clinging to others

Based on your answers, create a self-portrait of yourself under stress—in words or in a drawing, a cartoon figure, an emoticon, or a selfie. Create another image of yourself feeling strong, confident, and capable when confronting a stressor.

TECHNIQUE: Introductory Breathing Exercise

Breath brings life. Each inhalation draws energizing oxygen into your body; each exhalation releases the waste product carbon dioxide. As discussed in Chapter 12, certain breathing patterns serve as powerful tools for releasing stress. The following exercise introduces **diaphragmatic or abdominal breathing**, which balances the levels of oxygen and carbon dioxide in your blood and reduces muscle tension and anxiety.

Listen to the Introductory Breathing Exercise audio instructions in MindTap, read and record them yourself, or pair up with a classmate and take turns leading each other through this exercise.

- Choose a time and place where you will not be disturbed. Turn off cell phones, laptops, or any other device that may interrupt this calming exercise.

- Sit comfortably, with your eyes closed and your spine reasonably straight. Place one hand gently on your abdomen.

- Bring your attention to your breathing. Press your hand down on your abdomen as you exhale forcefully.

- Let your abdomen push up against your hand as you inhale.

- As you slowly inhale and exhale, pay close attention as each inhalation brings air first into your abdomen, then your middle chest, and finally your upper chest. Imagine filling a glass with water from bottom to top as you inhale.

- Once you establish a pattern of smooth deep breaths, you can slow your breath even more. Inhale through your nostrils and exhale through your mouth as if you were breathing out through a straw. With each breath, feel your abdomen lower and rise.

- Focus on the sound of your breaths as you become increasingly relaxed.

- If thoughts or feelings enter your consciousness, take note of their arrival and then return to focusing on your breathing.

- Repeat this basic breathing exercise for about five or ten minutes at least once a day. Gradually extend your time to fifteen and then twenty minutes.

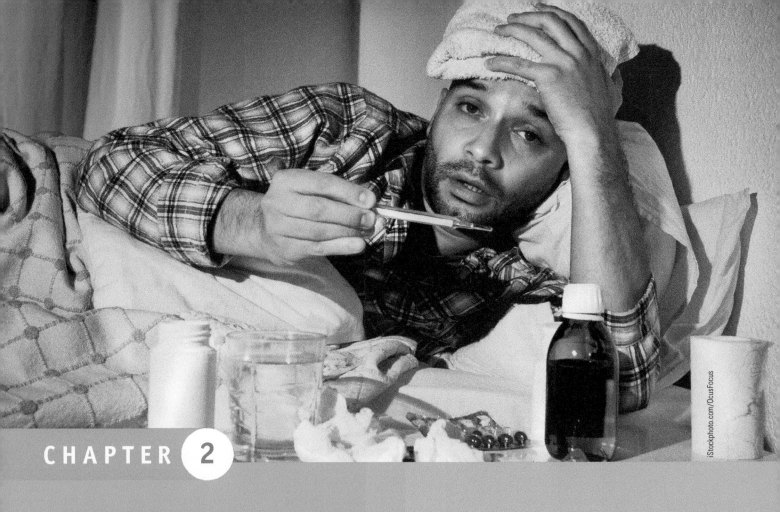

iStockphoto.com/OcusFocus

CHAPTER 2

Stress and Your Body

After reading this chapter, you should be able to:

2.1   Explain the biological responses to stress.

2.2   Describe stress and susceptibility in the context of the diasthesis stress model.

2.3   Discuss the physical and emotional impact of repeated or chronic stress.

2.4   Summarize the effects of stress on immunity.

2.5   Differentiate between the impact of acute, episodic, and chronic stress on the cardiovascular system.

2.6   List the physiological changes brought about by stress on the gastrointestinal system.

2.7   Describe the responses of skeletal muscles and smooth muscles to stress.

2.8   Relate the connection between stress and the skin.

2.9   Discuss sexuality and reproductive issues created by stress.

2.10   Assess the role of stress as a factor that causes cancer.

2.11   Explain the relationship between telomeres, telomerase, and aging.

2.12   Identify effective strategies to relieve stress.

_____ Take a few deep breaths.

_____ Focusing on your head, pay attention to your forehead, your eyes, your nose, your cheeks, your mouth, where your head meets your neck, your throat.

_____ Observe how your head and neck feel both on the surface and deep within. Take a moment to consciously explore every part.

_____ Now focus your attention on your shoulders and upper back. Explore how each of your muscles feels, how they connect with one another, how you are holding yourself.

_____ Notice any tension or tightness. Consciously release and relax this area.

_____ Gradually shift your focus to your midsection.

_____ How does your chest feel as you breathe in and out?

_____ How does your stomach feel? Your heart? Your mid- and lower back area? Your spinal column? Your sides?

_____ Pay attention to how each muscle, bone, and organ feels at this moment. Are you feeling comfortable, tense, anything noteworthy or out of the ordinary?

_____ Shift your attention to your arms and hands.

_____ Notice the weight of your arms, how your joints feel, the weight of your hands and the air between your fingers.

_____ Take a moment to think about the temperature, textures, and position of your arms and hands.

_____ Shift your attention to your legs and feet.

_____ Focus on how your bottom feels in your seat, then how your thighs and calves feel.

_____ Take note of your joints and any tension in the muscles of your lower body.

_____ Concentrate on your feet and toes, paying attention to how they feel against the ground or in the air.

_____ Be mindful of any tension in the muscles throughout your body, anything that feels good or that feels uncomfortable.

_____ Be mindful of your own skeletal structure and how your body connects together.

_____ Take a few more deep breaths and reflect on what you've noticed.

Record what you've observed about yourself in your journal.

When his throat started feeling scratchy during finals week, Kyle thought to himself, "I can't get sick—especially now." But he couldn't stop hacking and sneezing. He felt chilled one minute, sweaty the next. At the campus health center, a physician's assistant tried to console Kyle.

"It happens at the end of every term," she said. "Students get so stressed out that they get sick." Kyle found little comfort in the fact that he had inadvertently confirmed that during exam time, students are more susceptible to upper respiratory infections like colds and flu.[1]

The same thing can happen to any of us—and not just during tense times like finals. Stress affects multiple organ systems in the body, often in subtle ways. Over time people may become so conditioned to stress's impact that they no longer notice, yet this silent threat contributes to an estimated 50 percent of illnesses and as many as 80 percent of all visits to physicians.[2]

These risks are real, but they are not inevitable. Stress isn't necessarily or uniformly harmful. Its impact often depends on how individuals perceive and respond to it.

"Stress increases the risk of health problems, except when people regularly give back to their communities," notes psychologist Kelly McGonigal, author of *The Upside of Stress*. "Stress increases the risk of dying, except when people have a sense of purpose. Stressing increases the risk of depression, except when people perceive themselves as capable. Stress is debilitating, except when it helps you perform. Stress makes people selfish, except when it makes them altruistic. For every harmful outcome there is an exception that sometimes replaces the harm with an unexpected benefit."[3]

Remember: The stress response is normal—and useful. Yes, you may find it frightening to feel your heart beating faster when you're stressed. But your heart speeds up under all sorts of non-threatening circumstances—when you're jogging, for instance, or watching the final minutes in a tied championship game. As described in Chapter 1, the biology of stress is not different from the biology of excitement or even of courage. When you're riding a roller coaster, you think of your intense physical reaction as thrilling rather than threatening. Similarly, first-responders feel a surge of adrenaline when they run into a burning house or rescue a victim from raging flood waters. Like them, you can learn to recognize your physiological responses to stress as empowering rather than upsetting.[4]

Stress is most likely to take a toll on your health when you view it as harmful; when you do not think you have the capacity or resources to cope with it; when you see yourself as isolated from others; or when it feels utterly meaningless and involuntary. But you can take positive steps to lessen stress's toxic effects, enhance its benefits, and achieve homeostasis or balance in your body and in your life. In this chapter you'll learn more about what happens inside your body under stress, what makes certain people more susceptible to it, and its impact on various organ systems.

The Biology of Stress

You know how stress feels: the pounding heart, the dry mouth, the tense muscles. But your automatic stress responses also set off a cascade of physiological changes that you may not be aware of.

The Inside Story

Beyond the sensations you consciously feel, stress triggers a cascade of physiological processes (see Figure 2.1), including the following:

- Your mental and brainwave activity increase.
- Your heart rate, cardiac output (volume of blood pumped by the heart), and blood pressure increase.
- Your breathing rate increases, and your air passageways widen.
- Your metabolism speeds up.
- More oxygen flows to your brain.
- Muscle contraction increases, boosting your muscular strength.
- More blood flows to your muscles and limbs.
- Your blood thins (to reduce the risk of clots).
- Your body increases production and circulation of blood cholesterol and free fatty acids.
- Your liver releases more glucose (blood sugar) to nourish the muscles.
- Your pituitary gland releases endorphins.
- Your pupils dilate (widen).

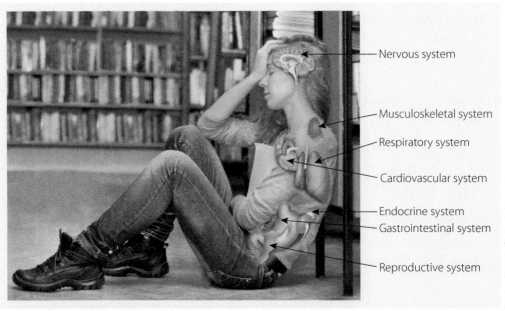

Nervous system

Musculoskeletal system

Respiratory system

Cardiovascular system

Endocrine system
Gastrointestinal system

Reproductive system

Ermolaev Alexander/Shutterstock.com

FIGURE 2.1 Stress triggers physiological changes that affect multiple systems within the body.

- You perspire more.
- Your body dampens or suppresses functions not essential for immediate action, including the immune, reproductive, and digestive systems.

The Key Players

The primary structures responsible for these physiological changes include the following (See Figure 2.2.):

- The **amygdala**, an almond-shaped structure within the brain, plays a critical role in processing emotions, particularly negative ones related to danger. When you encounter someone who's shouting in anger, for instance, the amygdala generates a sense of anxiety and fear.

- The **hypothalamus**, deep in the central region of the brain, functions like a command center.

- The **pituitary gland**, attached by a stalk to the base of the brain, regulates all hormonal functions in the body.

- The **adrenal glands**, located above the kidneys, consist of two parts: an inner section called the **adrenal medulla** and an outer layer called the **adrenal cortex**. The medulla produces **epinephrine** (also called adrenaline) and its metabolite **norepinephrine** (noradrenaline), powerful chemicals that increase blood pressure, stimulate heart muscle, and accelerate the heart rate so the heart pumps more blood. The cortex secretes **cortisol**, a hormone that spurs the metabolism of nutrients to provide energy and fuel for your body and brain.

- The **autonomic nervous system**, the branch of the nervous system responsible for functions such as digestion, blood pressure, and body temperature, controls essential involuntary body functions that occur without our thinking about them, such as breathing, blood pressure, heartbeat, temperature, appetite, and sleep cycles. It consists of two branches:

  - The **sympathetic nervous system**, which is responsible for initiating the fight-or-flight response, functions like a gas pedal in a car. In response to a possible threat, it provides a burst of energy so the body can respond to perceived dangers.
  - The **parasympathetic nervous system**, which returns the body to a state of homeostasis, acts like a brake. It promotes the "rest and digest" response that calms the body after the danger has passed.

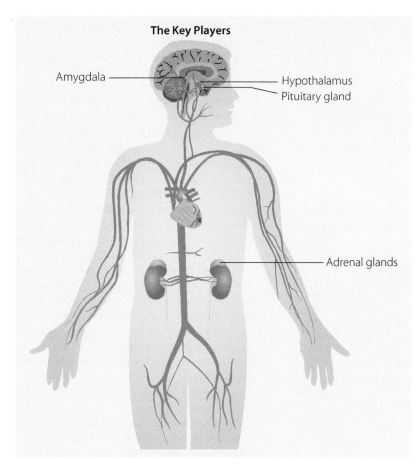

The Key Players

Amygdala

Hypothalamus
Pituitary gland

Adrenal glands

FIGURE 2.2 Structures within the brain and the endocrine system direct the body's physiological response to stress.

Sounding the Stress Alarm

The stress response begins in the brain. When you hear a footstep behind you on a dark street, your ears alert the amygdala; this stress sentry sends a distress signal to the hypothalamus, which activates the sympathetic nervous system by sending messages through the autonomic nerves to the medulla in each adrenal gland; the medulla immediately releases the stimulants epinephrine and norepinephrine into the bloodstream.

As a result, your heart rate, pulse rate, and blood pressure go up; you breathe more rapidly; the small airways in your lungs open wide so you can take in as much oxygen as possible with each breath; your blood carries extra oxygen to the brain, increasing alertness; your sight, hearing, and other senses become sharper; with the release of glucose (blood sugar) and fats from temporary storage sites in the body, nutrients flood into your bloodstream. As long as the control centers of the brain perceive the need for arousal, stimulation of the medulla continues—which can eventually fatigue this part of the adrenal gland.

These physiological responses begin before the brain's visual centers have even had a chance

amygdala An almond-shaped structure within the brain that plays a critical role in processing emotions, including anxiety and fear.

hypothalamus Chief region of the brain that acts as the command center for higher-order thinking.

pituitary gland The key regulator of all hormonal functions in the body.

adrenal glands Two triangle-shaped glands, one positioned on top of each kidney, that secrete stress hormones during the stress response.

adrenal medulla
Inner portion of adrenal glands, where epinephrine and norepinephrine are secreted.

adrenal cortex Outer portion of adrenal glands.

epinephrine
A powerful chemical, also called adrenaline, produced during the stress response that increases blood pressure, stimulates heart muscle, and accelerates the heart rate so the heart pumps more blood.

norepinephrine Also known as noradrenaline, a hormone that, together with epinephrine, brings about the changes in the body known as the fight-or-flight response.

cortisol A stress hormone produced by the adrenal cortex that spurs the metabolism of nutrients to provide energy and fuel for your body and brain.

autonomic nervous system The branch of the nervous system responsible for essential involuntary body functions that occur without our thinking about them, such as breathing, blood pressure, heartbeat, temperature, appetite, and sleep cycles.

sympathetic nervous system The branch of the autonomic nervous system responsible for initiating the fight-or-flight response.

to fully process what is happening; this is why people can jump out of the path of an oncoming car before they are fully aware of what they are doing.

As the initial surge of epinephrine subsides, the hypothalamus activates the second component of the stress response system: the HPA axis, which consists of the hypothalamus, the pituitary gland, and the adrenal glands. By means of chemical signals, the HPA keeps the sympathetic nervous system—the "gas pedal"—pressed down.

If the brain continues to perceive something as dangerous, the hypothalamus produces corticotropin-releasing hormone (CRH), which speeds to the pituitary gland, triggering the release of adrenocorticotropic hormone (ACTH). This hormone travels to the cortex of the adrenal glands, prompting them to release cortisol so the body stays revved up and on high alert. Cortisol affects metabolism (that is, total body processes) by increasing the availability of energy (mainly in the form of glucose), either for the stress response or for recovery from an extreme period of overactivity.

When a perceived threat passes, cortisol levels fall. The parasympathetic nervous system—the "brake"—then dampens the stress response and restores a state of homeostasis. Breathing and heart rate slow; blood pressure and body temperature drop; muscles relax; routine processes such as digestion, energy storage, tissue repair, and growth return to normal. Your body regenerates and restores itself.

Oxytocin, produced by the pituitary gland, plays a special role at this stage. The so-called "cuddle chemical" fine-tunes the brain's social network, increases empathy, and fosters willingness to help and support others. As an additional benefit, it protects the cardiovascular system by stimulating natural anti-inflammatory agents that help the heart regenerate and grow stronger. Oxytocin may also contribute to the behavioral response to stress dubbed "tend and befriend" (see Chapter 1) by increasing feelings of trust.[5] Women, in particular, may respond to stress by reaching out to others—both to care for those in need and to be cared for in return.

> **Stress Reliever:** Take a Breath!
>
> Whenever you feel the stress response kicking in, try this quick deep-breathing exercise developed by Harvard psychologist Alice Domar:
>
> • Sit or stand upright.

> • Place your hand just beneath your navel so you can feel the rise and fall of your belly as you breathe deeply through your nose.
>
> • As you inhale, count slowly, saying to yourself, "One, two, three, four."
>
> • Exhale slowly, counting back down from four to one.
>
> • Do this for one minute or longer, if possible.

Stress and Susceptibility

A group of individuals may survive the same harrowing experience—a devastating fire or tornado, for instance—yet some will react much more intensely and suffer long-term consequences while others recover quickly. Why? What makes certain individuals more susceptible to stress while others show remarkable resilience?

Psychologists explain such variability with a term initially used in medicine: diathesis, which means a predisposition that may stem from genetic, developmental, psychological, biological, or situational factors. According to the **diathesis stress model**, particular stressors have different effects on different people because of this variation in vulnerabilities. A diathesis does not in itself cause illness; a stressor—social, psychological, or physical—must occur to precipitate symptoms. However, the greater one's inherent vulnerability, the lower the threshold for problems to develop.

Psychological (see Chapter 3) and environmental factors (see Chapter 11) can affect stress-susceptibility. Other influences include:

Biological Sex

Stress affects men and women in different ways, with more women than men consistently reporting higher stress levels than men. Other differences include the following:

• Women respond more intensely to acute stressors. Their hearts race faster and their immune systems are more suppressed.

• Blood races to different regions of the brain in each sex, with men showing greater blood flow to the right prefrontal cortex, which functions as a command center, and women showing more activation of the limbic system, which regulates emotion.[6]

• In a study of young adults, men reacted more intensely to performance-oriented tasks while women showed greater increases in the stress hormone cortisol in response to social rejection.[7]

- Women adopt more coping strategies that buffer the impact of stress, including greater reliance on faith and religion.[8]
- In psychological experiments, men under stress display higher aggression (for example, delivering more shocks to another volunteer) than women. Women show more empathy, perhaps because of the different parts of the brain activated by the stress response.[9]

Race and Ethnicity

Race refers to genetic patterns, inherited characteristics, and physical traits, such as skin, hair, and eyes, shared by a unique population. **Ethnicity** describes the common heritage—the customs, language, history, and characteristics—of a certain group. For example, "Caucasian" indicates race, while the term "Latino" refers to the ethnicity of a person of Cuban, Mexican, Puerto Rican, South or Central American, or other Spanish culture or origin, regardless of race.

"Asian" is another broad term applied to individuals from a wide variety of racial and ethnic backgrounds. An Asian American may have ancestors from China, Japan, Korea, Mongolia, Tibet, Taiwan, Bangladesh, Bhutan, India, Nepal, Pakistan, Sri Lanka, Burma, Cambodia, the Philippines, Indonesia, Laos, Malaysia, Singapore, Thailand, or Vietnam, or be of Hmong or Mien descent.

The terms **biracial** and **multiracial** describe individuals who genetically belong to more than one race—for example, an individual with a Japanese biological parent and a Mexican biological parent. Just as individuals can identify with more than one race, it is also possible to identify with more than one ethnicity. According to the U.S. Census, multiracial Americans have the fastest percentage growth rate across the country.

While identity formation can be challenging for anyone, the experience of having different ethnocultural backgrounds can make it more complicated for multiracial individuals. "I don't fit into any of the usual categories," one multiracial undergraduate explains. "There isn't a single box for me to fill out on application forms. Strangers tell me I look 'exotic' and ask 'what' my parents were, as if they were freaks rather than human beings." Some individuals feel pressured by stereotypes and prejudices to identify with one "side" of their genetic heritage and guilty about rejecting others. Some sense that they don't truly belong to any of the racial groups from which they are descended. (See Chapter 4 for a discussion of minority stress on campus.)

Genes

Just as individuals may inherit a predisposition to conditions such as hemophilia, scientists have identified genes that correlate with mental disorders, such as depression and anxiety, that can make individuals more vulnerable to stress. Individuals who inherit a variation of a gene called RGS2, for instance, associated with a greater risk for anxiety, may be more sensitive to elevated stress levels.[10]

Although scientists long assumed that our genetic make-up remains largely unchanged over our lifetimes, this is not the case. Genes influence behavior—and behavior affects genes. As the emerging field of human social genomics has demonstrated, various influences, including social conditions and our subjective perceptions of them, can trigger changes in the expression of hundreds of genes.[11] Researchers have linked both acute stressors, particularly major life events involving rejection, and chronic social stressors, such as isolation, to changes in the immune system that increase vulnerability to disease.[12]

Family History

Genes are dramatically affected by the emotional environment in which an individual grows up. A nurturing childhood environment produces demonstrable, objective changes in the genes controlling certain molecules that play an important

Minority students may experience the stress of feeling isolated because of their race or ethnicity.

David Young-Wolff / PhotoEdit

parasympathetic nervous system The branch of the autonomic nervous system that returns the body to a state of homeostasis, or balance, after a danger has passed.

oxytocin A hormone (sometimes called the "cuddle chemical") produced by the pituitary gland that fine-tunes the brain's social network, increases empathy, fosters willingness to help and support others, and helps protect the cardiovascular system.

diathesis stress model The theory that a predisposition stemming from genetic, developmental, psychological, biological, or situational factors makes people more or less susceptible to stress.

race Genetic patterns, inherited characteristics, and physical traits, such as skin, hair, and eyes, shared by a unique population.

ethnicity The common heritage—the customs, language, history, and characteristics—of a certain group.

biracial and **multiracial** Terms used to describe individuals who genetically belong to more than one race.

role in regulating the emotions and in modulating the negative impact of stress hormones.

A stable, supportive family may better equip children to regulate their emotions and handle life's ups and downs. Growing up in families troubled by alcoholism, drug dependence, or physical, sexual, or psychological abuse may have a lifelong impact on youngsters and increase susceptibility to stress and its ill effects. Childhood abuse, as longitudinal studies have confirmed, causes abnormalities in physiological stress responses that alter immunity and put individuals at greater health risk throughout life.

Protective factors, such as a supportive network of family and friends, also make a positive difference. (See Chapter 5 for a comprehensive discussion of relationships.) Growing up in poverty, for example, has long been linked with greater vulnerability to ill health in adulthood. But as a recent study of young adults found, a mother's love matters, regardless of family income. Poor children whose mothers cared for them with great warmth showed fewer signs of impaired immunity in adulthood than those in the study who received less loving support.[13]

allostatic load The cumulative biological burden caused by daily adaptation to physical and emotional stress.

The Toll of Excess Stress

If you are juggling a lot of responsibilities or are constantly distracted by worry, your stress alarm system may be "on" most of the time—which means that it's harder to turn it down or shut it off. Chronic low-level stress keeps the HPA axis activated, much like a motor that is idling too high for too long. The body has to work so hard to adapt and maintain balance that it becomes exhausted.

Repeated stress of the same type—for example, subtle (or not-so-subtle) discrimination, power struggles at work, or conflict with a partner—teaches the neurons in the cortisol circuit to stop responding. At the same time, the hormone control system becomes hypersensitive and overreacts to other stressors, especially unpredictable or severe ones. At a molecular level, "cell stress," as scientists refer to it, may impose ever-increasing demands or **allostatic load**, the cumulative biological burden caused by daily adaptation to physical and emotional stress.[14] This is when chronic stress turns dangerous, even deadly (See Figure 2.3.).

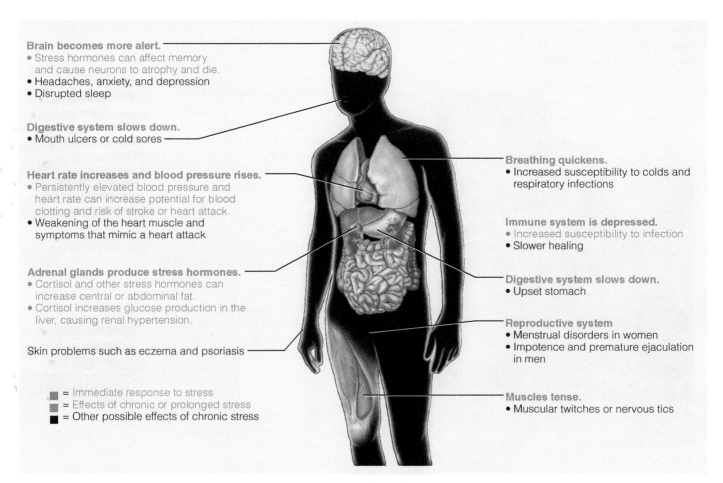

Brain becomes more alert.
- Stress hormones can affect memory and cause neurons to atrophy and die.
- Headaches, anxiety, and depression
- Disrupted sleep

Digestive system slows down.
- Mouth ulcers or cold sores

Heart rate increases and blood pressure rises.
- Persistently elevated blood pressure and heart rate can increase potential for blood clotting and risk of stroke or heart attack.
- Weakening of the heart muscle and symptoms that mimic a heart attack

Adrenal glands produce stress hormones.
- Cortisol and other stress hormones can increase central or abdominal fat.
- Cortisol increases glucose production in the liver, causing renal hypertension.

Skin problems such as eczema and psoriasis

■ = Immediate response to stress
■ = Effects of chronic or prolonged stress
■ = Other possible effects of chronic stress

Breathing quickens.
- Increased susceptibility to colds and respiratory infections

Immune system is depressed.
- Increased susceptibility to infection
- Slower healing

Digestive system slows down.
- Upset stomach

Reproductive system
- Menstrual disorders in women
- Impotence and premature ejaculation in men

Muscles tense.
- Muscular twitches or nervous tics

FIGURE 2.3 The effects of stress on the body.

Chronic stress, for instance, can be a risk factor for Type 2 diabetes (once known as adult-onset diabetes), a disease in which either the pancreas does not make enough insulin or the body is unable to use insulin correctly. Once rare, Type 2 diabetes now accounts for 90 to 95 percent of cases of diabetes and is becoming common in children and teenagers. Factors such as low socioeconomic status or a stressful work environment may contribute to this metabolic disorder by repeated and persistent activation of the physiological stress response.[15]

Over an extended period of time, the compounds produced by your body under stress can also increase the risk for several other leading causes of death and disability, including heart disease, accidents, cancer, liver disease, lung ailments, and suicide, as well as a host of other illnesses:[16] infections and autoimmune disorders, flare-ups of asthma[17] and allergies, cardiovascular disease, chronic pain, depression, gastrointestinal problems, infertility, and worsening of progressive diseases.[18]

Among the specific effects of stress on the body are:

- Persistent surges of epinephrine damage blood vessels and arteries, increasing blood pressure and raising the risk of heart attacks or strokes.

- Elevated cortisol levels create physiological changes designed to replenish the body's energy stores. This can contribute to the buildup of fat tissue by storing unused nutrients as fat and to weight gain through increased appetite.

- Muscle mass decreases because cortisol breaks down proteins to generate energy.

- With a weakened anti-inflammatory response, toxic chemicals rise within cells.

- Since the immune system is compromised, you become more vulnerable to infections.

- The levels of stress hormones in fat cells rise, increasing fat deposits and the likelihood of type 2 diabetes and cardiovascular disease.

In addition to affecting how you feel, excess stress affects how you behave. In a study of college students, researchers found that in times of stress undergraduates fall back on familiar habits, both good (such as working out regularly) and bad (smoking).[19] If you find that you are comforting yourself with indulgences like cookie dough ice cream or pints of Guinness, stop and take stock of what is going on in your life. The relaxation techniques described in Chapter 12 can help.

 Stress Reliever: Put on the Brakes

Think of something that caused you stress yesterday or today—perhaps a good friend not returning your urgent texts. What thought went through your head? What could you have said to yourself that might have put the brakes on the way you reacted? Would you have gotten so upset if you had realized that your friend's phone battery was dead?

In your Journal, reflect on other ways in which you might slow down your stress response to unexpected or frustrating occurrences.

Stress and the Immune System

✔ **Check-in:** Cold case.

When was the last time you had a cold? What do you remember about what was going on in your life? Could stress have played a role?

Does it take longer for you to recover from a cold or a cut during high-stress times like finals?

The following section explains how stress affects immunity.

Various parts of your body safeguard you against infectious diseases by providing immunity, or protection, from health threats. Your immune system includes structures of the lymphatic system, such as the spleen, thymus gland, and lymph nodes, and more than a dozen different types of white blood cells (lymphocytes) that act together like an internal police force.

Psychoneuroimmunology is a multidisciplinary field that studies the interaction between psychological processes and the nervous and immune systems—in other words, the ways in which the brain and the immune system communicate.[20] As classic laboratory experiments in the 1970s showed, a painful stressor can, via signals transmitted by the central nervous system, turn down or suppress the immune system. Scientists have since discovered that specific neuropeptides and neurotransmitters (chemicals produced by the brain) act directly on the immune system,

psychoneuroimmunology
A multidisciplinary field that studies the interaction between psychological processes and the nervous and immune systems.

indicating that emotions and immunity are deeply interconnected.[21]

The hormones released during the stress response dampen the immune system's ability to produce and maintain lymphocytes (the white blood cells that kill infection) and natural killer cells (specialized cells that, because they seek out and destroy foreign invaders, are crucial in the fight against disease and infection). The longer that stress persists, the more the immune system shifts from potentially adaptive changes to potentially harmful ones.

Various stressors—from a troubled marriage to unemployment—diminish the body's ability to ward off disease and to heal after injury. Positive interventions, including relaxation and meditation, bolster its defenses. Uncontrollable stressors so profound and persistent that they seem without end suppress immune responses the most. The stress of losing a loved one through death or divorce, for instance, can impair immunity for a year or longer.

Chronic psychosocial stressors, such as loneliness or academic pressure, also disrupt the body's defensive mechanisms and contribute to a range of physiological issues, including infections, flare-ups of allergies and asthma, slower healing of cuts or other injuries, and the development of autoimmune disorders such as rheumatoid arthritis. Stress has a greater impact on women's immune and inflammatory reactions, which may initially help protect them from trauma and infection. However, it may contribute to the higher prevalence of stress-related autoimmune or allergic disorders among women.[22]

Effects of Acute Stress:

Suppression of the body's protective mechanisms; reduced production of lymphocytes; increased production of agents that cause inflammation.

Effects of Episodic Stress:

Increased susceptibility to infection; slower healing of wounds; diminished response to vaccination.[23]

Possible Effects of Chronic Stress:

Greater risk of infections; development of autoimmune disorders; worsening of chronic illnesses such as allergy and asthma.

🔧 **Stress Reliever:** Sigh!

As tension builds within your body, you can take a time-out from stress with an exaggerated sigh:

- Sit or stand up straight.

- Sigh deeply. As the air rushes out of your lungs, let out a sound of deep relief.

- Let your lungs refill with air slowly and effortlessly.

- Repeat several times.

Stress and the Cardiovascular System

✔ **Check-in:** Listen to your heart.

Does your heart race when you are called on in class or when you have to speak in public?

Does it seem to skip beats when you're stressed?

Do you feel a surge of heat or perspiration when under pressure?

Read the following section to find out what may be behind these sensations.

The cardiovascular system consists of the heart—a fist-sized, hollow, muscular pump—and of the vessels that transport blood and oxygen throughout the body. Stress can affect this complex network in various ways. A short-term or acute stressor, such as an angry outburst, initiates the release of hormones that cause the blood vessels to constrict, blood pressure to rise, cholesterol

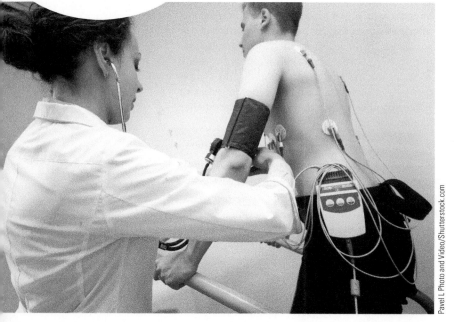

Cardiac monitoring during the stress of exercise can reveal potential health dangers.

Pavel L Photo and Video/Shutterstock.com

and clotting factors in the blood to increase, and the force and speed of the heart's contractions to intensify.[24]

These changes can trigger a heart attack in individuals with underlying coronary artery disease.[25] Hot-tempered, ever-harried "Type A's" may be especially susceptible. In some people, just thinking about a stressful experience, such as an angry confrontation, can raise blood pressure days or even weeks later.[26] Stressed individuals often are prone to heart-harmful behaviors. Men and women with high stress levels tend to smoke more and exercise less—and to have higher rates of heart attacks, strokes, and bypass surgeries.

Episodic acute stress, such as a volatile relationship that erupts into periodic angry confrontations, may contribute to chronic low-grade inflammation, which can increase the build-up of sludge-like plaque within the arteries.[27] Chronic daily stressors or severe psychological trauma increases the risk of developing (and dying from) cardiovascular disease (CVD).

Stress may be as great a threat for cardiovascular disease as smoking, hypertension, and other major risk factors, depending on how individuals respond to a stressor. According to a recent large-scale longitudinal study, men with low stress resilience in adolescence faced a greater danger of cardiovascular illness in middle age—perhaps because of unhealthy habits they acquired at an early age or because of inadequate coping skills.[28]

Psychological stressors have been implicated as a cause of myocardial ischemia (inadequate blood supply to the heart) in an estimated 30 to 70 percent of patients with CVD. Mental stress does not normally produce chest pain or other typical symptoms, but it increases the risk of a potentially fatal heart attack.[29]

Elevated cortisol, which spikes during chronic psychosocial stress, raises the risk of hypertension (high blood pressure) and may elevate levels of C-reactive protein, an indicator of inflammation.[30] Stress also slows the clearance of triglycerides, a type of fat linked to heart disease, from the bloodstream.

The way individuals perceive and respond to stressful events also affects their hearts—and may vary in men and women.[31] For instance, women are more likely to engage in **rumination**, or persistent repetitive, intrusive, negative thinking (see Chapter 3) that may delay or impair the body's recovery after stress so blood pressure remains elevated for a long period. Depression, anxiety, and stress often occur together and take a cumulative toll on the cardiovascular system.

Effects of Acute Stress:
Heart rate increases; blood pressure rises.

Effects of Episodic Stress:
Elevated blood pressure; faster heart rate; increased potential for blood clotting; greater risk of heart attack or stroke in individuals with underlying cardiovascular disease.

Possible Effects of Chronic Stress:
Weakening of the heart muscle, worsening hypertension, high cholesterol, and atherosclerosis (narrowing of the arteries).

Stress and the Gastrointestinal System

✔ **Check-in:** Listen to your gut.

Do you get butterflies in your stomach the first day of class?

Have you ever felt that you wanted to throw up after seeing an embarrassing photo online?

Do you lose your appetite before an interview or a big game?

The following section explains why.

The "brain-gut axis," as gastroenterologists call it, links the brain with the organs involved in digesting food as it enters your mouth, moves down the esophagus to the stomach, passes through the small and large intestine, and finally exits through your rectum and anus. During the stress response, the body diverts blood and nutrients away from the digestive system to more critical functions. This may lead to the following effects:

- Decreased saliva so your mouth becomes dry (a frequent occurrence under the stress of speaking in public).

- Contractions in the esophagus that interfere with swallowing.

- Increased levels of hydrochloric acid in the stomach.

- Constricted blood vessels in the digestive tract.

- Altered rhythmic movements of the small and large intestines necessary for the transport of food (leading to diarrhea if too fast, or constipation if too slow).

- Blockage of the bile and pancreatic ducts.

- Increased risk of pancreatitis (inflammation of the pancreas), ulcerative colitis, and irritable bowel syndrome.[32] See Chapter 9 for more on nutrition and stress, including foods that may increase digestive problems.

rumination Persistent repetitive, intrusive, negative thinking

Ulcers

For many years, stress alone was blamed for causing stomach ulcers, but scientists have since discovered that a bacterium, *Helicobacter pylori*, infects the digestive system and sets the stage for ulcers. Yet this finding doesn't rule out stress as a culprit. In a recent 12-year study of more than 3,000 healthy adults, those who scored high on stress assessments were more likely to develop ulcers than those with the lowest scores.[33] Doctors theorize that stress may increase susceptibility by reducing the protective mucous lining of the stomach so ulcers can develop more readily.

Weight Gain

Cortisol, produced during the stress response, increases appetite and stores unused nutrients as fat. Stress also affects what researchers call our "drive to eat." Stressed individuals eat more, binge more, and choose "palatable non-nutritious foods" (better known as junk foods) like candy and cookies rather than healthier options.[34] The reason may be that foods high in sugar and fat target pleasure centers in the brain and provide temporary comfort and relief. However, sweet treats can send blood sugar levels on a roller coaster—up one moment and down the next—so you plunge from a brief sugar rush to a sugar "crash." (See Chapter 9 for a discussion of stress and weight management.)

Belly or Visceral Fat

Even if they don't consume more calories, some people, perhaps those genetically sensitive to cortisol, put on "belly" or visceral fat (deposited deep within the central abdominal area of the body) when stressed. This type of fat poses a greater health threat than subcutaneous (under-the-skin) fat because it enters the bloodstream more readily, raises levels of harmful cholesterol, and heightens the risk of diseases such as diabetes, high blood pressure, and stroke.

Digestive Disorders

With other chronic digestive diseases, such as **GERD (gastroesophageal reflux disease)** and irritable bowel syndrome, stress can be both a contributor and a consequence, causing or worsening symptoms that in turn intensify stress.

Effects of Acute Stress:
Slowing of digestive system; dry mouth.

Effects of Episodic Stress:
Upset stomach; nausea; heartburn; acid reflux; abdominal cramps; diarrhea.

GERD (gastroesophageal reflux disease) A digestive disorder characterized by the return (reflux) of the contents of the stomach to the esophagus.

skeletal muscles The muscles that are attached to bones within the body

bracing Chronic tensing of muscles.

Possible Effects of Chronic Stress:
Weight gain, flare-ups of irritable bowel syndrome, GERD, pancreatitis, ulcerative colitis.

> **Stress Reliever:** Soothing a Stressed Stomach
>
> Some simple strategies can help prevent stress-related digestive problems.
>
> - Drink plenty of water to avoid dry mouth and dehydration, both common when stressed.
> - Eat fiber-rich foods to counteract stress-induced constipation or cramping.
> - Don't skip meals. If you do, you're more likely to feel fatigued and irritable.
> - If you have difficulty eating, choose comfort foods such as warm cereal or soups.
> - Slow down, and chew your foods thoroughly. Eating too much too fast increases abdominal pressure.
> - Chew gum to lower your overall sense of stress and lessen the temptation to comfort yourself by "stress eating." (Don't try this if you suffer from jaw pain or temporomandibular disorder (TMD).)

Stress and the Muscles

✔ **Check-in:** Do you squeeze your pen when writing an essay on a test? Clench your jaw when frustrated? Tighten your grip on the steering wheel when driving in a storm?

The following section explains why.

During stress, your brain signals your **skeletal muscles**, those attached to bones, to prepare for action, so they contract (shorten). If the stress is physical—such as lifting a heavy barbell or sprinting for a bus—your muscles contract fully to accomplish the task. If there is no physical challenge, your muscles contract partially, resulting in tension. Chronic muscle tension is called **bracing** and can lead to fatigue, pain, and health problems.

The stress response also affects the smooth muscles that control the contraction of your internal organs. When the smooth muscles within your blood vessels contract, your blood pressure rises. When those within the stomach wall contract, you may get a stomachache. Other common stress-related muscle problems include headaches, backaches, and **temporomandibular disorder (TMD)**.

Headache

Stress can cause involuntary contractions of the muscles of the eyes, forehead, neck, and jaw, leading to tension headaches so severe that they interfere with study, work, and other normal activities. Treatments include medication (such as aspirin or ibuprofen), heat, or massage. Stress management techniques, such as relaxation (see Chapter 12) and biofeedback (see Chapter 14), also can reduce the frequency and intensity of tension headaches.

Temporomandibular Disorder (TMD)/Bruxism

Five muscles and several ligaments (short bands of connective tissue) coordinate the operation of the temporomandibular joint, which connects the upper and lower jaw. The most common cause of its malfunctioning is clenching or grinding of teeth (**bruxism**) as a result of stress. Symptoms include facial pain, clicking or popping sounds when the mouth opens and closes, migraine headaches, earaches, ringing in the ears, dizziness, and sensitive teeth.

Treatment may consist of a "mouthguard" (a protective device worn at night, or, in some cases, 24 hours a day) and dental procedures to adjust the bite. Stress reduction techniques, such as biofeedback (see Chapter 14), have helped TMD sufferers to relax their jaws and reduce tooth grinding.

Backache

The average person has an 80 percent chance of experiencing back pain in the course of a lifetime. You are at greater risk if you are overweight, out of shape, or overstressed. Most backaches stem from muscular weakness or "bracing," which causes muscles to lose elasticity and fatigue easily. The result can be a muscle spasm or soreness, particularly in the lower back. Because of fear of worsening the pain or risking injury, people often limit their daily activities. As a result, their muscles become weaker, leading to more pain and stress.

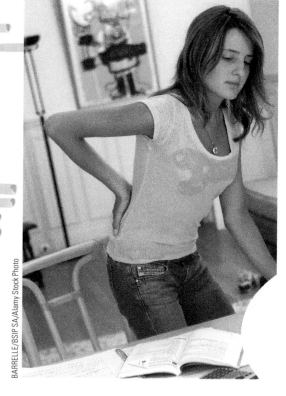

BARRELLE/BSIP SA/Alamy Stock Photo

The average person has an 80 percent chance of experiencing backpain in the course of a lifetime.

According to physician John Sarno, stress-related back and neck pain, which he calls **tension myositis syndrome (TMS)**, is caused by unconscious emotions such as anger. It is most likely to develop when individuals with certain personality characteristics, such as being self-motivated, driven to succeed, highly self-critical, and perfectionistic, are dealing with stressful life situations. Their unconscious tension causes constriction of the blood vessels and reduced flow to the muscles, tendons, ligaments, and nerves of the back. The decreased supply of oxygen, and the subsequent buildup of biochemical waste products in the muscles, result in spasms and pain.[35]

Focusing on psychological rather than physical causes, Sarno's approach to back pain emphasizes stress reduction and psychotherapy to deal with unconscious issues. His theory, which has not been tested in large, well-controlled research studies, remains controversial in the medical community.

More widely endorsed is a multidisciplinary approach to stress-related back pain that encompasses physical therapy and/or pain medications, diagnosis and treatment of mental disorders such as depression or anxiety, and reduction of stress with cognitive and behavioral approaches (described in Chapters 3 and 8) and mind-body exercises such as yoga or Pilates (see Chapter 14).

temporomandibular disorder (TMD) A malfunctioning of the joint that connects the upper and lower jaw.

bruxism Clenching or grinding of teeth as a result of stress.

tension myositis syndrome (TMS) A term coined by Dr. John Sarno for the unconscious tensing of muscles caused by repressed emotions that constricts blood vessels, reduces the supply of oxygen, and causes pain in the back or neck.

To lower the physical stress on your back:

- Because sitting is more stressful than standing, get up from your seat every 20 to 30 minutes to stretch or walk around.

- When standing in place, shift your weight from one foot to another. Hold in your stomach, tilt your pelvis toward your back, and tuck in your buttocks to provide crucial support for your lower back.

- Whenever possible, sit in a straight chair with a firm back.

- Avoid slouching in overstuffed chairs or dangling your feet in midair.

- When driving, keep the seat forward so your knees are raised to hip level; your right leg should not be fully extended. Use a small pillow or towel to support your lower back.

- When lifting, bend at the knees, not from the waist.

trichotillomania A mental disorder characterized by pulling out chunks of hair from the scalp or elsewhere on the body.

Stress can increase self-consciousness and lead to nervous habits such as picking at the skin.

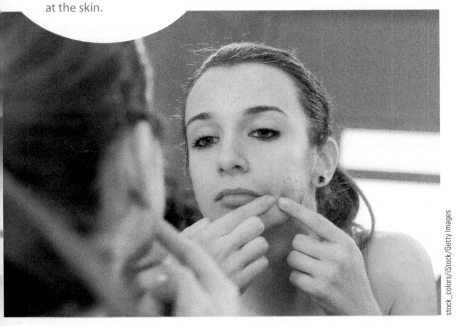

stock_colors/iStock/Getty Images

Stress and the Skin

✔ **Check-in:** Do you "wear" your stress on your skin?

Does your face break out before a big social event?

Do you get a rash during finals?

This section explains why.

Experts in "psycho-dermatology" have identified what they call the "brain-skin axis," made up of nerve cells, immune cells, skin cells, and signaling mechanisms involved in the cross talk between the brain and the skin. Stress, as numerous studies have confirmed, can aggravate many skin conditions, including acne, atopic dermatitis (rash), eczema, pruritis (itching), hair loss, and rosacea (enlarged facial blood vessels that produce flushing).[36]

Stress can also lead to nervous habits, sometimes called self-soothing, such as picking at your skin or tugging at strands of hair. What may begin as pulling out a hair or two when stressed may escalate into pulling out chunks of hair from the scalp or elsewhere on the body in a short period of time. This condition is a diagnosable mental disorder called **trichotillomania**. Scratching or rubbing your skin also may be soothing under stressful conditions, but when it causes bruising, scarring, or tissue damage, it meets the diagnostic criteria for Skin Picking Disorder (SPD) or Excoriation Disorder.

One of the most visible—and stressful—skin conditions is psoriasis, a chronic disease that speeds up the growth cycle of skin cells to cause itchy spots, red patches, and thick flaky lesions. Day-to-day stressors, such as losing something important to you or embarrassing yourself in public, can lead to an increase in psoriasis symptoms—but only in patients who worry or scratch a lot (possible indicators of greater perceived stress).[37]

Effects of Acute Stress:
Pimples; acne breakouts; rash; picking at skin; pulling out hair.

Effects of Episodic Stress:
Flare-ups of psoriasis, eczema, and other chronic skin disorders.

Possible Effects of Chronic Stress:
Increasing self-consciousness and stress over appearance, worsening of chronic skin problems, hair graying or loss, trichotillomania (hair-pulling), skin picking disorder.

Stress Reliever: Yawn!

Like a sigh, a yawn can release some tension when you're stressed. Try these simple steps:

- Open your mouth wide.

- Lift your arms above your head, and stretch.

- Yawn—be as loud as you can.

- Repeat several times.

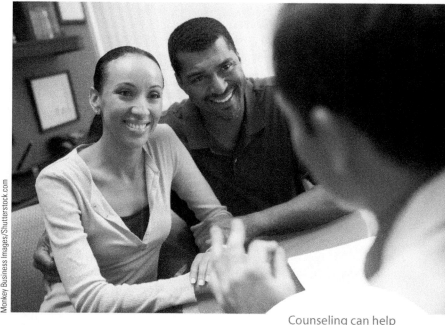

Counseling can help couples if chronic stress causes sexual difficulties or fertility problems.

Stress and the Reproductive System

Regardless of whether it is acute, episodic, or chronic, stress can affect every phase of sexual response by:

- lowering or blocking sexual desire, so individuals fantasize and think about sex less and feel less motivated to engage in sexual activity.

- interfering with sexual arousal and excitement. Women may be unable to attain or maintain sufficient vaginal lubrication, making intercourse painful. Men may experience erectile disorder (ED), previously called impotence, and be unable to attain or maintain an adequate erection for completion of sexual activity.

- impairing ability to achieve orgasm. Even when stimulated, men and women may not be able to reach orgasm.

- contributing to sexual pain disorders, such as dyspareunia (genital pain that may occur before, during, or after intercourse in men and women) and vaginismus (involuntary contractions of the vagina during attempted penetration, causing tightness, pain, and cramping).

The profound physiological changes triggered by stress may lower levels of testosterone, the key hormone linked to sexual desire in men and women. Research studies have correlated stress with low levels of testosterone and diminished sexual arousal and desire in both sexes.[38] Stress also has been implicated as a contributor to infertility. A man's ability to handle stress may affect production of healthy sperm.[39] Chronic stress may interfere with a woman's ability to conceive and may increase the risk of complications during pregnancy and delivery.[40]

The hormonal changes caused by stress may intensify symptoms of premenstrual syndrome (PMS), although the precise mechanisms involved are not well understood. Stress-management techniques, such as meditation and breathing exercises, have proven helpful as part of comprehensive treatment programs for women with premenstrual syndrome (PMS).[41]

Effects of Acute Stress:
Diminished sexual desire; reduced vaginal lubrication in women; impaired ability to attain and maintain an erection in men; impaired ability to reach orgasm in both sexes.

Effects of Episodic Stress:
Pain during or after intercourse; loss of interest in sexual activity; possible intensification of PMS symptoms.

Possible Effects of Chronic Stress:
Sexual disorders; impaired intimacy with a partner; infertility; increased risk of pregnancy complications and preterm labor.

Stress and Cancer

The rates of new cancers and of cancer deaths have declined significantly in the last decade, and the number of survivors living with cancer in the United States has soared. Cutting-edge research has not only transformed cancer treatments but has also deepened understanding of the role of psychosocial factors, including stress, in vulnerability to and recovery from cancer.[42]

Psycho-oncology, the field that combines medical and psychological approaches to cancer, has documented some of the ways in which stress affects cancer risk and prognosis:

- Stress-related abnormalities in cortisol, inflammation, and the sympathetic nervous system can affect cancer growth.[43]

- Stressful life experiences and depression are associated with poorer survival and greater mortality from various types of cancer, including breast, lung, and head and neck tumors.

- Stress may have a greater impact on the vulnerability of persons who have what has been dubbed a "Type C," or cancer-prone, personality. Although they appear quiet and introspective, Type C individuals live with great frustration, repress feelings rather than become angry, and appease others even if they have to sacrifice their own needs and desires.

- Social relationships (or a lack thereof) have a greater effect on the risk of cancer patients' dying than physical inactivity and obesity. Perceived loneliness or isolation predicts greater risk of complications and death in patients of all ages, while a greater sense of social attachment lowers their likelihood.

- Psychosocial support improves quantity as well as quality of life in patients with cancer. In fifteen studies of group therapy for patients with various cancers, eight showed a lengthening of survival time. Additional benefits included less distress, depression, and pain, as well as better coping and life satisfaction. With psychosocial support and improved coping skills, even terminally ill patients live better at the end of life—and in some cases they live longer as well.[44]

Stress and Aging

From the moment we are born, we start getting older—a process regulated by our genes, which are located inside chromosomes (double-stranded molecules of DNA). At the tips of the chromosomes are protective strips of DNA called **telomeres**, often compared to the plastic wrappers on the end of shoelaces, that keep the chromosomes from shredding.

Each time a cell divides, telomeres get shorter, but the enzyme telomerase keeps them from wearing down too much. However, as cells split repeatedly, telomerase activity declines, the telomeres shorten, and the cells age.[45] Eventually they can no longer divide and deteriorate into a state called senescence. Stress may accelerate the aging process by shortening telomeres and lowering levels of telomerase. Shorter telomeres are associated with aging, age-related diseases such as cancer, stroke, cardiovascular disease, obesity, osteoporosis, and diabetes, and a higher risk of death.

Stress-related changes in telomeres may be reversible. In a five-year study by Dr. Dean Ornish, a leader in preventive medicine, men with prostate cancer who engaged in meditation, breathing exercises, and yoga-based stretching to reduce stress—along with regular exercise, a plant-based diet, and group support—showed a significant

telomeres Protective strips of DNA at the ends of chromosomes that prevent the chromosomes from shredding.

Stress can influence whether individuals of the same age remain active and independent or are limited by disabilities and frailty.

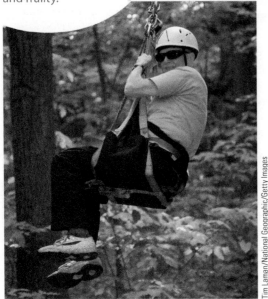

Tim Laman/National Geographic/Getty Images

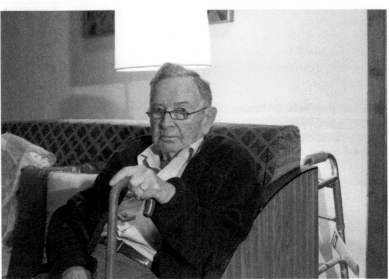

eddtoro/Shutterstock.com

increase in their telomere length compared with those who did not make lifestyle changes.[46] Other researchers have reported increases in telomere length and telomerase expression in individuals who practiced various forms of meditation, including mindfulness and "Loving Kindness" meditation.[47] (See Chapter 13.)

Rx: Relax

Excess stress, as you've learned, can undermine the body's natural defenses, narrow arteries, tighten muscles, upset the digestive system, irritate the skin, and accelerate aging. But you can take steps to counter these harmful effects. One of the most effective is deep relaxation, the physical and mental opposite of stress. (See Chapter 12 for an in-depth discussion of relaxation.)

We are not talking about the sort of "relaxing" you do when you hang out with friends or go to the beach, but about step-by-step, scientifically tested techniques that can counter the wear and tear of life's challenges. Among the other health dividends of relaxation are fewer physical symptoms, such as headaches and back pain; less anger and frustration; more energy; improved concentration; enhanced immunity; and a healthier heart.

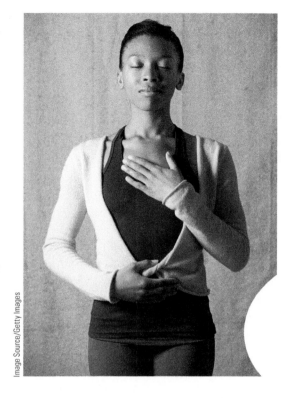

Image Source/Getty Images

Deep breathing and other relaxation techniques can counter the harmful effects of stress.

Do you think of yourself as relaxed? Before you answer, read the questions in the Reflection exercise at the end of the chapter. Then try the introductory relaxation exercise on page 37.

Chapter Summary

- An individual's susceptibility to stress depends on many factors, including diathesis, a predisposition that may stem from genetic, developmental, psychological, biological, or situational factors.

- According to the diathesis-stress model, particular stressors have different effects on different people because of this variation in vulnerabilities. Other factors that affect stress susceptibility are gender, race and ethnicity, genetics, and family history.

- Your body's automatic stress responses set off a cascade of physiological changes, including increases in heart rate, blood pressure, breathing, muscle contraction, blood flow, metabolism, perspiration, and production of glucose to nourish the muscles. The structures within the brain orchestrating these changes include the amygdala, which processes emotions; the hypothalamus, which functions like a command center; and the pituitary gland, which regulates hormonal functions.

- In response to stress, the adrenal glands produce the hormones epinephrine (adrenaline) and its metabolite norepinephrine (noradrenaline), which increase blood pressure, stimulate heart muscle, and accelerate the heart rate, and cortisol, which spurs the metabolism of nutrients to provide energy for body and brain.

- The sympathetic nervous system triggers the fight-or-flight response, providing the body with a burst of energy, while the parasympathetic nervous system calms the body down after the danger has passed. Oxytocin, produced by the pituitary gland, plays a special role at this stage by increasing empathy and fostering willingness to reach out to others, part of the behavioral response to stress dubbed "tend and befriend."

- Repeated or chronic stress may impose ever-increasing demands or allostatic load, the cumulative biological burden caused by daily adaptation to physical and emotional stress. Over an extended time the compounds produced under stress can increase the risk for several leading causes of death—heart disease, accidents, cancer, liver disease, lung ailments, and suicide—as well as infections and autoimmune disorders, flare-ups of asthma and allergies, cardiovascular disease, depression, diabetes, gastrointestinal problems, and infertility.

- Although the health risks are real, the biology of stress is not different from the biology of excitement or even of courage. You can learn to recognize your physiological responses to stress as empowering rather than upsetting.

- Chronic psychosocial stressors, such as loneliness or academic pressure, can disrupt the immune system and contribute to type 2 diabetes, infections, flare-ups of allergies and asthma, slower healing of cuts or other injuries, and the development of autoimmune disorders such as rheumatoid arthritis.

- Stress triggers changes in the cardiovascular system that can increase the risk of hypertension, atherosclerosis, heart attack, and stroke.

- Stress can disrupt the gastrointestinal system and cause a range of problems, including upset stomach, nausea, heartburn, acid reflux, abdominal cramps, diarrhea, weight gain, and flare-ups of digestive disorders such as irritable bowel syndrome, GERD, pancreatitis, and ulcerative colitis.

- Common stress-related muscle problems include headaches, backaches, and temporomandibular disorder (TMD).

- Stress can aggravate many skin conditions, including acne, atopic dermatitis (rash), eczema, pruritis (itching), hair loss, rosacea (enlarged facial blood vessels that produce flushing), psoriasis, and picking or pulling the skin, scalp, or hair.

- In both men and women stress can diminish sexual desire, impair ability to reach orgasm, contribute to pain during or after intercourse, and increase the risk of infertility, pregnancy complications, and preterm labor.

- Stressful life experiences and depression are associated with poorer survival and greater mortality from various types of cancer, including breast, lung, and head and neck tumors. Individuals with a "Type C" or cancer-prone personality, who repress their anger and frustration, may be especially vulnerable.

- Stress may accelerate the aging process by shortening telomeres and lowering levels of telomerase—changes that may be reversed by various forms of meditation.

- Step-by-step, scientifically tested relaxation techniques can counter the harmful effects of excess stress. Their benefits include fewer physical symptoms, such as headaches and back pain; less anger and frustration; more energy; improved concentration; enhanced immunity; and a healthier heart.

 ## STRESS RELIEVERS

Take a Breath!

Whenever you feel the stress response kicking in, try this quick deep-breathing exercise developed by Harvard psychologist Alice Domar:

- Sit or stand upright.

- Place your hand just beneath your navel so you can feel the rise and fall of your belly as you breathe deeply through your nose.

- As you inhale, count slowly, saying to yourself, "One, two, three, four."

- Exhale slowly, counting back down from four to one.

- Do this for one minute or longer, if possible.

Put on the Brakes

Think of something that caused you stress yesterday or today—perhaps a good friend not returning your urgent texts. What thought went through your head? What could you have said to yourself that might have put the brakes on the way you reacted? Would you have gotten so upset if you'd realized that your friend's phone battery was dead?

In your Journal, reflect on other ways in which you might slow down your stress response to unexpected or frustrating occurrences.

Sigh!

As tension builds within your body, you can take a time-out from stress with an exaggerated sigh:

- Sit or stand up straight.

- Sigh deeply. As the air rushes out of your lungs, let out a sound of deep relief.

- Let your lungs refill with air slowly and effortlessly.

- Repeat several times.

Soothing a Stressed Stomach

Some simple strategies can help prevent stress-related digestive problems.

- Drink plenty of water to avoid dry mouth and dehydration, both common when stressed.

- Eat fiber-rich foods to counteract stress-induced constipation or cramping.

- Don't skip meals. If you do, you're more likely to feel fatigued and irritable.

- If you have difficulty eating, choose comfort foods such as warm cereal or soups.

- Slow down, and chew your foods thoroughly. Eating too much too fast increases abdominal pressure.

- Chew gum to lower your overall sense of stress and lessen the temptation to comfort yourself by "stress eating." (Don't try this if you suffer from jaw pain or temporomandibular disorder (TMD).)

Give Your Back a Break

To lower the physical stress on your back:

- Because sitting is more stressful than standing, get up from your seat every 20 to 30 minutes to stretch or walk around.

- When standing in place, shift your weight from one foot to another. Hold in your stomach, tilt your pelvis toward your back, and tuck in your buttocks to provide crucial support for your lower back.

- Whenever possible, sit in a straight chair with a firm back.

- Avoid slouching in overstuffed chairs or dangling your feet in midair.

- When driving, keep the seat forward so your knees are raised to hip level; your right leg should not be fully extended. Use a small pillow or towel to support your lower back.

- When lifting, bend at the knees, not from the waist.

Yawn!

Like a sigh, a yawn can release some tension when you're stressed. Try these simple steps:

- Open your mouth wide.

- Lift your arms above your head, and stretch.

- Yawn—be as loud as you can.

- Repeat several times.

⊖ YOUR PERSONAL STRESS MANAGEMENT TOOLKIT

REFLECTION: How relaxed are you?

Ask yourself the following questions, and write down your reflections in the book, a journal, or in MindTap:

- Can you completely relax your muscles? Can you allow them to go completely limp? Try it with your forehead, your face, your biceps, and your leg muscles. When you feel you are as relaxed as possible, check or have someone else check your neck and shoulders with a very gentle squeeze of the hand to see whether your muscles are soft or stiff. _____

- Rate how completely you relaxed your body on a scale of 1 (dry spaghetti) to 10 (overcooked spaghetti): _____

- Can you relax or stop your mind? Check the time. Close your eyes, sit comfortably, and breathe deeply and evenly. Banish all thoughts. As soon as a random thought—even one about how well or poorly you are doing at this exercise—flickers into your consciousness, open your eyes and check the time. _____

- Rate your ability to clear your mind on a scale of 1 (less than five seconds) to 10 (more than 30 seconds): _____

- Can you be in the here and now and stay in the moment? Pause, sit comfortably, and breathe deeply. Tune in to each part of your body, noting the slightest sensation—an itch, an ache, a feeling of warmth. Rate your ability to tune in to bodily sensations on a scale of 1 (numb) to 10 (supersensitive): _____

- Can you focus your attention as a means of letting go? Select the simple image of a candle flame. Set a timer for 10 minutes. Sit quietly, breathe deeply, close your eyes, and focus on this image. If thoughts enter your mind, think of them as breezes that make the candle flicker. Keep the flame as steady as possible in your mind. Rate the difficulty of this focusing exercise on a scale of 1 (easy) to 10 (excruciating): _____

- Review your personal ratings, and write a brief description of your ability to relax in your journal.

TECHNIQUE: Tense and Relax Exercise

Every thought you have creates a response in the body. Most of these responses involve subtle muscular tension. Therefore, being able to maintain even brief thought-free periods is deeply relaxing to body and mind.

This basic technique, a variation on progressive or deep muscle relaxation (see Chapter 12), involves alternate tensing and relaxing of various muscle groups in the body. You focus your attention on a specific muscle group, such as the arm muscles. You tense them tightly and then release them.

These tension-release exercises are often used to help people with headaches and other stress-related maladies; they become more effective the more you use them, and you become progressively more relaxed in less time. They also teach you to recognize what your body feels like when its muscles are very tense and very relaxed. Focusing your attention on this process becomes relaxing in itself. Listen to the Tense and Relax Exercise audio instructions in MindTap or pair up with a classmate and take turns leading each other through this exercise.

- Sit comfortably in your quiet place. Turn off your digital devices.

- Begin with your major muscle groups, starting by clenching your fists as tightly as possible and then letting the tension go. Then move elsewhere as the instructions indicate.

- When you tense your muscles, do so vigorously, but not so much that you develop a cramp. Hold the muscle in its tensed position for five to seven seconds, count "one thousand one, one thousand two, one thousand three," and so on, to time the contraction. Relax for 15 to 20 seconds.

- Concentrate on what is happening. Feel the buildup of tension; notice the tightening of the muscles; feel the strain and then the release; relax and enjoy the sudden feeling of limpness.

- You will be tensing and relaxing each muscle group twice. If any specific part of your body still feels tense after completing the exercises, go back and tense and relax these muscles again.

- Keep all other muscles relaxed as you work on specific muscle groups. This is challenging at first, but you will soon become adept.

- To begin, take three deep breaths, holding each one for five to seven seconds.

- Clench your dominant fist (right, if you're right-handed; left, if left-handed). Hold and count for five to seven seconds; relax. Repeat.

- Flex your dominant bicep. Tense, relax, tense, relax.

- Clench the fist of your non-dominant hand; relax. Repeat. Proceed to the non-dominant bicep. Take a couple of deep breaths, and notice how relaxed and warm your arms feel. Enjoy the feeling.

- Tense the muscles of your forehead by raising your eyebrows as far as you can. Hold for five seconds. Relax. Repeat. Let a wave of relaxation cover your face.

- Close your eyes very tightly. Release and notice the relaxation. Repeat.

- Clench your jaws very tightly. Make an exaggerated smile. Release and repeat.

- Take a couple of deep breaths, and notice how relaxed the muscles of your arms and head feel.

- Take a deep breath, and hold it for a few seconds. Release slowly. Repeat.

- Try to touch your chin to your chest but use your neck muscles to keep it from touching. Release and repeat.

- Try to touch your back with your head, but use your neck muscles to push the opposite way. Notice the tension building up. Release quickly. Repeat and let your neck become completely relaxed.

- Push your shoulder blades back and try to make them touch. Notice the tension across your shoulders and chest. Relax and repeat.

- Try to touch your shoulders by pushing them forward as far as you can. Hold, relax, and repeat.

- Shrug your shoulders, trying to touch them to your ears. Hold, relax and repeat.

- Take a very deep breath. Hold for several seconds, and release slowly. Do this again, noticing a wave of relaxation overtaking your body.

- Tighten your stomach muscles and hold for several seconds. Release. Notice the relaxation in your abdomen. Repeat.

- Tighten your buttocks. Hold, release, and repeat.

- Tense your thighs, release quickly. Repeat.

- Point your toes away from your body. Notice the tension. Return to a normal position. Repeat.

- Point your toes toward your head; return to normal position. Repeat.

- Point your feet outward, release quickly. Repeat.

- Point your feet inward; hold. Relax and repeat.

- Just let your body relax for a few minutes. Notice and enjoy the good feeling.

- Practice this or another relaxation exercise from Chapter 12 at least once a day. Do not rush. Complete each step, skipping none.

(See Chapter 12 for more relaxation exercises.)

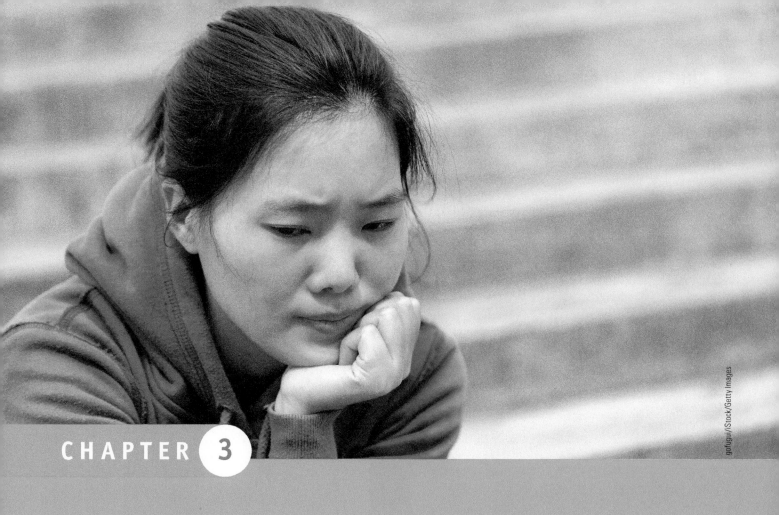

gofugui/iStock/Getty Images

CHAPTER 3

Stress and Your Mind

After reading this chapter, you should be able to:

3.1 Discuss the key features of psychological health.

3.2 Describe the anatomy, function, and development of the brain.

3.3 Compare the four perception-based theories of stress.

3.4 Describe cognitive-behavior therapy as a basis for the management of stress.

3.5 Summarize effective strategies to "talk back to stress."

3.6 Assess the potential impact of acute, episodic, and chronic stress on mental health.

3.7 Identify the causes and symptoms of stress-related mental disorders.

3.8 Analyze the reasons for the prevalence of suicide.

3.9 Describe the benefits of techniques that can be used to effectively manage stress.

PRE-CHAPTER CHECK-IN: ARE YOU IN BALANCE?

The goal of stress management is balance—of mind as well as body. Take inventory of your psychological balance by answering the following items on a scale of 0 to 10 for how they describe you in general. Assign a score of 5 if you feel that your current situation is one of perfect balance. Scores below 5 indicate a deficit or lack in this area compared to what would be ideal for you. A score of 4 indicates a mild deficit; a score of 0 indicates an extreme one. Scores above 5 indicate a surplus of something in your life compared to what would be ideal for you.

How balanced do you feel? Identify the aspects of your life that need adjustment. Reflect on ways you might improve your psychological balance in your journal.

Psychological Balance Inventory

	0	1	2	3	4	5	6	7	8	9	10	
Bored												Overstimulated
Sleep-deprived												Sleepaholic
Inactive												Hyperactive
Not challenged												Burned out
Underachieving												Maxed out
Isolated												Too social

Mei's mother used to say she was a born worrier. Night and day, worrisome thoughts—of assignments to finish, work hours to submit, a dental appointment to make, an aunt's birthday to remember—race through Mei's mind. Lying awake at night, she recalls the chemistry quiz she barely passed or the snarky comment her ex-boyfriend tweeted. Whenever she thinks of all the people and pressures in her life, Mei feels overwhelmed.

"If I don't get my grades up, I'll lose my scholarship," she frets. "Then I'll have to drop out of school. What would I do then? Where would I find a job? What would my parents say? What would my old friends from high school think?" Increasingly she wonders if it is "just stress" or something more serious that is affecting the way she thinks about herself and her life. You may have asked yourself similar questions.

As you've already learned, stress starts in the brain, the amazing information-processing machine that combines the analytic capacity of a computer, the organizational skills of a filing system, and the communications ability of a wireless network. Every day you use your brain to gather, process, and act on information; to think through your values; to make decisions and set goals; and to figure out how to handle problems or challenges.

Stress also has a profound impact on your mind, the sense of consciousness and choice that arises out of the workings of the brain. Your brain keeps you alive; your mind fills your life with meaning. No machine or invention, however sophisticated, can match its unique ability to laugh at a punchline, dream of daffodils, believe in the unknown, fall in and out of love—or learn how to manage stress.

Your mind produces the perceptions and thoughts that set the stress response in motion. If distorted, irrational, or biased, they can prolong cortisol release, elevate blood pressure, promote inflammation, and delay or impair the body's recovery after stress.[1] However, you have the ability to change the way in which you monitor, evaluate, and process your perceptions, thoughts, and language so they promote rather than sabotage your mental health. This chapter will show you how.

Psychological Health

Psychological health encompasses brain and mind, thoughts and feelings. Mental health generally refers to our ability to perceive reality as it is, to respond to its challenges, and to develop rational strategies for living; emotional health includes feelings and moods. Together they enable an individual to live an effective life, find satisfaction in life, and enjoy genuine happiness.

The key features of psychological health include:

- Determination and effort put forth to be healthy and happy.
- Flexibility and adaptability to a variety of circumstances, however stressful.
- Realistic perceptions of the motivations of others.
- Rational, logical thought processes.
- Compassion for others and the capacity to be unselfish in serving or relating to others.
- Establishment of close relationships that are deep and satisfying.
- Acceptance of the limitations as well as the possibilities that life has to offer.
- A sense of meaning and purpose that makes the routines and responsibilities of daily life seem meaningful and worthwhile.
- The ability to cope with stress in a way that allows for emotional stability and growth.

Psychological well-being is not a fixed state of being, but a process driven by your thoughts, including the ways you perceive and respond to stress. Faced with a challenge, you can choose to catastrophize (assume that the worst can and will happen), or you can remind yourself of past achievements; you can anxiously anticipate the coming of some unknown disaster, or you can cultivate hope and optimism as you look to the future. When faced with an upsetting situation,

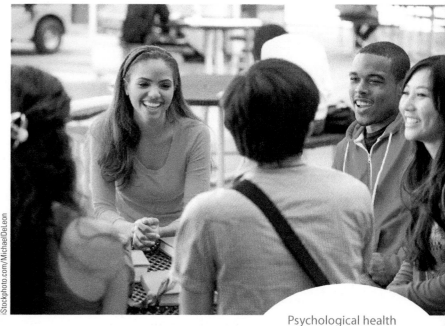

Psychological health includes the ability to establish close relationships that are deep and satisfying.

you can fly off the handle, or you can learn to achieve and maintain a state of internal calm.

Stress and the Brain

The key regions of the brain involved in responding to the many stressors you encounter every day include the following (see Figure 3.1):

- **prefrontal cortex** in the frontal lobe; this regulates cognitive processes such as planning and problem-solving and functions as the center for postponing gratification, self-discipline, and emotional regulation. Because this is the last part of the brain to mature fully, stress may have a greater impact on the prefrontal cortex of those under age 25. At any age, stress affects both the structure and function of the prefrontal cortex by causing neurons to atrophy and by disconnecting circuits.
- hypothalamus, located above the brain stem; the hypothalamus links the body's nervous and endocrine (hormone-producing) systems.
- amygdala, which plays a role in processing emotions such as anxiety or fear. Stress feeds the amygdala so it actually gets bigger and produces a larger, more intense fear response.
- hippocampus, which is located just below the amygdala; the hippocampus is involved in memory. Chronic stress kills neurons and causes the hippocampus to atrophy.

psychological health The ability to perceive reality as it is, to develop rational strategies for living, and to keep feelings and moods in balance.

prefrontal cortex The part of the frontal lobe in the brain that regulates cognitive processes such as planning and problem solving and functions as the center for postponing gratification, self-discipline, and emotional regulation; may not mature fully until age 25, making younger individuals more vulnerable to stress.

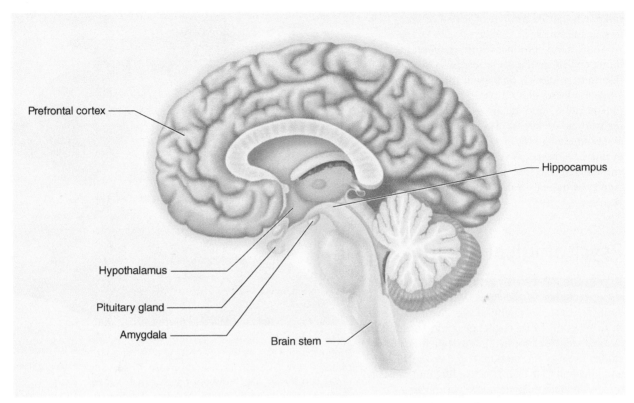

FIGURE 3.1 These are the key regions of the brain involved in responding to the stressors you encounter every day.

Your perceptions determine whether you view new places and experiences as stressful or stimulating.

- locus coeruleus, located in the brain stem; the locus coeruleus synthesizes the neurotransmitter norepinephrine and stimulates the fight-or-flight response.

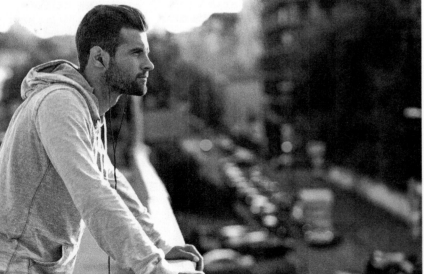

- pituitary gland, which is located under the hypothalamus; the pituitary gland releases various hormones, including oxytocin, that maintain homeostasis or equilibrium in the body.

Just as acute stress mobilizes the body for action, it also maximizes the workings of your brain by:

- enhancing awareness
- speeding up reflexes and thinking
- boosting cognitive ability
- sharpening memory so you can retrieve crucial information
- motivating greater effort (for instance, to meet a deadline)
- improving performance (as in a game or competition).[2]

Once a challenge or potential threat passes, the brain restores its internal balance. But if it persists, stress can impair learning and memory, disrupt sleep, and cause symptoms such as headaches. If stress becomes chronic, brain cells atrophy or die. The **synapses** (the connections by which neurons transmit electrical impulses) between neurons weaken, impairing communication within the brain. Levels of **dopamine**, a neurotransmitter involved in reward and pleasure, fall, and the risk of mental disorders (such as anxiety and depression) increases.[3] Long-term stress also causes disconnections of circuits in the prefrontal cortex, the part of the brain involved in emotional regulation, long-term planning, self-discipline, and decision-making.

Scientists once considered such damage irreparable because they believed that no new neurons or synapses formed in the brain after birth; they were wrong.[4] As we now know, the brain continues to produce new neurons and synapses throughout life in a process called **neuroplasticity**. Specific, learnable techniques, such as meditation (see Chapter 13), can tap into this innate flexibility and help the brain "armor up" for stress by generating new cells, creating and strengthening connections between neurons, and compensating for damage caused by stress, injury, and disease.

Perception-Based Theories of Stress

Every day we view the world and our lives through various "lenses" that affect how we evaluate and respond to stress. As you read through the following section, ask yourself if you've ever looked at yourself and your circumstances through any of these psychological filters. Keep in mind that even when we cannot change the things that cause stress, we can change our perceptions of them—and this changes how we respond to stress itself.

Locus of Control

Decades ago in a university laboratory, volunteers played a game in front of a panel containing three buttons; below the buttons was a round hole from which marbles rolled into a small trough. Their goal was to try to win as many marbles as possible by pressing the buttons on the panel. Some "contestants" were told this was a game of chance, and it made no difference which buttons they pressed; others were told that this was a game of skill, and their strategic pushing of the buttons would determine the outcome. The volunteers didn't know that, no matter which buttons they pressed in which order, they all received marbles in the same fixed, predetermined sequence. At some point, the marbles stopped coming.

What happened next? The volunteers who thought they were engaged in a game of chance played for a while and then quit. What was the point of continuing? Those told the game depended on their skill not only kept playing but also repeatedly changed tactics and tried complicated strategies, as if trying to remember which actions had produced marbles before.

Psychologist Julian Rotter, who devised this now-classic experiment, wondered whether the results might tell us something about people's conceptions about life in general. Some people, he theorized, go about life as if they received "skill" instructions for it, while others feel nothing they do will make any difference. His hunch was that if people viewed outcomes as directly related to their efforts, they would persist longer, try harder, and apply their intelligence to solving a problem—just like the participants in his game of marbles.

Rotter's observations led to more than 30 years of research into **locus of control**, an individual's sense of the forces that determine what happens in life. "Internals" assume they are personally responsible. If, for instance, they get an "A" on a test, they credit their hard work and understanding of the material. "Externals" view their lives as governed by luck or fate. If they get a good grade, they assume the teacher was an easy grader or used a curve. In general, Internals act more independently, enjoy better health, and are more optimistic about their future. Externals find it harder to cope with stress and feel increasingly helpless over time.

An internal locus of control also is related to higher self-esteem—and self-esteem has to do not just with feeling good about yourself, but also with achieving results. You cannot and do not achieve results if you do not act and if you are not able to manage stress. On the other hand, you will not exert effort unless you have a reasonable expectation of being able to succeed. An internal locus of control sets up a positive spiral that builds on itself; an external one freezes you in place. (Complete the "Are You Internal or External?" self-assessment on page 59 at the end of this chapter to evaluate your locus of control.)

Self-Efficacy

Managing stress goes hand in hand with belief in your ability to do so. As psychologist Albert Bandura demonstrated in his ground-breaking research, the individuals most likely to achieve a goal or accomplish what they set out to do are those who believe that they can. Your judgment of your own "**self-efficacy**" (belief in your ability to accomplish a goal or change a behavior)

synapses The connections by which neurons transmit electrical impulses.

dopamine A neurotransmitter involved in reward and pleasure.

neuroplasticity Ability of the brain to produce new neurons and synapses throughout life.

locus of control The sense of whether external or internal influence determines what happens in life.

self-efficacy Belief in one's ability to accomplish a goal or change a behavior.

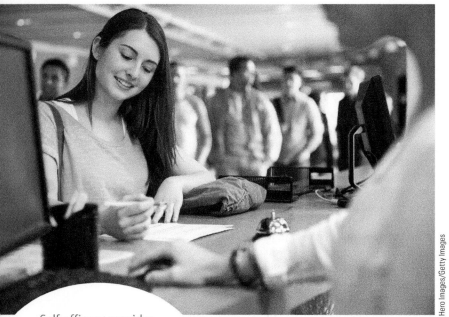

Self-efficacy provides the confidence needed to apply for a competitive internship or job.

helps determine whether you undertake particular goal-directed activities, as well as how hard and how long you work to accomplish them. Although it may sound similar to internal locus of control, self-efficacy is different because it is task-specific. An individual might have high self-esteem, an internal sense of control, and high self-efficacy in managing money, but poor self-efficacy in meeting deadlines or eating a healthy diet.

Self-efficacy influences how you perceive a potential stressor, what actions you take, and the amount of energy and time that you commit to them. Individuals with little faith in their abilities to cope are more likely to panic, assume the worst possible outcome, and become extremely anxious. By comparison, those who have confidence in their ability to handle stress focus on planning and taking effective action to deal with the problem at hand. A strong sense of self-efficacy provides another bonus: It keeps fear and hopelessness at bay to calm you in threatening or hazardous situations.

Expectations

Think ahead to your next big test. What do you expect will happen? Do you anticipate studying hard and acing the exam? Or do you look ahead to a frantic, late-night cramming session and blanking out when you look at the questions? All too often expectations turn into self-fulfilling prophecies, in part because they filter what you notice or ignore in daily life.

As psychologists have shown, we base expectations on past experiences. If you recently put in four hours of study for an earth science quiz and four hours of study for a sociology exam, and you did well in both, you might expect that four hours of studying will yield a good grade on your upcoming statistics test. If this doesn't happen, you feel out of control and uncertain about what to expect in the future. Your stress response automatically kicks in, and anxiety, fear, and unease increase.

Other people can also influence your expectations. Say you are in a class with 300 other students, most of whom received average or poor grades on the last test. You may overhear them complaining about how hard the class is and how unlikely it is for anyone to do well. Influenced by their comments, you may expect that you, too, will perform poorly. Rather than studying more, you may ask, "What's the use? No one gets this stuff." Your stress increases, and you are less likely to do well on the test.

Expectations also affect your relationships because they announce to the world what you anticipate, which affects how others respond to you. People assume that you know yourself better than anyone. If you're self-confident, they let you take the lead. If you seem passive and compliant, someone will rush to exert control over you.

 Stress Reliever: Take Control

Identify the circumstances in which you feel most and least in control. Are you least stressed on the basketball court but anxious on a date? Can you work out a dispute with your friends without stress, yet fall apart when a landlord refuses to refund your security deposit?

Look for ways in which you can exert more influence in situations where you once yielded to external pressures.

Attributions

Another way we try to make sense of why things happen and why people do the things they do is by attributing events and behaviors to various causes. Often people explain others' behavior by attributing it to internal factors, such as personality traits. If someone explodes in anger, for example, we may attribute the rage to a bad temper. When we interpret our own behavior, we tend to make external attributions to situational or environmental factors. If you lash out at a waiter who knocks over a glass of water, you may attribute your outburst to the server's clumsiness rather than your irritability.

In various studies, undergraduates attributed their performance on an actual exam, computer game, or anagram to a variety of factors, including their ability, the effort they expended, the teacher's effectiveness, their concentration during the test, and luck. Often students credited their success to an internal cause, making comments such as, "I aced the test because I was well-prepared," but attributed failure to external causes, such as "The professor was biased." When other students did better than they had, students were more likely to give external attributions, such as "The instructor likes them" or "They got lucky."

Students who thought they performed poorly because they hadn't studied enough were motivated to study more for the next test; those who blamed their failure on a lack of ability were likely to put in the same or even less effort than in the past and to experience more distress in the future.

··

✔ **Check-in:** Grade your attributions.

··

Think back to the best test grade you got this semester. What did you attribute it to?

··

What was the worst grade you've gotten this semester? What did you attribute it to?

··

How did each attribution affect your stress level at the time? Did it influence your preparation for future tests?

··

Taking Charge of Your Thoughts

One of the most important psychological breakthroughs of the last half-century was the discovery that thoughts create feelings and drive behavior. This concept is the foundation of **cognitive behavioral therapy (CBT)**, which targets irrational or inaccurate thoughts or beliefs to help individuals break out of a distorted way of thinking.

Initially used for mental disorders such as depression and anxiety disorders, CBT has become one of the mainstays of stress management. Many techniques in this book are based on CBT, including identification of self-sabotaging beliefs and attitudes, recognition of toxic thought patterns, and mastering alternative ways of thinking. These approaches can help free you from the distortions and negative thoughts that create or intensify stress.

Thought Awareness

Every day each of us thinks about sixty thousand different thoughts as we plan, evaluate, judge, interpret, and remember. Most of our thoughts are mundane, focused on the petty details of daily life. But some—fears, insults, doubts, catastrophic expectations, illogical leaps—can flit into your consciousness, wreak psychological havoc, and disappear without your even realizing what's happening. A small setback blows up into a major disaster. An embarrassing blunder brands you as a loser. Whatever goes wrong, you're sure that it must be your fault.

Since you do not take the time to notice these intruders, their sinister messages—however incorrect and absurd—go unchallenged in your mind. Over time they can sabotage your confidence, undermine your performance, and paralyze your mental skills. You cannot counter irrational automatic thoughts until you recognize them. In essence, you have to learn how to read your own mind.

Thought awareness is the process of observing your thoughts and becoming aware of what is going through your head, particularly during stressful situations.

··

✔ **Check-in:** Eavesdrop on yourself.

··

Throughout the day, pause and listen in to your internal dialogue without judgement. Each evening, reflect on what you heard: Are your thoughts encouraging or critical? Positive or negative? Are you talking to yourself the way a loving friend would?

··

If not, ask yourself: What triggered these thoughts? Are they rational? Are they based on facts or fears?

··

As you begin monitoring your mental processes, you will become more conscious of the words and phrases you use to talk to yourself when stressed. You will step back and "see," perhaps for the first time, the ways in which faulty thinking patterns and fruitless worries add stress to your life. If your negative thoughts have some basis in reality, take appropriate action. If, for instance, you really do procrastinate and miss important deadlines, follow the advice on time management in Chapter 6. If there is no rational basis for your distorted thoughts, let them move through your consciousness and out of your mind. The following exercise can help.

cognitive behavioral therapy (CBT)
A form of psychotherapy that targets irrational or inaccurate thoughts or beliefs to help individuals break out of a distorted way of thinking.

Imagine sitting on top of a hill, looking down on a railroad track. Picture a train moving across the valley. As you see each car pass, think of it as one of your thoughts. Without jumping onto the train, notice each thought as it goes by.

If one thought keeps popping up, you might say, "Oh, here it comes again," and watch it leave. If you find yourself jumping on the train, gently return to the top of the hill.

Cognitive Restructuring/ Reframing

Stress begins with **cognition**, the mental process that consists of thinking and reasoning. Cognitive distortion occurs when you fall into faulty thinking patterns, such as assuming responsibility for things that are beyond your control or magnifying a mistake or setback out of proportion to its seriousness. Such distortions often lead to or intensify stress.

Cognitive restructuring or reframing, a technique used in cognitive behavioral therapy, refers to the mental act of changing the meaning or interpretation of self-sabotaging thoughts. You start by noticing self-criticisms such as "I will never understand this material" or "No one wants to talk with me." You then challenge such thoughts with positive statements such as, "I felt the same way in microbiology, but after working with a volunteer tutor, I did well in the course" or "I'm going to smile and start a conversation with someone who looks friendly."

The following exercise provides other examples you can try:

Stress Reliever: Tell Yourself...

I am going to be all right. My thoughts are not always rational, but I know that everything will be all right.

Right now I am having some thoughts that I don't like. They're really just ghosts and they are fading away. I will be fine.

These thoughts are not helpful. I'm going to focus on _____.

I have more control than I once imagined. I'm going to focus on something more positive.

I'm choosing to move in a better direction.

I've done this before; I know I can do it again.

Rational Emotive Behavior Therapy

Rational Emotive Behavior Therapy (REBT), developed by psychiatrist Albert Ellis, a pioneer in cognitive behavioral therapy, is based on the premise that stressors alone do not cause anxiety, anger, or depression. What fuels stress and negative feelings are irrational thoughts. Among the most common are:

- **I must be loved and appreciated by every significant person in my life.** In fact, pleasing all the people in your life is impossible. This irrational belief is one of the most common causes of stress and misery.

- **In order to feel worthwhile, I must be competent, successful, and almost perfect in every aspect of life.** No human being can live up to this standard, which leads to stress, self-blame, and lower self-esteem. Simply strive to do your best and learn from your failures.

- **Some people are evil and wicked and should be punished severely.** While certain behaviors may be inappropriate or antisocial, it is not up to you to judge or punish others. Only they can change the way they act.

- **Not having things go the way I want is catastrophic and awful.** Therapists call this the "spoiled-child syndrome." Having a tantrum every time you don't get what you want accomplishes nothing more than stressing yourself and irritating others.

- **People cannot control their happiness or unhappiness.** You may have limited control over external events and other people, but you can control your own thoughts, emotions, and behavior.

- **One should keep dwelling on the possibility that something terrible may occur.** Constant anxiety about the unknown or uncertain has no impact on what actually happens and adds unnecessary stress to your life.

cognition The mental process that consists of thinking and reasoning.

cognitive restructuring or reframing An approach to changing the meaning or interpretation of stressors.

rational emotive behavior therapy (REBT) Treatment based on the theory that irrational, self-defeating thoughts and behaviors that cause stress can be challenged and changed.

- **It is easier to avoid life's difficulties than tackle them head on.** Ducking responsibility may seem easier than dealing with problems in the short run but it only leads to greater stress in the long term.

- **Your past behavior determines how you behave now and in the future.** You may habitually act or react a certain way, but you can identify the behaviors that didn't serve you well in the past and learn from them.

- **You absolutely need something or someone stronger than you to rely on.** Rather than protecting you from stress, total dependence on others makes you feel weak and vulnerable.[5]

REBT counters these irrational beliefs with a series of steps dubbed the ABCDE approach:

- **A:** an *activating* external or internal event.

- **B:** your *beliefs* about the world around you.

- **C:** the *consequences* of how your beliefs interpret events. Irrational or distorted beliefs lead to negative consequences and feelings.

- **D:** *disputing* irrational beliefs to avoid their negative impact.

- **E:** the *effects* of challenging irrational beliefs, such as lowering stress, overcoming self-blame, and feeling less anger, guilt, and frustration.[6]

If, for example, your bike is stolen (the activating event) and you feel this is unfair and catastrophic (your beliefs), you become angry, fearful, and stressed (the consequences). If you tell yourself that bike thefts occur every day on campus and that you can take the shuttle to get around (disputing), you may still be irritated but you won't feel victimized and angry (effects).

The following section includes common irrational thoughts and beliefs targeted by cognitive behavioral therapy.

Thinking Traps

Some of our thoughts are as precise and logical as mathematical equations. Others are misleading, inappropriate, or so corrosive that they undermine peace of mind and erode our ability to take stress in stride. "Stinking thinking," according to an apt nickname that therapists use, can take many forms, including:

- *All-or-nothing thinking*: You look at life in "black-or-white" categories. If something is less than perfect, you see it as a total failure.

If you get three A's and a B minus, for instance, you conclude that you've gotten a terrible report card.

- *Over-generalizing*: You think of a single negative event as a never-ending pattern. If you stumble as you rush across the quad, you are sure the entire student body thinks you're a klutz.

- *Catastrophizing*: You're sure that the worst-case scenario will inevitably happen. If a classmate turns down your invitation to hang out, you're convinced that you are doomed to be an outcast for life.

- *Mind-reading*: You assume that others are thinking badly of you. If a casual acquaintance glances away during your conversation, you assume he or she is bored and wants to get away from you.

- *"Gloomy glasses"*: Nothing sunny can penetrate your dark lenses. You see only the negative, the hurtful, and the hopeless and completely miss or dismiss any positive achievements or compliments coming your way. If you stumble during a presentation, you ignore the praise of your classmates and remember only your mistake.

- *Emotional reasoning*: You assume that the way you feel reflects the way things actually are. If you're feeling frustrated and incapable, you assume that a project is stupid or requires too much effort or that you're not smart enough to complete it.

- *Comparing and despairing*: You look at your Facebook friends, who all seem happier and more successful than you, and conclude that you are worse off and less worthy.

- *Molehills into mountains*: You exaggerate any risk, danger, or misstep. You react to a late notice on a forgotten bill as if you were on the brink of bankruptcy.

- *Shoulds*: You believe you *should* be able to do it all—that, for instance, everyone expects you to ace every test, organize every friend's birthday celebration, and coordinate all family outings.

- *Personalizing*: You see yourself as responsible for events that have little or nothing to do with you. If the person next to you at a café spills their drink on you, you apologize.

- *Compensating*: You believe that you are inadequate as you are, so you inflate your achievements with claims that, for instance, you qualified for the Olympics but chose to stay in college or created a popular app but never got credit.

Whenever you find yourself falling into a thinking trap, stop and ask: "Is this true? Where is the evidence?" Remind yourself that your distorted thoughts aren't carved in stone or supported by any facts; then let them go.

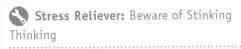
Why Worry?

What if you've studied the wrong material for tomorrow's test? What if the bus is late? What if your mother hates the birthday present you bought her? What if the newest computer virus wipes out your hard drive? What if your boss blames you for the screwed-up order? What if a meteor crashes into the earth and destroys the planet?

The better question to ask: Why worry about things you can't control? (See Figure 3.2.)

rumination The continuous processing of negative thoughts and feelings.

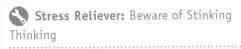

FIGURE 3.2 Creating a worry tree can help you let go of worries you can't change or take action to deal with an issue effectively.

Worrying can be helpful if it spurs you to take action and solve a problem. However, chronic worrying is a destructive mental habit that can sap your emotional energy, spike your anxiety, and interfere with your daily life. It also takes a toll on your health by increasing levels of the stress hormone cortisol and keeping them high.

Everyday worrying can intensify into **rumination**, the continuous processing of negative thoughts and feelings. It may start with a simple "why"—as in "Why is this happening to me?" or "What did I do to deserve this?" Ultimately, rumination creates more problems than it solves because:

- It focuses on causes and consequences instead of solutions.
- It emphasizes what has gone wrong and fosters negative thinking.
- It can lead to or intensify depression.
- It can encourage inactivity and avoidance of problem solving.

If you find yourself dwelling on difficulties and things that upset you, thinking repeatedly about things that went wrong in the past, or so preoccupied with a problem that you can't get it out of your mind, you may be caught in a rumination loop. In order to break out, switch to more "how" questions:

- How can I get out of this situation?
- How can I handle this better?
- How can I get the help I need?
- How can I make things better?

Other stress management strategies can also help ease nagging worries, keep you in the moment with your immediate experience, and prevent stress-induced symptoms. When researchers, for example, have taught volunteers "attentional" skills such as focused breathing (Chapter 12) and meditation (Chapter 13), their levels of the stress hormone cortisol fell—and continued to drop as they became more adept at focusing on the moment and the task at hand.

Talking Back to Stress

Language has the power to paralyze or inspire, mire you down or move you forward. Because your choice of words, spoken or unspoken, can either intensify or ease stress, pay attention both to *what* you say and *how* you say it. What kind of language are you using in day-to-day situations, both with yourself and with others?

Self-Talk

Self-talk describes the messages you send to yourself. Many of us don't realize that our internal dialogue may be sabotaging our self-esteem because we are so used to making negative judgments about ourselves that we begin to believe they are true. If this applies to you, one way to change how you talk about yourself in your head is to imagine that you are talking to a friend you care about and whose feelings you don't want to hurt.

As you eavesdrop on your self-talk, watch for stress-inducing statements, such as "I hate working out," or "I can't learn Mandarin Chinese." Comments like these not only make you feel bad about yourself but also severely limit your sense of personal efficacy. Positive self-talk, in contrast, can improve self-esteem and eliminate the chronic, nagging self-doubt that destroys people from the inside out.

To improve your self-talk, shift tenses from the present to the past. Rather than thinking, "I can't control my temper," say "I used to have problems controlling my temper." Instead of "I always screw-up my relationships," you can reflect, "I used to have problems maintaining good relationships."

When you move negative habits or characteristics into the past, you avoid hanging onto them. Changing the tense also helps you differentiate between what you once did from what is possible now. By editing your comments, you remind yourself that you have changed, are changing, or at the least are capable of change. Here is another exercise that can help:

🌀 **Stress Reliever:** Go for the Positive

Another gentle but effective tool that decreases stress and changes your supposed limits is being positive about your possibilities. For instance, instead of saying, "I hate exercise," say, "I am learning to enjoy exercise." Instead of "I'll never figure out how to do spreadsheets on Excel," switch to "I haven't learned how to do spreadsheets on Excel yet."

Hear and feel the difference in the following statements:

"I'm terrible at languages"—"It's harder for me to learn languages than some other subjects."

"I always feel awkward at parties"—"Tonight I'll try smiling at someone I don't know and maybe even start a conversation."

"I'm never going to figure out photo editing"—"If I keep at it, I'll get the hang of it."

"Things never work out for me; I'm such a loser"—"Things didn't work out this time. Next time I'll..."

Negate the Negatives

Some people constantly replay scenes from their lives, fretting about what they should or could have done differently. Others criticize or belittle themselves, magnifying the most minor of faults or failures into monstrous proportions and feeding anxiety and tension. You don't have to tolerate such self-sabotaging thoughts. Here are some suggestions for clearing them from your mind:

- For each negative, give yourself two positives. This counteracts the common tendency to remember negative statements longer. If you find yourself saying, "I screwed up again," remind yourself that you have a brown belt in karate and can speak two languages.

- Take a few deep abdominal breaths, then go deeper, and ask: Do I really want to do this to myself? Do I really want to keep feeling the way these statements make me feel?

- When a derogatory statement forms in your brain, say firmly, "Stop!"

- If you keep calling yourself an idiot or berating yourself for an insensitive comment, write the thought on a piece of paper and shred, burn, or crumble it and throw it away. This symbolic gesture will remind you to get rid of all the negative thoughts that creep into your head.

- If you are in a situation in which you cannot or do not wish to reverse a negative statement aloud (in a classroom, for instance), do it in your head by saying to yourself "delete" or "cancel."

- To break a barrage of negative thoughts, distract yourself with simple mind exercises, such as reciting the alphabet backwards or starting at 100 and subtracting by 4 all the way back to zero.

Self-talk The internal messages you send to yourself

Affirm Yourself

In the early 1920's Émile Coué, a French therapist, developed a technique called "conscious autosuggestion," which required repeating the phrase "Every day in every way, I'm getting better and better" twenty times on awakening and twenty times before retiring. Through the years, researchers around the world have confirmed that repeating a positive statement affects self-perceptions and self-esteem. Frequent repetition of an "**affirmation**," a positive statement that you repeat to yourself for emotional encouragement and support, has become a fundamental part of cognitive behavioral therapy and a powerful tool for stress management.

As research has confirmed, affirmations can improve problem solving, self-worth, and self-regulation.[7] When you are feeling stressed, repeating an affirmation is one of the fastest ways to restructure your thought patterns, develop new pathways in your brain, and change your mindset. Within a short time, you'll find that you no longer recycle the old habitual put-downs. As you keep repeating your affirmation, you'll feel a greater desire to stick with your new behavior.

It's useful to recite your affirmations several times a day and to repeat your affirmation as soon as you start to engage in a negative thought or behavior. The affirmations you choose to repeat should be phrases that are meaningful to you. They become more powerful when you say them out loud, especially while looking in the mirror.

affirmation A positive statement repeated to oneself for emotional encouragement and support.

Affirmations can change the thought patterns in your brain and boost your sense of self-worth.

 Stress Reliever: Affirm Yourself

- I am confident and capable.
- I can handle this situation.
- I am a valuable and special person.
- Write several affirmations for yourself. Repeat them when you brush your teeth, shower, get dressed, gel your hair, walk to class, ride an elevator, or wait for your computer to boot. The more time you devote to your affirmations, the more dramatic a difference you'll feel.
- Continue repeating affirmations at least five times first thing in the morning and last thing at night.
- Be creative and send affirmations to yourself in e-mails, reminders, and text messages. Celebrate the best in you.

Stress and Mental Health

Stress in itself usually doesn't cause a psychological problem, but it can increase vulnerability. Acute stress can trigger negative feelings, such as anger, worry, and irritability, as well as problems sleeping. When stressed, people often stop the healthy coping strategies that usually keep their moods on track. They may not go to yoga class or read before bed or catch up with close friends. They may snap at roommates or pull away from family. Small mistakes, such as misplacing a flash drive, multiply.

Episodic acute stress may lead to insomnia, loss of appetite, lack of enjoyment in things that once brought pleasure, and increased physical symptoms, such as muscle aches or digestive problems. The long-term effects of chronic stress include serious mental illness—a diagnosable mental, behavioral, or emotional disorder that interferes with one or more major activities in life, like dressing, eating or working—as well as increased risk of self-harm and suicide.

As many as 50 percent of undergraduates may have a diagnosable mental disorder, but fewer than 25 percent of these individuals ever seek help (See Table 3.1.). For them, the consequences of untreated mental disorders include poorer academic performance and increased likelihood of dropping out before graduation.

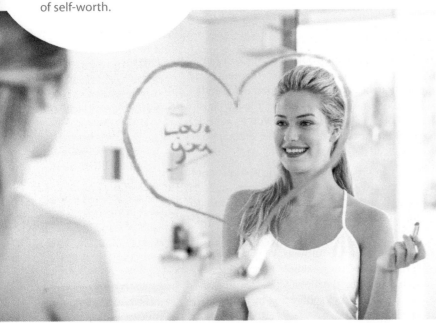

Wavebreak Media/AGE Fotostock

TABLE 3.1 Mental Disorders on Campus

Student mental disorders diagnosed and treated by a professional within the last 12 months:			
Condition	**Percent (%)**		
	Male	**Female**	**Average**
Anxiety	10.3	20.5	17.3
Depression	9.0	16.8	14.5
Both	6.1	12.9	10.9

Source: American College Health Association. American College Health Association-National College Health Assessment II: Reference Group Executive Summary Fall 2015. Hanover, MD: American College Health Association, 2016.

🌐 Stress Reliever: Do You Know Where to Turn for Help?

Check out the counseling services at your school. Is there a peer-counseling program? Can you set up an appointment with a mental health professional through the health center? Call a local helpline or a national support center such as the National Alliance on Mental Health hotline.

There are also numerous online sites, including support groups and chat rooms through hubs such as PsychCentral.com, CrisisChat.org, and WebMD.com. Is there a support group at your school?

TABLE 3.2 Recognizing Anxiety

The characteristic symptoms of generalized anxiety are:

- faster heart rate
- sweating
- increased blood pressure
- muscle aches
- intestinal pains
- irritability
- sleep problems
- difficulty concentrating.[8]

some point within the last twelve months that it was difficult to function.[9] Some paid less attention to their day-to-day needs; others neglected their responsibilities, stopped communicating with friends and family, or lost interest in activities they previously enjoyed (see Table 3.3).

Anxiety

Anxious people often describe themselves as "stressed," but a true anxiety disorder is more profound and persistent (see Table 3.2). Chronically anxious individuals worry, not just some of the time and not just about the stresses and strains of ordinary life, but constantly, about almost everything: their health, families, finances, marriages, potential dangers. Their constant state of arousal may cause prolonged activation of the HPA (hypothalamus-pituitary-adrenal) axis described in Chapter 2 and increase their risk of both psychological and physical problems.

Depression

Stress and depression often occur together, with both contributing to symptoms such as irritability, poor sleep, and impaired concentration. In a nationwide survey, 35.5 percent of all students—29.4 percent of men and 37.6 percent of women—reported feeling so depressed at

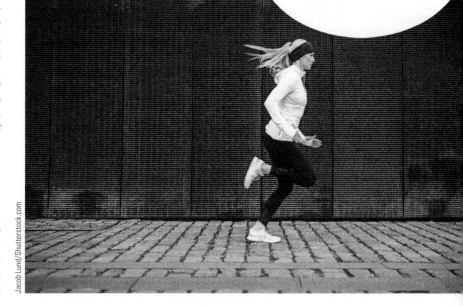

Jacob Lund/Shutterstock.com

Exercise is one of the best ways to reduce stress and symptoms of anxiety and depression.

TABLE 3.3 Recognizing Depression

The characteristic symptoms of major depression include:

- Feeling depressed, sad, empty, discouraged, tearful most of the day, nearly every day.

- Loss of interest or pleasure in previously enjoyable activities.

- Eating more or less than usual and either gaining or losing a significant amount of weight.

- Having trouble sleeping or sleeping much more than usual.

- Feeling slowed down or restless and unable to sit still.

- Lack of energy or fatigue nearly every day.

- Feeling helpless, hopeless, worthless, inadequate, or inappropriately guilty.

- Difficulty thinking or concentrating; indecisiveness.

- Persistent thoughts of death or suicide.[10]

Stress may put women at greater risk of depression, particularly if they experienced major stressful life events in adolescence and young adulthood. Men are more likely than women to become depressed following a breakup, divorce, job loss, or a career setback. Rather than becoming sad, they may feel a sense of being dead inside or of worthlessness, hopelessness, and helplessness.[11]

Stress-Related Mental Disorders

The stress of some events and life challenges can trigger specific psychological problems, including adjustment disorder, acute stress disorder, and post-traumatic stress disorder (PTSD).

Adjustment Disorder

An **adjustment disorder** refers to the development of emotional or behavioral symptoms within three months of an identifiable stressor, whether a single event (such as being robbed) or multiple or recurrent stressors (such as conflict with a roommate or partner). Stressors can involve specific developmental events, such as going to school, leaving or returning to a parental home, getting married, or having a baby.

Individuals with an adjustment disorder suffer greater-than-ordinary distress that significantly impairs their ability to function at home, work, school, or another important area of their lives. They feel down, tearful, hopeless, worried, and jittery. Most people seeking treatment for adjustment disorders are in their twenties and benefit from talk therapy. Putting painful fears and feelings into words reduces the pressure caused by the stressor and enhances the individual's ability to cope.

Here is another specific strategy that can help when you're going through a challenging time:

adjustment disorder Development of mild to moderate emotional or behavioral symptoms within three months of an identifiable stressor, whether a single event (such as being robbed) or multiple or recurrent stressors (such as conflict with a roommate or partner).

acute stress disorder Development of disabling symptoms, such as recurrent and intrusive distressing memories or dreams related to the trauma, within three days to a month after exposure to a traumatic event.

 Stress Reliever: Schedule Your Stress

Just as you schedule classes and appointments, try scheduling your stress:

- Designate 15–30 minutes of your day just for stressing. You have to be present and engaged during this time. Push yourself to process all your stresses, worries, and fears. When your appointed time is over, tell yourself that you're done with your stressful thinking for the day.

- If stressful thoughts come into your mind (which is natural and normal), remind yourself, "I'll think about this during my scheduled stress time." Acknowledge the stress, but remember that you will think about it in depth soon, and refocus your attention.

- Practice breathing exercises (See Chapter 12) and with each exhalation, use your breath to release your stress and push the thoughts away. Until the appointed time, refocus your attention to the present and continue on with your day.

Acute Stress Disorder

In **acute stress disorder**, disabling symptoms occur within three days to a month after exposure to a traumatic event. These may include recurrent and intrusive distressing memories or dreams related to the trauma; flashbacks, in which individuals feel that the traumatic event is recurring; inability to experience positive emotions; efforts to avoid distressing reminders, memories, or thoughts related to the event; sleep disturbances; irritable behavior and angry outbursts; problems with concentration; and an intensified startle response.

Acute stress disorders interfere with the ability to work, study, relate to others, or maintain usual routine and social activities. People with an acute stress disorder initially need protection, consolation, assurance of safety, and assistance with decisions and plans. The greatest help of all may be the support of those closest to them. Supportive psychotherapy, with a focus on working through emotional responses to trauma or stress, also can be beneficial.

Post-Traumatic Stress Disorder (PTSD)

In the past, **post-traumatic stress disorder (PTSD)** was viewed as a psychological response to truly out-of-the-ordinary stressors, such as kidnapping or combat. However, more common experiences—a life-threatening accident, a natural disaster, sexual assault, gun violence—can also forever change the way people view themselves and their world. More than half of people experience traumatic events, but far fewer—an estimated

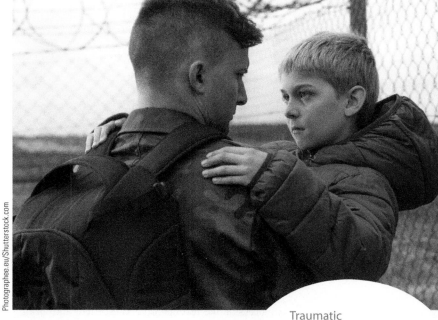

Photographee.eu/Shutterstock.com

8.7 percent of American adults—develop PTSD in their lifetime. Although men experience more traumatic events, PTSD is twice as common in women, most often as a consequence of sexual abuse and assaults.[13] The disorder tends to be more severe and longer lasting when the stressor is not an act of fate or bad luck but instead involves deliberate human malice (See Table 3.4.).[14]

Traumatic experiences, including deployment in a war zone, increase the risk of PTSD.

TABLE 3.4 Recognizing PTSD

Symptoms of PTSD, which usually begin within months after a trauma, include:

- Recurrent, involuntary, and intrusive distressing memories of the traumatic event.

- Recurrent distressing dreams related to the trauma.

- Flashbacks

- Intense or prolonged psychological distress.

- Strong physiological reactions to "cues" that symbolize or resemble some aspect of the traumatic event.

- Avoiding or attempting to avoid distressing memories, thoughts, or feelings and/or reminders related to the trauma.

- Inability to remember an important aspect of the trauma.

- Persistent and exaggerated negative thoughts, expectations, or beliefs about oneself, others, or the world.

- Persistent feelings of guilt, shame, anger, horror, fear, or other negative emotions.

- Diminished interest or participation in once-valued activities.

- Persistent inability to experience positive emotions such as happiness and loving feelings.

- Irritable behavior and angry outbursts.

- Reckless or self-destructive behavior.

- Hypervigilance (a state of heightened reactivity).

- Problems concentrating.

- Problems falling or staying asleep and other sleep disturbances.[12]

post-traumatic stress disorder (PTSD) A psychological response to a trauma such as a life-threatening accident, a natural disaster, sexual assault, or gun violence that leads to repeated reliving of the incident and persistent psychological symptoms that interfere with normal functioning.

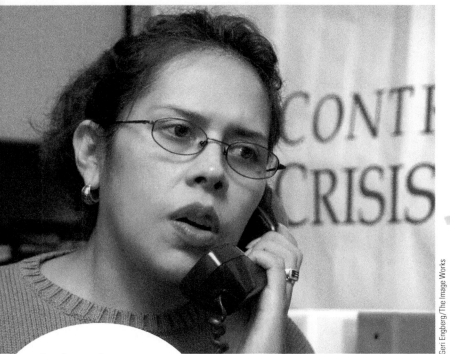

Students who are considering suicide can find help and hope from crisis hotlines.

Geri Engberg/The Image Works

Suicide

Suicide can be difficult to think or talk about, especially when a young person "with everything to live for" takes his or her own life. Although not in itself a mental disorder, suicide can be the tragic consequence of emotional and psychological problems that often are intensified by stress. Because it carries such stigma, desperate individuals who find themselves thinking of killing themselves feel ashamed and terribly alone as they struggle with unbearable pain.

The suicide rate among 10- to 24-year-old young Americans has increased steadily since 2007 to 11.1 deaths per 100,000.[17] More than 1,100 college students commit suicide every year. According to the National College Health Assessment, about 10 percent say they have considered suicide; 1.4 percent attempted suicide but survived.[18] (See Table 3.5.)

Task forces investigating suicides at various campuses have identified a common underlying stressor: the pressure to be—or at least to seem to be—perfect. (See "The Duck Syndrome" in Chapter 4 on "Students Under Stress.") Struggling to meet the high expectations of parents and teachers, some students feel devastated if they aren't as smart, accomplished, attractive, or popular as they feel they should be—or as the classmates radiating happiness on social media seem to be. Some turn to substances such as drugs or alcohol. Students who binge drink are significantly more likely to contemplate suicide, to have attempted suicide in the past, and to believe they would make a future suicide attempt than non-binge drinkers.

Untreated depression is the most significant reason that individuals consider or attempt suicide. (See Table 3.6.) Two thirds of those who kill themselves experienced depressive symptoms at

Some people may be especially vulnerable to PTSD because of genetics, childhood exposure to traumatic experience, family and peer problems, poverty, and mental disorders. During the first days after a trauma, protection, reassurance of safety, help with decisions and plans, and the support of those closest to them can be most significant in easing distress. Certain approaches, such as immediate "debriefing" to release emotions or treatment with anxiety-reducing medications, have been found to be ineffective and may even hinder long-term recovery.[15] What has proven helpful is cognitive behavioral therapy along with stress reduction techniques such as mindfulness and meditation (see Chapter 13).[16]

TABLE 3.5 Suicide on Campus

Percentage of Students Who Seriously Considered Suicide			
	Male	**Female**	**Total**
Anytime in last 12 months	8.0	9.9	9.6
Never	78.9	74.6	75.6

Percentage of Students Who Attempted Suicide			
	Male	**Female**	**Total**
Anytime in last 12 months	1.4	1.5	1.6
Never	92.5	89.6	90.2

Source: American College Health Association. American College Health Association-National College Health Assessment II: Reference Group Executive Summary Fall 2015. Hanover, MD: American College Health Association, 2016.

TABLE 3.6 Risk Factors for Suicide

- Depression or depressive symptoms.
- Family history of mental illness.
- Suicide of a family member or friend.
- Personality traits such as hopelessness, helplessness, impulsivity, and aggression.
- Alcohol use and binge drinking. Among college students, binge drinkers are significantly more likely to contemplate suicide, to have attempted suicide in the past, and to believe they would make a future suicide attempt than non-binge drinkers.[19]
- Ineffective problem solving and coping skills.
- Recent sexual or physical victimization; being in an emotionally or physically abusive relationship.
- Family problems.
- Trauma or chronic stress.
- Feelings of loneliness or social isolation.
- Harassment because of sexual orientation.

the time of their deaths, particularly a profound sense of helplessness. When hope dies, people expect the worst possible outcomes for their problems. Given this way of thinking, suicide may seem a reasonable response to a life seen as not worth living.

Although many schools offer counseling and crisis services, less than a quarter of students who die by suicide have ever sought help. Often they don't know where to turn when they feel hopeless or are thinking about suicide. Do you know what types of counseling are available on your campus?

Stress Reliever: If You Ever Start Thinking about Taking Your Life:

- Talk to a mental health professional. If you have a therapist, call immediately. If not, call a suicide hotline. The national suicide hot line number is 1 (800) 273-TALK (8255).

- Find someone you can trust and talk honestly about what you're feeling.

- If you suffer from depression or another mental disorder, educate friends or relatives about your condition so they are prepared if called upon to help.

- Write down some uplifting thoughts, or spend time looking at loved ones (pet included) on your phone or tablet. Even if you are despondent, you can help yourself by focusing on positive thoughts or memories.

- Avoid drugs and alcohol. Most suicides are the result of sudden, uncontrolled impulses, and drugs and alcohol can make it harder to resist these destructive urges.

- Go to the hospital. Hospitalization can sometimes be the best way to protect your health and safety.

Harnessing the Powers of Your Mind

Stress is not a uniquely human phenomenon. Animals experience and respond instinctively to stressors such as hunger or danger. Yet only humans have the mental capacity to not only think through the most effective strategies to cope with a current stressor, but also to learn from past experiences and to prepare for future challenges.

As you deal with life's inevitable stresses, your mind can be either your worst enemy or your staunchest ally. If you allow it to bombard you with toxic thoughts and distorted perceptions, you will feel more anxious and discouraged. But if you consciously take charge of the

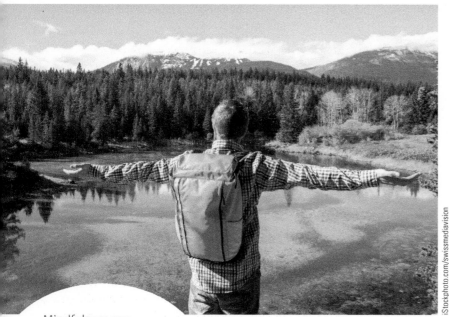

Mindfulness can enhance your ability to make the most of relaxing moments in nature.

mindfulness
A modern form of concentration that involves maintaining awareness in the present moment.

mindfulness-based stress reduction
A program based on mindfulness meditation that uses awareness techniques to reduce stress and promote wellness.

ways you think and reason, you can effectively manage stress on a day-to-day basis as well as master techniques that will enhance every aspect of your life.

As researchers have documented, increases in stress hormones can impair memory and other functions essential for thinking and problem solving. However, specific techniques can counter their negative impact. One of the most powerful is **mindfulness**, based on a psychological technique derived from Tibetan Buddhism that involves maintaining awareness in the present moment.[20] (See Chapter 13 for a comprehensive discussion of mindfulness, and try the Mindfulness Meditation exercise on page 59 at the end of this chapter.)

Mindfulness enhances your ability to pay attention to and accept whatever thoughts, sensations, and emotions are happening in the here and now. **Mindfulness-Based Stress Reduction**, which focuses on progressive development of mindful awareness, has been used for patients with a wide variety of medical problems as well as for healthy people coping with daily stress.[21] Even brief sessions of mindfulness can increase awareness, decrease symptoms of anxiety and depression, and relieve symptoms such as back pain.[22] Mindfulness-based stress reduction and meditation increase the brain's plasticity, or ability to change and boost resilience (discussed in Chapter 10)[23] Other psychological benefits include greater self-compassion, decreased absent-mindedness, less difficulty regulating emotions, and reduced fear of emotion, worry, and anger.

> **Stress Reliever:** Engage Your Mind
>
> Make a purposeful decision to interpret an obstacle or difficulty in your life as a challenge and as a teacher. Consciously decide that nothing will crush you. Stay in charge of your thoughts despite any adversity you might encounter.
>
> Take a position of no surrender. This is not a position of stubborn stupidity or inflexibility, but of resourcefulness and determination that you will accept no other outcome. If one path does not work, discard it and find another.
>
> Develop the stress-resistant attitude that rough experiences are the source of valuable lessons.
>
> Purposely cultivate an internal perspective on stress that is oriented to learning and coping rather than feeling victimized and blaming circumstances or others.
>
> If you are momentarily thrown off by setbacks, obstacles, or adversity, talk and coach yourself back to this perspective. Resolve to learn from your setback, make the necessary adjustments, and continue, knowing you are the stronger for it.

Chapter Summary

- Acute stress can enhance awareness, speed thinking, sharpen reflexes, and improve performance. Ongoing stress, even if time-limited, can impair learning and memory, disrupt sleep, and cause headaches. Chronic stress can cause brain cells to atrophy or die and can impair the ability to feel enjoyment and increase the risk of depression and anxiety.

- Worry, blame, criticism, and rumination can hijack the mind, prolong cortisol release, keep blood pressure elevated, promote inflammation, and delay or impair the body's recovery after stress. Individuals who block negative thoughts, draw on positive emotions, and seek support from others return more quickly to a state of balance.

- A sense of self-esteem, of belief or pride in ourselves, provides confidence to handle the stress of taking on new challenges at school or work. One of the most useful techniques for bolstering self-esteem is developing the habit of positive thinking and positive self-talk (how you address yourself in your thoughts).

- Locus of control (the sense of who or what determines what happens in life) affects your perceptions of stress and its health implications. "Internals," who see themselves as in charge of their well-being, take better care of themselves than "externals," who feel that stress or other factors most influence health.

- Self-efficacy (a belief in your ability to handle a specific challenge or change) affects how you respond to a stressor. Individuals with a strong belief in their capabilities feel less fear and focus on taking effective actions to handle a stressor.

- Changing your perception of stress can change the way you respond to it. Catastrophizing (assuming that the worst will happen), expecting failure, attributing performance to factors beyond your control, and projecting your own weaknesses onto others can

influence how much stress you experience in a challenging situation.

- Stress in itself usually doesn't cause a psychological problem, but it can increase vulnerability to a diagnosable mental, behavioral, or emotional disorder that interferes with one or more major activities in life.

- An acute stress disorder, characterized by recurrent, distressing memories, dreams, and flashbacks and other disabling symptoms, may occur within three days to a month after exposure to a traumatic event. Supportive psychotherapy can be beneficial.

- An estimated 20 to 50 percent of survivors of a traumatic experience may develop post-traumatic stress disorder (PTSD) and re-experience their terror and helplessness again and again in their thoughts or dreams. Some engage in aggressive, reckless, or self-destructive behavior. Others enter a state of emotional numbness and no longer can respond to people and experiences the way they once did. Individuals with PTSD may require different types of help at different stages.

- Mindfulness, a psychological technique that maintains awareness in the present moment, has proven one of the most successful approaches to helping people cope with daily stress. Its psychological benefits include greater self-compassion, decreased absentmindedness, less difficulty regulating emotions, and reduced depression, anxiety, and anger.

🌐 STRESS RELIEVERS

Take Control

Identify the circumstances in which you feel most and least in control. Are you least stressed on the basketball court but anxious on a date? Can you work out a dispute with your friends without stress, yet fall apart when a landlord refuses to refund your security deposit?

Look for ways in which you can exert more influence in situations where you once yielded to external pressures.

The Thought Train

Imagine sitting on top of a hill, looking down on a train track. Picture a train moving across the valley. As you see each car pass, think of it as one of your thoughts. Without jumping onto the train, notice each thought as it goes by. If one thought keeps popping up, you might say, "Oh, here it comes again," and watch it leave. If you find yourself jumping on the train, gently return to the top of the hill.

Tell Yourself...

- I am going to be all right. My thoughts are not always rational, but I know that everything will be all right.

- Right now I am having some thoughts that I don't like. They're really just ghosts and they are fading away. I will be fine.

- These thoughts are not helpful. I'm going to focus on _____.

- I have more control than I once imagined. I'm going to focus on something more positive.

- I'm choosing to move in a better direction.

- I've done this before; I know I can do it again.

Beware of Stinking Thinking

Have you ever fallen into any of the thought traps described in this chapter? When and how? Record your observations.

Go for the Positive

Another gentle but effective tool that decreases stress and changes your supposed limits is being positive about your possibilities. For instance, instead of saying, "I hate exercise," say, "I am learning to enjoy exercise." Instead of "I'll never figure out how to do spreadsheets on Excel," switch to

"I haven't learned how to do spreadsheets on Excel yet." Hear and feel the difference in the following statements:

- "I'm terrible at languages"—"It's harder for me to learn languages than some other subjects."

- "I always feel awkward at parties"—"Tonight I'll try smiling at someone I don't know and maybe even start a conversation."

- "I'm never going to figure out photo editing"—"If I keep at it, I'll get the hang of it."

- "Things never work out for me; I'm such a loser"—"Things didn't work out this time. Next time I'll…"

Affirm Yourself

- I am confident and capable.

- I can handle this situation.

- I am a valuable and special person.

- Write several affirmations for yourself. Repeat them when you brush your teeth, shower, get dressed, gel your hair, walk to class, ride an elevator, or wait for your computer to boot up. The more time you devote to your affirmations, the more dramatic a difference you'll feel.

- Continue repeating affirmations at least five times first thing in the morning and last thing at night.

- Be creative and send affirmations to yourself in e-mails, reminders, and text messages. Celebrate the best in you.

Do You Know Where to Turn for Help?

Check out the counseling services at your school. Is there a peer-counseling program? Can you set up an appointment with a mental health professional through the health center? Call a local helpline or a national support center such as the National Alliance on Mental Health hotline.

There are also numerous online sites, including support groups and chat rooms through hubs such as PsychCentral.com, CrisisChat.org, and WebMD.com. Is there a support group at your school?

Schedule Your Stress

Just as you schedule classes and appointments, try scheduling your stress:

- Designate 15–30 minutes of your day just for stressing. You have to be present and engaged during this time. Push yourself to process all your stresses, worries, and fears. When your appointed time is over, tell yourself that you're done with your stressful thinking for the day.

- If stressful thoughts come into your mind (which is natural and normal), remind yourself, "I'll think about this during my scheduled stress time." Acknowledge the stress, but remember that you will think about it in depth soon, and refocus your attention.

- Practice breathing exercises (See Chapter 12) and with each exhalation, use your breath to release your stress and push the thoughts away. Until the appointed time, refocus your attention to the present and continue on with your day.

If You Ever Start Thinking about Taking Your Life:

- Talk to a mental health professional. If you have a therapist, call immediately. If not, call a suicide hotline. The national suicide hot line number is 1 (800) 273-TALK (8255).

- Find someone you can trust and talk honestly about what you're feeling.

- If you suffer from depression or another mental disorder, educate friends or relatives about your condition so they are prepared if called upon to help.

- Write down some uplifting thoughts, or spend time looking at loved ones (pet included) on your phone or tablet. Even if you are despondent, you can help yourself by focusing on positive thoughts or memories.

- Avoid drugs and alcohol. Most suicides are the result of sudden, uncontrolled impulses, and drugs and alcohol can make it harder to resist these destructive urges.

- Go to the hospital. Hospitalization can sometimes be the best way to protect your health and safety.

Engage Your Mind

- Make a purposeful decision to interpret an obstacle or difficulty in your life as a challenge and as a teacher. Consciously decide that nothing will crush you. Stay in charge of your thoughts despite any adversity you might encounter.

- Take a position of no surrender. This is not a position of stubborn stupidity or inflexibility, but of resourcefulness and determination that you will accept no other outcome. If one path does not work, discard it and find another.

- Develop the stress-resistant attitude that rough experiences are the source of valuable lessons.

- Purposely cultivate an internal perspective on stress that is oriented to learning and coping rather than feeling victimized and blaming circumstances or others.

- If you are momentarily thrown off by setbacks, obstacles, or adversity, talk and coach yourself back to this perspective. Resolve to learn from your setback, make the necessary adjustments, and continue, knowing you are the stronger for it.

REFLECTION: Are You Internal or External?

Answer the following questions by checking "a" or "b".

1. a. _____ Many of the unhappy things in people's lives are partly due to bad luck.
   b. _____ People's misfortunes result from the mistakes they make.

2. a. _____ One of the major reasons why we have wars is because people don't take enough interest in politics.
   b. _____ There will always be wars, no matter how hard people try to prevent them.

3. a. _____ In the long run, people get the respect they deserve in this world.
   b. _____ Unfortunately, an individual's worth often passes unrecognized no matter how hard he tries.

4. a. _____ The idea that teachers are unfair to students is nonsense.
   b. _____ Most students don't realize the extent to which their grades are influenced by accidental happenings.

5. a. _____ Without the right breaks, one cannot be an effective leader.
   b. _____ Capable people who fail to become leaders have not taken advantage of their opportunities.

6. a. _____ No matter how hard you try, some people just don't like you.
   b. _____ People who can't get others to like them don't understand how to get along with others.

7. a. _____ I have often found that what is going to happen will happen.
   b. _____ Trusting to fate has never turned out as well for me as making a decision to take a definite course of action.

8. a. _____ In the case of the well-prepared student, there is rarely, if ever, such a thing as an unfair test.
   b. _____ Many times exam questions tend to be so unrelated to coursework that studying is really useless.

9. a. _____ Becoming a success is a matter of hard work; luck has little or nothing to do with it.
   b. _____ Getting a good job depends mainly on being in the right place at the right time.

10. a. _____ The average citizen can have an influence in government decisions.
    b. _____ This world is run by the few people in power, and there is not much the little guy can do about it.

11. a. _____ When I make plans, I am almost certain that I can make them work.
    b. _____ It is not always wise to plan too far ahead because many things turn out to be a matter of luck anyway.

12. a. _____ In my case, getting what I want has little or nothing to do with luck.
    b. _____ Many times we might just as well decide what to do by flipping a coin.

13. a. _____ What happens to me is my own doing.
    b. _____ Sometimes I feel that I don't have enough control over the direction my life is taking.

Based on J.B. Rotter (1966). "Generalized Expectancies for Internal versus External Control of Reinforcement." *Psychological Monographs 80:* (1, Whole No. 609).

Give yourself one point for every "a" answer you gave to questions 1–4 and 8–13 and for every "b" answer you gave to questions 5–7. A high score indicates an internal locus of control; a low score, an external locus of control. If you score as an "external," don't accept your current score as a given for life. If you want to shift your perspective, you can. Stretch beyond your comfort zone, and practice taking more of an active role in situations where you once were passive or submissive.

TECHNIQUE: Mindfulness Meditation

In this exercise, you tune in to each part of your body, scanning from head to toe, noting the slightest sensation, and allowing whatever you experience—an itch, an ache, a feeling of warmth—to enter your awareness. Then you open yourself to focus on all the thoughts, sensations, sounds, and feelings that enter your awareness without getting caught up in them.

Listen to the Mindfulness Meditation audio instructions in MindTap, or pair up with a classmate and take turns leading each other through this exercise.

- Sit comfortably, with your eyes closed and your spine reasonably straight.

- Bring your attention to your breathing. Take a deep breath in through your nostrils. Hold the breath inside. Then slowly exhale through your mouth.

- Imagine that you have a balloon in your stomach. Every time you breathe in, the balloon inflates. Each time you breathe out, the balloon deflates.

- Notice the sensations in your abdomen as your inner balloon inflates and then deflates. Be mindful of your abdomen rising as you inhale, the fullness within you as you hold the breath, and the experience of release as you exhale.

- Thoughts will come into your mind, and that's okay, because that's what the human mind does. Simply notice these thoughts and bring your attention back to your breathing.

- You may notice sounds, physical feelings, emotions. Again, just bring your attention back to your breathing.

- Be mindful of the rhythm you create as you inhale deeply through your nose and slowly exhale through your mouth.

- You don't have to follow thoughts or feelings that pop into your mind; don't judge yourself for having them, or analyze them in any way. It's okay for the thoughts to be there. Just notice these thoughts, and let them drift on by.

- Keep bringing your attention back to your breathing.

- Whenever you notice that your attention has drifted off and is becoming caught up in thoughts or feelings, simply note that the attention has drifted, and then gently bring the attention back to your breathing.

- Continue to fill your inner balloon with air; be aware of the oxygen filling your body, and be mindful of the slow release of your breath.

- By concentrating on your breathing, you can stay "present" in the moment rather than being distracted by regrets from the past or worries about the future.

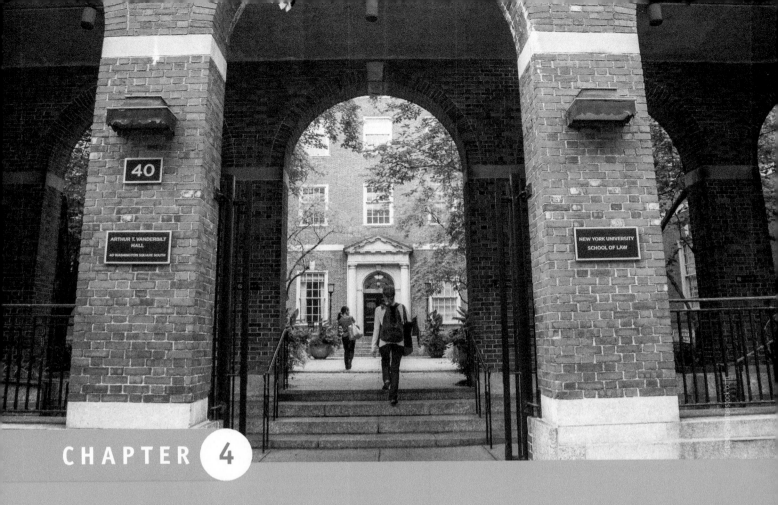

CHAPTER 4

Stress on Campus

After reading this chapter, you should be able to:

4.1 Discuss the effects of college stressors on the dimensions of health and on students of different genders, ages, races, and ethnicities.

4.2 Describe how study techniques and test-taking strategies can reduce academic stress.

4.3 Identify other common stressors on college campuses.

4.4 Develop effective strategies to reduce and cope with campus stress.

The Student Stress Scale, an adaptation of Holmes and Rahe's Life Events Scale for college-age adults, provides a rough indication of stress levels and possible health consequences. Each event, such as beginning or ending school, is given a score that represents the amount of readjustment a person has to make as a result of the change. In some studies, using similar scales, people with high scores were more likely to develop serious illnesses.

To determine your stress score, add up the number of points corresponding to the events you have experienced in the past 12 months.

Death of a close family member	100
Death of a close friend	73
Divorce of parents	65
Jail term	63
Major personal injury or illness	63
Marriage	58
Getting fired from a job	50
Failing an important course	47
Change in the health of a family member	45
Pregnancy	45
Sex problems	44
Serious argument with a close friend	40
Change in financial status	39
Change of academic major	39
Trouble with parents	39
New girlfriend or boyfriend	37
Increase in workload at school	37
Outstanding personal achievement	36
First quarter/semester in college	36
Change in living conditions	31
Serious argument with an instructor	30
Getting lower grades than expected	29
Change in sleeping habits	29
Change in social activities	29
Change in eating habits	28
Chronic car trouble	26
Change in number of family get-togethers	26
Too many missed classes	25
Changing colleges	24
Dropping more than one class	23
Minor traffic violations	20

Total Stress Score _____

If your score is 300 or higher, you're at high risk for developing a health problem. If your score is between 150 and 300, you have a 50-50 chance of experiencing a serious health change within two years. If your score is below 150, you have a one-in-three chance of a serious health change.

If your score on the Student Stress Scale is high, think about the reasons your life may be in turmoil. Of course, some stress-inducing events, such as a robbery or a beloved grandparent's death, are beyond your control. Even so, you can respond to such stressors with coping techniques that will protect your long-term well-being.

Source: Mullen, Kathleen, and Gerald Costello. *Health Awareness Through Discovery*. Minneapolis: Burgess Publishing Company, 1981.

Jared, 29, who served two tours of duty in Afghanistan, says adjusting to civilian life is his number-one stressor; for Yuko, 19, who had never gotten a grade lower than a B until her stats course, it's academics; for Varun, a 21-year-old transfer student, it's the transition from a junior college to a big university. Child care ranks at the top of a long list of stressors for Krista, 31, a single mother of two; Xian, 23, struggles with English as his second language; Shanya, 26, finds it hard to fit her online course work in between shifts at the call center where she works; Sam, 20, living on 99-cent burritos and Ramen noodles that he eats straight from the Styrofoam cup, is stressed about yet another tuition hike.

You may be enrolled in a two-year college, a four-year university, or a technical school; your classrooms may be in a bustling city or a sleepy small town—or exist solely online; you may be pursuing a career in business or graphic arts, music or medicine, kinesiology, or computer science. But there is at least one thing you have in common with these undergraduates: stress.

Campus stress is unique because college is a unique microcosm. Regardless of how old you are, whether you're at a small private school, a community college, or a huge state university, whatever your ethnic background or economic status, a campus can seem a foreign universe. Surrounded by strangers, eating unfamiliar foods in unfamiliar places, you may still be figuring out how to cut across campus to get to class in time or how to fit in with dorm dwellers, townies, Greeks, geeks, jocks, and party animals.

No one—parent, teacher, or advisor—is micromanaging your life. College may have brought greater freedom than you have ever known. It's up to you to find positive ways to meet academic and social goals and to deal with emotional reactions to both success and disappointment. You may have—or may have seen others—respond by experimenting with new behaviors, including some, such as drug and alcohol use (discussed in Chapter 8), with potential consequences that create more stress. Keep in mind that the choices you make—to spend hours on fantasy football or following celebrity tweets, for example, rather than finishing an assignment—have consequences that can make your life more or less stressful.

College represents a new chapter in your life. Most people in your classes never met you before. They don't know or care whether you were always the shortest kid your age or the winner of the junior high science fair, whether you spent two years serving in the military or every summer at computer camp. They see you as you are today, and they judge you by what you do here and now. Your college experience, the dividing line between what was and what will be, provides the perfect opportunity to grow, experiment, question, learn, connect—and practice and build your stress management skills.

Students under Stress

The number of students attending American colleges and universities has increased to some 20.2 million, the largest and most diverse national collegiate student body ever.[1] Today's undergraduates include more women, more nontraditional-age men and women, and more minorities (see Figure 4.1).

They are also the first generation of "digital natives," who have grown up in a wired world, both more connected and more isolated than their predecessors, with a "tribe" of friends, family, and acquaintances. More of them are working and working longer hours, taking fewer credits, requiring more time to graduate, and leaving college with larger student loan debts.

Students also are more stressed than previous generations. In the American College Health Association (ACHA) annual survey, stress outranks

Here is a statistical profile of the 20.2 million students attending American colleges and universities:

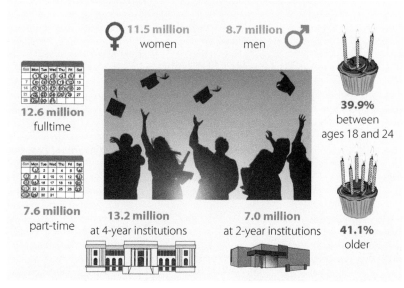

FIGURE 4.1 Today's undergraduates make up the largest and most diverse student body in history.

Source: National Center for Education Statistics. http://nces.ed.gov/programs/digest

illness, sleep problems, and relationship difficulties as the number-one barrier to academic performance.[2] About 9 in 10 students rate the overall level of stress they experienced in the previous 12 months as "average," "more than average," or "tremendous." (See Table 4.1) More than eight in ten—76 percent of men and 90 percent of women—report feeling overwhelmed by all they had to do at some point in the past 12 months.[3]

Undergraduates respond to stress in ways that affect every dimension of their health:[4]

- Physiologically—by sweating, stuttering, trembling, consuming more junk food and losing sleep, exercising less, or developing physical symptoms ranging from headaches or digestive problems to itching, rashes, or hair loss[5]. Perceived stress also undermines students' immunity, increasing their susceptibility to infectious illnesses.[6]

- Emotionally—by becoming anxious, fearful, angry, guilty, or depressed and feeling less satisfaction with life.

- Behaviorally—by crying, eating, smoking, being irritable or abusive, or engaging in behaviors that can harm their health, including smoking, excessive drinking, and substance abuse.

- Cognitively—by finding it difficult to pay attention and concentrate, ruminating about stressful situations, falling into the "thinking traps" described in Chapter 3.

TABLE 4.1 Stressed-Out Students

Stress levels reported by students within the past 12 months	Percent (%)		
	Male	**Female**	**Average**
No stress	4.0	0.9	2.0
Less than average	12.8	4.9	7.5
Average	37.7	35.3	35.9
More than average	36.8	46.3	43.1
Tremendous	8.7	12.6	11.4

How would you rate your stress? Average? Less than average? More than average? Tremendous?

Source: American College Health Association. American College Health Association-National College Health Assessment II: Reference Group Executive Summary Fall 2015. Hanover, MD: American College Health Association; 2016.

✔ **Check-in:** Are you feeling the impact of college stress?

Take the Self-Survey in the Personal Stress Management Toolkit on page 78 at the end of this chapter.

Like other forms of stress, campus stress is always personal, varying with gender, age, ethnicity, economics, background, social support, and psychological make-up.[7] Freshmen and first-generation students rate their stress significantly higher than seniors. Athletes and students taking more than 18 credit hours or working more than four hours a week also report greater stress. Those who pray daily say they experience less stress than those who never pray.[8] Other factors also influence student stress levels, including the following.

Gender Differences

In college surveys, women consistently rate their perceived stress higher than men.[9] If you're a woman, you're more likely than your male classmates to feel stressed about finances, social relationships, and daily hassles. In the national ACHA survey, more female than male students reported feeling hopeless, overwhelmed, or exhausted (but not from physical activity). Women also felt more stressed than men about having too many things to do at once, being separated from people they care about, financial burdens, and important decisions about their education.[10]

Differences in lifestyle may explain some of this gender gap. College men spend significantly more time doing things that are enjoyable and relaxing: exercising, watching TV, and playing video games. Women, on the other hand, typically study more, volunteer more, and handle more household and child-care chores.

There are also gender differences in coping with stress. Female students engage in more emotionally expressive coping behaviors by seeking social support—talking with family members and close friends, for instance, or using social media. Men handle stress through more solitary activities, such as exercise[11] and (less adaptively) drinking. They are also more prone to avoid dealing with a problem directly and to take impulsive measures.[12]

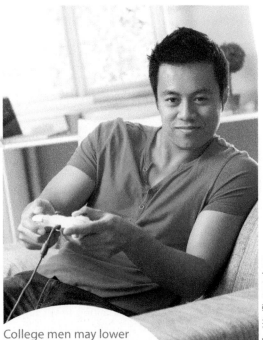

College men may lower their stress levels by playing video games or other enjoyable activities.

StockLite/Shutterstock.com

Students under Age 25

If you are entering college in your late teens or early twenties, you have to deal with the stresses traditional-age students have always faced: being on your own for the first time, feeling pressure to drink, party, or use drugs, balancing academic and leisure pursuits. You also may feel stressed about getting along with a difficult roommate, missing old friends, or living up to your parents' and teachers' expectations. As you adjust to campus life, you may experience the ongoing stress of forging a new identity and finding a place for yourself in various social hierarchies.

Those of you between the ages of 18 and 25 are in the life stage termed "emerging adulthood." During this potentially challenging transition period, young men and women are more likely to engage in behaviors that can increase stress and imperil health, such as eating more junk food, smoking, not exercising, and putting on weight. Most "emerging adults" do not get regular physical or dental exams and do not seek health care when they need it. Drug abuse, unprotected sex, and sexually transmitted infections (STIs) are common.

Although you may feel fully capable of making mature decisions and coping with stress as well as older adults, the scientifically documented fact is that your brain remains a work in progress. Its development continues throughout the first quarter-century of life, and this affects cognitive and problem-solving skills.

In dealing with daily stressors, for instance, a teenaged or twentysomething brain relies more on the amygdala, the small almond-shaped region in the medial and temporal lobes that processes emotions and memories and, as you learned in Chapter 3, alerts the brain and body to a potential threat. This is one reason why any stressor—a lost sweater or a snarky tweet, for instance—can feel as intensely upsetting as a major crisis. As individuals age, the frontal cortex, which governs reason and forethought, plays a greater role and helps put challenges into perspective.

A young or "maturing" brain does not necessarily lead to poor judgments and risky behaviors. However, if you are under 25, be aware that your brain may not always grasp the long-term consequences of your actions, set realistic priorities, or restrain potentially harmful impulses. You can learn to center yourself with the breathing and relaxation techniques described in Chapter 12 and by seeking the counsel of others. Be cautious of drugs and alcohol, which are especially toxic to the developing brain and can lead to risky behaviors that add to the stress in your life.

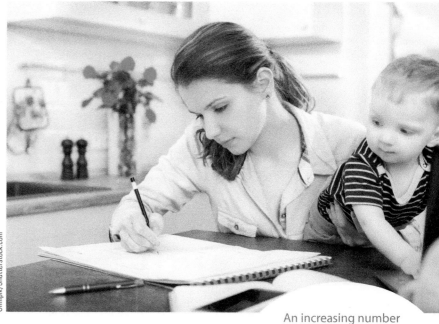

An increasing number of undergraduates are juggling the multiple demands of being parents as well as students.

Nontraditional-Age Students

The number of older undergraduates is skyrocketing. Many of these students, often parents with full- or part-time jobs, are entering or returning to higher education with a different set of adult life experiences than younger classmates.[13] Most have no interest in getting wasted, hooking up, or partying—and not just because they don't have the time, money, or energy for such pursuits.

Older students often find themselves playing multiple roles—as students, workers, parents, caretakers—and facing multiple stressors, including pressure to perform well to qualify for a better job or graduate school. Veterans may still be adjusting to civilian life after service in distant and dangerous lands and may feel disconnected from campus life.[14] Time management and finances are huge sources of stress, and many worry about the costs of housing and child care and fear incurring additional debt.[15]

Yet despite the fact that they deal with more stressors, older students generally report less school-related stress compared to traditional students—perhaps a payoff of lessons acquired with age and experience[16] as well as greater emotional intelligence, the ability to understand, express, and regulate feelings, discussed in detail in Chapter 8.[17]

In research on women returning to school, family emerges as the greatest source of both stress and support. On the one hand, women feel stressed about not earning more money, missing special occasions like their children's softball games or school plays, and keeping up with endless household chores. On the other hand, they

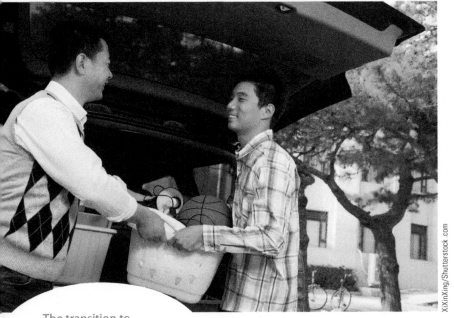

The transition to college brings many changes and challenges for entering freshmen.

believe that their short-term sacrifices will pay off in greater long-term security for their families. Single mothers face the most acute stressors, such as not being able to complete an assignment on time because they have to care for a sick child.

Entering Freshmen and First-Generation College Students

The first year of college is the most stressful for undergraduates. Many report loneliness, homesickness, conflict, relationship problems, and symptoms of depression. Interventions, such as orientation programs that promote psychological wellness and teach stress management skills, have proven effective in helping freshman through this transition.[18]

First-generation college students—those whose parents never enrolled in college for at least one full year—encounter more difficulties with social adjustment than freshmen whose parents attended college. They are less likely to share details of campus life and course work with their families, who may not be able to relate to and understand college stressors. This lack of social support itself adds to students' stress levels because they have no experience, even vicarious, to draw from as they negotiate the transition to university life.

First-generation students often see themselves in the challenging position of being trailblazers and role models in addition to handling the usual academic and personal demands. Expectations are often greater and more stressful for those who are the first in their families to attend college. At some schools, first-generation students

have united in groups such as Harvard's First Generation Student Union and Princeton's Hidden Minority Council, to provide support, information, and peer mentoring.[19] Are such programs available at your school?

Students whose parents and perhaps grandparents attended college may have several advantages, including a clearer picture of what they are embarking on, more knowledge of college life, greater social support, more preparation for college in high school, a greater focus on college activities, and more financial resources. However, some report increased stress because of the high expectations of their college-educated parents.[20]

The expectations that freshmen bring with them to college also can add to their stress.[21] In one study, students who categorized their expectations as "fearful" reported more stress, depression, and poorer university adjustment than did individuals with "optimistic," "prepared," or "complacent" expectations.[22]

 Stress Reliever: Change One Thought

Under the right circumstances, changing one simple thought can make a big difference. If you find yourself thinking "I'm lonely," for example, change that thought to "I am loved by someone."[23] The emotional impact can be dramatic.

Minority Students

Americans of all backgrounds often see a college education as the key to opportunity, and campuses reflect our society's rich mix of races, cultures, and creeds. Regardless of your race or ethnic background, college may bring culture shock. You may never have encountered so much diversity in one setting. You meet students with different values, unfamiliar customs, entirely new ways of looking at the world—experiences you may find both stimulating and stressful.

Undergraduates who feel different from most of their peers in any way may feel isolated and anxious. Some may have ambivalent, even conflicting feelings about whatever makes them different—proud to be Korean, for instance, but embarrassed that their parents don't read and write English, or excited to come out but nervous about homophobia or rejection on campus and at home.

Minority stress refers to the unique stresses experienced by students in any racial, ethnic, or gender minority that interfere with their adjustment and integration into the university

minority stress The unique pressures experienced by students in any racial, ethnic, or gender minority that interfere with their adjustment and integration into the university community.

community. Often they see few students like themselves in their classrooms and have few, if any, instructors, mentors, or role models from their own group. Some feel invisible; others face subtle and not-so-subtle discrimination or stereotypes about their academic expectations and ability. Feeling isolated and perceived as academically inferior increases the likelihood that minority students will drop out of college without obtaining a degree.[24]

······································

✔ **Check-in:** How do you identify racially? Ethnically?

······································

Has your racial or ethnic background affected your personal stress level?

······································

In an ideal world, prejudice would not exist. In a diverse world, it undeniably does—often stemming from ignorance and fear. The belief that any person is inferior or superior feeds prejudice, and prejudice breeds stress. Perceived discrimination and racism have been identified as key factors in chronic stress-related health disparities, such as increased hypertension,[25] diabetes,[26] cardiovascular disease,[27] adverse birth outcomes,[28] and mental disorders among minority groups, including African Americans, Filipinos, Latino Americans,[29] and Native Hawaiians.[30] Factors such as economics, education, geography, neighborhood, environment, lower-quality health care, and inability to navigate the health system also contribute to stress—and stress intensifies their negative impact on health.

Acculturative Stress

Minority students face "minority status stress," above and beyond general stress, in part because of the demands of **acculturation**, a complex psychosocial process in which an ethnic minority changes, both as individuals and as a group, as a consequence of contact with the ethnic majority. Predominantly white campuses can seem hostile, alienating, and socially isolating, and nonwhite students often report estrangement from the campus community, including faculty and peers.

In studies of minority freshmen, Asian, Filipino, African American, and Native American students all felt more sensitive and vulnerable to the college social climate, to interpersonal tensions between themselves and non-minority students and faculty, to experiences of actual or perceived racism, and to discrimination.

The stress of adapting to the orientation and values of the dominant culture can have an influence on many physical and mental health conditions, including hypertension, depression, substance dependence, and anxiety disorders.[31] Perceived

social support may make a difference in easing acculturative stress for international students.[32]

Male African-American students who have experienced higher levels of lifetime discrimination report more negative moods and more alcohol use—alone rather than in social settings.[33] Race-related stress also may affect minority students' choices of majors and careers. Because of the many perceived racial barriers to success, African-American students who overcome these barriers to enter college may seek out a career in a field with excellent job prospects, such as engineering.[34]

······································

✔ **Check-in:** Have you experienced acculturative stress?

······································

Have you felt conflicted over beliefs or practices that you grew up with and differing ones you have recently faced?

······································

How would you describe it to your classmates?

······································

Stereotypes and Stress

Different minority students confront specific stereotypes—for instance, that Asian Americans are quiet and passive or that Latinos entered the country illegally. Black male college students, particularly at mainly white universities, report a sense that other students or the college administrators want them to fail.[35] Many say that they are watched with hypervigilance by police on and off campus and treated as if they are "out of place" and "fitting the description" of intruders into a campus community. Black men may experience psychological stress responses symptomatic of what some refer to as "racial battle fatigue": frustration, shock, anger, disappointment, resentment, anxiety, helplessness, hopelessness, and fear.[36]

Students from racial minorities, despite scoring above the national average on the SAT, have reported not feeling accepted as legitimate undergraduates and sensing that others viewed them as unworthy beneficiaries of affirmative action initiatives. Students who have recently immigrated to the United States report feeling ostracized by students of similar ancestry who are second- or third-generation Americans.

In the last decade, there have been reports of more acts of hate on college campuses, such as vandalism of minority students' meeting places or painting of swastikas or racist words on walls. To counteract this trend, many schools have set up programs and classes to educate students about each other's backgrounds and to make campuses less alienating and more culturally and emotionally accessible to all.

Racism and prejudice can be hard to deal with individually. By banding together, however, those

acculturation
A complex psychosocial process in which an ethnic minority changes, both as individuals and as a group, as a consequence of contact with the ethnic majority.

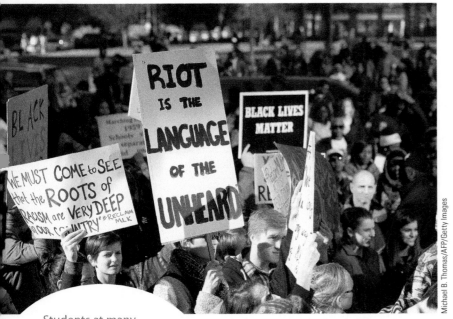

The perpetrators of microaggressions may be unaware of the hidden messages that they transmit and that, even when inadvertent, foster negative stereotypes. In classic experiments, African Americans and women performed worse on academic tests when primed with stereotypes about race or gender. Women told that many females have poor math aptitude, for instance, typically do worse on math tests than those given positive encouragement. African Americans' intelligence test scores may plunge when they're primed with messages of inferior intelligence.

✔ **Check-in:** Microaggression on campus

If you are an ethnic, racial, gender or sexual minority, have you experienced any form of microaggression? Write or share with your classmates a brief reflection about its impact.

If you are Caucasian, do you think you have ever—consciously or not—acted in ways that were demeaning to minorities? Have you become more aware of the impact of such behavior?

Students at many campuses have banded together to challenge discrimination and bigotry.

who experience discrimination can take action to protect themselves, challenge the ignorance and hateful assumptions that fuel bigotry, and promote a healthier environment for all.

Microaggressions

While many minority students say that overt prejudice is rare and relatively easy to deal with, everyday insults, indignities and demeaning messages, called **microaggressions**, can undermine their academic confidence and their ability to bond with the university. They can take several forms:

microaggressions
Subtle pressures that may undermine minority students' academic confidence and their ability to bond with the university.

microassaults
Conscious and intentional actions or slurs, such as using racial or sexual epithets or showing preferential treatment to non-minority customers at shops and restaurants.

microinsults Verbal and nonverbal communications that subtly convey rudeness and insensitivity and demean a person's racial heritage or identity.

microinvalidations
Communications that subtly exclude, negate, or nullify the thoughts, feelings or experiential reality of an individual.

- **Microassaults**: conscious and intentional actions or slurs, such as using racial or sexual epithets or showing preferential treatment to non-minority customers at shops and restaurants.

- **Microinsults**: verbal and nonverbal communications that subtly convey rudeness and insensitivity and demean a person's racial heritage or identity, for example, comments that a Hispanic student speaks English without an accent or that an individual doesn't look or dress "gay."

- **Microinvalidations**: communications that subtly exclude, negate, or nullify the thoughts, feelings, or experiential reality of an individual. For instance, white people may ask Asian Americans where they were born, conveying the message that they are perpetual foreigners in their own land, or may ask someone of mixed-race background "what" he or she is.[37]

Academic Stress

How long have you been going to school? Twelve years? Fourteen years? Longer?

How many subjects have you studied? How many classes have you attended? Hundreds, for sure.

How many books have you read? How many papers have you written? How many tests have you taken? We're talking thousands.

After so much experience, you've figured out how to "do" school. You wouldn't be enrolled in this college, taking this course, or reading this text if you hadn't proven—time and time again—that you are qualified and capable. So why do students rate academics as their greatest stressor?

The reasons vary. You may have sailed through high school without breaking a sweat but are now finding college courses much more challenging. You may have a learning disability, get tongue-tied every time you're called on in class, or freeze during exams. Maybe you're a whiz at coding but struggle to compose a coherent three-paragraph essay. You may have children or a job and find it hard to put in the hours needed to keep up with assignments.

Perhaps you love everything about psychology but drift off reading 18th-century poetry or listening to lectures on macroeconomics. English may be your second (or third) language. Or you may be feeling the stress of working part-time, looking for a summer job, doing well at an internship, or preparing to apply for jobs after college.

Inside Academic Stress

It's normal for students to feel both eustress and distress. Positive stress motivates you to persevere, work harder, stretch your limits, and achieve at your highest level. Negative stress sabotages your efforts with self-doubt, criticism, and anxiety.

Academic stressors such as the following can produce chronic distress and its harmful health effects[38]:

- An **acute academic stressor** is a short-term, immediate obstacle or threat to a goal, such as a group assignment with a tight deadline.

- An **anticipatory academic stressor** is a long-term event that has the potential to influence a major goal in the future, such as finishing a portfolio of art for an end-of-semester critique or preparing for a graduate school admissions test.

- **Test anxiety** is a negative emotional state that can cause physiological and cognitive changes before, during, and after an exam.

Some students respond to academic stressors so intensely that their blood pressure spikes, increasing their risk of hypertension and cardiovascular disease later in life.[39] If you experience high levels of academic anxiety, remember that anything the mind can learn, it can also unlearn and replace. You can get rid of toxic thoughts and self-sabotaging behaviors and replace them with new ones, particularly feelings of hope and optimism (discussed in Chapter 8) that boost your confidence and reduce worries.[40]

The key is getting at the basis of academic stress, which—as with any stress—is fear. You feel stressed because you perceive that you are not up for the challenge and so you are afraid of a negative outcome, whether it's failing or just not getting an excellent grade. The antidote to fear is knowledge. But locus of control and self-efficacy are also crucial. Students who score high in academic self-efficacy have an internal orientation and believe the intelligence is not a given, but determined by effort. Believing that they have the ability to improve their grades, they monitor and self-regulate their impulses, work hard, and persist in the face of difficulties.[41]

Students with a sense of **academic entitlement**, the belief that they are owed more in an academic environment than is merited by their effort, blame external factors, such as unfair tests or inadequate teaching, for their academic anxiety. Colleges have found that programs that emphasize personal responsibility for academic performance and teach effective time and study skills can boost students' academic self-efficacy—and their performance.[42]

Did you rank as an "external" in the self-survey in Chapter 3? If so, stop and take stock. If you continue to view external forces as determining how well you do in school, you give away your power and experience a sense of helplessness that can create disabling anxiety. But if you cultivate the skills described in the following sections, you can boost your academic self-efficacy and take charge of how well you perform in college.

Your Study Style

The first step to overcoming academic stress is knowing and mastering a subject. Even then, you need to control the way you think about and talk to yourself about learning. Rather than worrying, shift your attention to studying and the pleasure of acquiring new information and insight. Rather than reminding yourself of classes that derailed you in the past, train yourself to ace courses in the future. Approach your education with curiosity and optimism. Remember that you have the ability to do well in school. You just need to use all of your resources—especially your thoughts and your behaviors. Start by analyzing the way you approach your studies.

Because of our different temperaments, talents, and experiences, we all develop a certain orientation or characteristic approach to study and work. Some of us tend to love rolling up our sleeves and digging deeply into a challenge. Others have a tendency to move away from situations that require intensive work.

....
✔ **Check-in:** What is your work/study orientation?
....
Are you self-directed? Do you get going without someone else's prodding?
....
Do you take initiative, or are you passive? When do you take initiative and when do you not?
....
Are you realistic about what will be required to accomplish tasks?
....

acute academic stressor A short-term, immediate threat to a goal, such as a zoology test or a presentation in an urban studies class.

anticipatory academic stressor A long-term event that has the potential to influence a major goal in the future.

test anxiety A negative emotional state that can cause physiological and cognitive changes before, during, and after an exam.

academic entitlement Students' belief that they are owed more—more attention from instructors, easier assignments, higher grades on papers and tests, etc.— in an academic environment than is merited by their effort.

Do you sidestep the fundamentals by getting lost in busy work?

Do you skip steps you consider unpleasant?

Keep your view of your study style in mind as you read the following sections.

Your Essential Study Skills

Perhaps you've studied a martial art. Or maybe you've learned to play a musical instrument or dance ballet. Whenever you've applied yourself to such pursuits, you had to rely on a set of skills that will also serve you well academically. Any "discipline" requires just that: self-control, commitment, and the willingness to put in whatever it takes to achieve mastery and excellence. Here are some of the most critical skills to apply to your studies:

Focus

All of us—not just students diagnosed with an attention disorder—have problems paying attention. This is no accident. The capacity to be distracted may have saved our species. If our prehistoric ancestors, as they gathered berries or tended a fire, weren't distracted by nearby twigs snapping under the weight of a predator's footsteps, we wouldn't be here today.

Undergraduates rank social distractions as the greatest barrier to effective study.[43] That's not surprising. Every day you can find ingenious and mundane ways to pass—and waste—time. Activities like computer games or binge-watching entire seasons of a favorite series can seem like the perfect antidote to stress—but lead to more stress in the long run due to missed study time. This alone is one reason to cultivate your ability to focus your attention.

You already know how to focus attention on things that are exciting or enticing. Your mind doesn't wander when you're gaming with your friends or, for that matter, when you're kissing. If your attention lapses when you're memorizing chemistry formulas, however, you may blame boredom. Actually it's the other way around. Boredom is often a sign that you have withdrawn your attention. This can be dangerous—particularly if you're behind the wheel and suddenly realize you've driven for miles without noticing your surroundings.

The mind craves use in the same way that muscles crave activity. When you are not paying attention, you are not utilizing your highest brain functions, not developing your highest capacities, not cashing in on the benefit of your evolutionary heritage—and not handling stress as well as

you might. The more that you learn to focus and stay on task, the more efficient you become at everything from homework to housework. You don't want to spend your time at the library reading and rereading the same page from *Intro to Biology* for twenty minutes. If you finish your work in an intensive, streamlined fashion, you will have more guilt-free time for hanging out with friends or going to a Zumba class.

Persistence

Persistence means continuing to work and to keep moving forward, even when stressed. A lack of persistence leads to the failure of many worthwhile ventures that, if only given more time, would eventually have borne fruit.

You do not go from photography student to Pulitzer Prize winner in a year. You do not go from sketching a skirt to launching your own clothing line in eighteen months. You need to persist long enough to give new and creative ideas sufficient time to take root. With persistence, you can overcome obstacles, accomplish great things, improve your problem-solving ability, meet your goals, and boost your self-esteem.

You would not be reading this if not for your proven persistence. How many times did you stumble over words before you could pronounce and understand them? Before that, how many times did you fall on your bottom before you could toddle across a room? Hundreds. It was no big deal. You just kept falling and failing until you got the hang of upright locomotion.

Problems with persistence crop up later in life, after your ego gets attached to not making mistakes or not wanting to humiliate yourself by failing yet again. The more skills you accumulate and the more you become accustomed to success, the more allergic you can become to feeling inadequate or unskilled—sensations that provoke stress.

Because stress can feel scary, you need persistence to pull you through what ski instructors call "the valley of doom." Novice skiers often observe that after taking a lesson devoted to learning a new technique, they actually ski worse for a while. The reason is that they are leaving behind the familiar groove of automatic habits and having to "think."

Stress produces the same effect. If you don't recognize this, you may abandon an assignment or project because your initial efforts seem to be setting you back rather than moving you forward. But if you do not persist, you will remain stuck where you are. If you do not continue to work towards your goals, you can even experience greater stress. This is why persistence is so essential.

persistence Continuing to work and to keep moving forward, even when stressed.

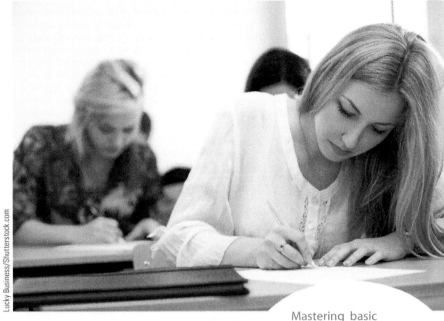

Lucky Business/Shutterstock.com

Mastering basic study and test-taking skills can reduce stress during examinations.

Consistency

While all-nighters are one approach to deadlines and exams, every scientific study of learning has demonstrated that regular, consistent, spaced intervals of practice produce the greatest gains. Inconsistent effort usually yields haphazard results. At times you may need a big burst of effort—or more than one—to push through and complete a project. But individuals who consistently achieve usually develop a methodical set of routines that enable them to make and keep making a consistent effort over time.

The words "kung fu" translate into "consistent practice over time." A tennis serve or a brush stroke in painting can be kung fu because they are the products of repeated practice. Even the most creative artists and writers—and certainly dancers and athletes—know that they have to put in regular effort to stay at the top of what they do. To learn new skills, to face and manage stress, requires the same. It is as simple as that. If you want to produce quality changes with the least amount of total effort, you must master the skill of consistency.

Repetition

When you learned to direct a soccer ball with a header or successfully make a backward somersault off the high dive, you practiced repetitively even if you did not think of it that way at the time. If you pursued tango or gymnastics, you likewise engaged in intense repetitive practice. If you practiced because you took personal pleasure from getting better, you undoubtedly progressed faster.

Repetition is not a matter of forcing yourself to repeat an action, but of tuning into the process. Much impatience stems from focusing on endpoints and outcomes rather than the steps leading to them. When things are worth doing well, all of the parts are worth doing. You do not go to a concert to hear the encore, but you're probably going to be pretty glad you stayed for it. If you persist at anything, you increase your ability to persist, tolerate frustration and monotony, and continue to work despite setbacks.

Since learning new skills requires repetition, learn to love it. Although it is thrilling to grasp things quickly and do remarkable things effortlessly, skills that demand repetition yield a different kind of pleasure. Do not miss out on it. If you duck language labs or hockey practices, you cheat yourself of opportunities to master repetition and practice. By taking pleasure in these sessions, you will progress more rapidly. Try, and see for yourself.

Developing patience through repetition is the equivalent of physical reps in the weight room. Each delivers the cumulative power of small repeated actions. If you consider small acts trifles that are not worthy of the bother, you will remain unable to do large things. You must get in shape and build emotional endurance. Repetition builds internal muscle, which you can engage whenever you need to learn something new.

Test Stress

✔ **Check-in:** Test yourself

Analyze the last three tests you took. Pay no attention to the grade. Your job is to reconstruct how you prepared and deconstruct how you felt.

How much time did you spend preparing?

How long before the test did you start studying?

How many hours did you put in every day?

How did you study?

Did you eat balanced meals?

Did you exercise?

Did you stay up late to cram? Did you pull an all-nighter?

How did you feel the day of the test? How did you cope with this feeling?

What did you say to yourself before and during the test? Did you attack yourself, criticize yourself, or tell yourself you were stupid or worse? Did you say, "Oh no, here it (meaning text anxiety, a blank mind, or a major panic attack) comes again!"

What did you do when you came to a question that stumped you?

Did you become more or less anxious as time went on?

On a scale of 1 (no sweat) to 10 (heart-thumping terror), how would you rate your test stress on each of your last three tests? If your stress differed on the three, analyze why. Aside from the three most recent tests, what has been your general test stress level in the past? Read through your answers again, and put a + next to the behaviors that had a positive impact on your grade and your stress levels.

Smarter Test Preparation Strategies

The following recommendations will give you a better sense of control over your test preparation, your self-talk, and your mood before and during a test.

- Look ahead to your next scheduled tests. Set aside time on your schedule to start studying today and continue studying daily. Depending on when the exam is scheduled, you can spend as little as 30 minutes. Block out study times every day until the day of the test. Do this for every scheduled test in every class this term.

- Quiz yourself. Students who take brief quizzes at the beginning of every class retain

more material, attend class more regularly, and get better grades than those taking fewer tests. You can try this strategy on your own. At the end of each study session, write down five or six questions about the material. Also go back to a previous unit or test and add a question based on something you didn't fully comprehend or got wrong on an exam.

- The evening before the test, complete your review. Practice your test visualizations, and enjoy a good meal.

- Go to bed at your usual time—or earlier. Getting a good night's sleep before a test gives you double the bang for your buck. You feel more rested and relaxed, and the brain consolidates new information as you sleep so you'll remember more and perform better. As you nod off, remind yourself that your brain will be working all night long.

Smarter Test Taking Strategies

Get up 15 minutes early for a last review. Eat a good breakfast or lunch. Make sure it includes protein for stamina and brain energy. Get to the classroom early so you can choose your seat and settle in. Visualize yourself acing the test. Imagine yourself working through potentially problematic questions with confidence and persistence. Now get started:

- Breathe easily and calmly, and tell yourself, "I have a lot of information that I will be able to express on this exam." When you read through the questions, say, "This is not a big deal. This is what the instructor said would be on the test. I reviewed this last night." If you start to tense up, become your own cheerleader. Tell yourself, "I can do this!"

- As you proceed through the test, direct your unconscious (think of it as "the back of your mind") to work on questions you don't know while you consciously focus on the ones you do. Return to the harder questions after you've gained confidence from answering all the ones that you could answer most easily.

- If this is an essay test and you feel confident, write the essay that you think will take the most time or the one that counts for the most points first. If you are stumped, write the easiest essay first, and come back to the harder ones. Very important: Focus on what you can say about a topic rather than struggling to remember a particular fragment of information. No one fact or date is going to make all the difference. See the test and each question as an opportunity to demonstrate what you do know.

- Once you've completed the exam, allow yourself the sweet pleasure of relief that it's over.
- Learn from your tests. When you get a test back, use it to prepare for the next test. What types of questions were asked? Are a lot of the questions about dates? Are they mainly problems? How many key terms did you have to recognize? Analyze your answers. What did you do right and well? How can you modify your study and test-taking strategies to do even better? Did going to the class review help? What about studying with a classmate? Making up your own study guide? Did studying in the library work better than staying in your room? What study style did you use and was it helpful?

Common Campus Stressors

As shown in Table 4.2, almost half of undergraduates in the United States report having experienced three or more very challenging stressors in the previous year. Academics tops the list, followed by finances and intimate relationships. A review of 40 studies conducted in various countries over more than a decade identified similar

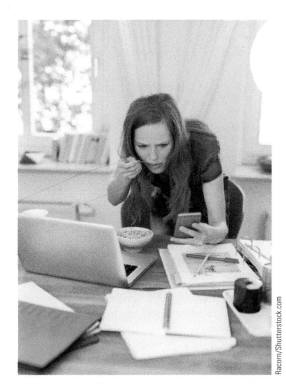

Trying to do several things at once can make busy students feel even more stressed.

Racorn/Shutterstock.com

stressors on campuses around the globe, with academics and relationships consistently near the top of every list.[44]

You may find other issues particularly stressful, such as choosing a major, getting into required

TABLE 4.2 Ten Top Student Stressors

Within the last 12 months, students found the following traumatic or very difficult to handle:	
Stressor	**Percent**
Academics	44.3
Finances	35.9
Intimate relationships	29.7
Sleep difficulties	28.9
Family problems	27.4
Personal appearance	26.8
Other social relationships	25.4
Career-related issue	23.8
Personal health issue	20.9
Health of family/partner	19.6
3 or more	49.0
2	12.2
1	12.7
None	26.0

Source: American College Health Association. American College Health Association-National College Health Assessment II: Reference Group Executive Summary Fall 2015. Hanover, MD: American College Health Association; 2016.

classes, or worry about family or friends. Although there are many stressors you can't avoid, you can take steps to avoid or lessen additional ones.

Problematic Smart Phone and Internet Use

✔ **Check-in:** How wired are you?

How much time do you spend on a computer or mobile device on a typical day? What would you do with that time if you weren't connected?

Walk into any residence hall, cafeteria, or classroom on campus, and you're likely to see the same thing: Students on their smartphones or tablets. College students often consider social networking and other online activities a "guilty pleasure."[45] Most can't imagine a life unconnected to friends, family, and everyone else on the world wide web. As discussed in Chapter 6, virtual relationships and Internet communities can be enjoyable and enriching—but not when they become a form of escapism.[46]

How much tech time is too much? That depends. If online poker, Vine videos, snapchat, and tweets interfere with other responsibilities, it's time to cut back. Another sign of excessive digital dependence: feeling stressed whenever you have to go offline or disconnect from your mobile devices.

On average, students report spending 279 minutes—almost 5 hours—on their cell phones and send 77 text messages a day. Stress increases along with time online.[47] High-frequency cell phone users (those on their phones 10 or more hours a day) report greater stress and anxiety, less satisfaction with life, and lower grades than peers who use their cell phones three hours a day or less.[48]

In the ACHA survey, 10 percent of students—more than the percentage citing relationship difficulties or depression—ranked Internet use/computer games as having a negative impact on their academic performance.[49] Like other addictions, "problematic" Internet use may lead to preoccupation, withdrawal, difficulty with control, disregard for harmful consequences, loss of other interests, desire for escape, hiding the behavior, and harmful effects on relationships or work- or school-related performance. Adverse physical effects include carpal tunnel syndrome, dry eyes, headaches, and altered sleep patterns.

Risky Behaviors

College is a time when students want to experiment, enjoy, stretch, and take some risks. But there is a difference between the risks of underage drinking or illicit drug use and the risks of

snowboarding or forming a band. Illegal activities can get you in serious trouble in the short term and cause adverse health consequences in the long run. Challenges—physical or creative—impart the thrill that comes with trying something difficult and mastering new skills.

This sort of stimulation differs from substance use: One is real; the other chemical. With one, you're in control; with the other, you're not. Addictive behaviors and substances may seem like quick escapes from stress, but ultimately they consume ever-increasing amounts of time, energy, and money, intensify the stress in your daily life, and create unforeseen and unpredictable new stresses.

Alcohol

Away from home, many for the first time, undergraduates are often excited by and apprehensive about their newfound independence. When new pressures and stressors seem overwhelming, when they feel awkward or insecure, when they just want to let loose and have a good time, they drink. Some students start drinking—and drinking heavily—when they arrive on campus, particularly during the first six weeks and during big weekends and Spring breaks. Alcohol consumption generally declines over the course of an undergraduate education, but a substantial number of students continue binge-drinking, often with highly stressful consequences. (See Chapter 8 for more on alcohol use and abuse).

Drugs

One of the most common reasons that college students turn to drugs, including prescription and illegal drugs, is to relieve stress. They don't think they'll ever lose control because they're too smart, too strong, or too lucky to get caught or hooked. However, over time any addiction or addictive behavior can produce changes in body, brain, and behavior that can lead to enormous stress as well destructive and even deadly consequences.

Illness and Disability

Whenever we come down with the flu, pull a muscle, or get an infection, we feel the stress of not functioning at our best. When the problem is more serious or persistent—a chronic disease like diabetes, for instance, or a lifelong hearing impairment—the emotional stress of daily coping is even greater. Stress also affects and is affected by pain, which may interfere with an individual's ability to perform certain roles and obligations, which in turn increases both stress and the risk of depression.[50]

Learning disabilities, which affect one of every ten Americans, are a common source of stress for college students. Most people with a learning disorder have average or above-average intelligence, but they rarely live up to their ability in school. Some have only one area of difficulty, such as reading or math. Others have problems with attention, writing, communicating, reasoning, coordination, and social skills. Yet not all students with learning disabilities experience greater stress. In some studies, they score significantly higher in resiliency and initiative in solving problems and working toward goals.

 Stress Reliever: Restore Yourself

Even when dealing with pain, discomfort, and limitations, you can consciously make a place for the things that make you feel good. Here are some ideas. Add to this list with your own favorites:

Watch a funny clip on YouTube

Listen to your favorite song

Call someone you like

Hang out with a friend

Spend time in nature

Read for pleasure

Do a puzzle

Savor a chocolate

Meditate

Make a list of people you admire

Take some photographs

Sing

Play a game

Have a dance party—by yourself or with friends

Violence and Crime

✔ **Check-in:** Do you feel safe on your campus? In your community?

According to the Bureau of Justice Statistics, college students are victims of almost half a million violent crimes a year, including assault, robbery, sexual assault, and rape. While this number may seem high, the overall violent crime rate has dropped from 88 to 41 victimizations per 1,000 students in the last decade. In the ACHA's national survey, 87 percent of undergraduates felt "very" safe on campus during the day, 33 percent at night, 56 percent in their community during the day, and 19 percent in their community at night.[51]

More than half of crimes against students are committed by strangers. Nine in ten occur off campus, most often in an open area or street, on public transportation, in a place of business, or at a private home. In about two thirds of the crimes, no weapon is involved. Most off-campus crimes occur at night, while on-campus crimes are more frequent in the day.

 Stress Reliever: A Do-It-Yourself Security Program

• Avoid walking alone in the evening or night. Take advantage of campus shuttle or escort services. If none is available, stick to well-lit routes.

• Train yourself to be aware of your surroundings and the people around you. Visualize potential exit routes in case of an emergency.

• Always carry your cell phone and enough money so that you can get a ride home if you find yourself in a dicey situation.

• Program the campus security number into your cell phone's speed dial numbers so you can access it with a single key stroke.

• Always lock your doors and any first- and second-floor windows at night. Don't compromise your safety for a roommate or friend who asks you to leave the door unlocked.

• Never leave your ID, wallet, checkbook, jewelry, cameras, and other valuables in open view.

• Be careful what information and which photographs you post online on social networking sites. You never know who will see them.

Coping with Campus Stress

The stressors you encounter in college present opportunities to develop and hone your stress-management skills. From this perspective, every experience—good or bad, uplifting or disheartening—becomes an opportunity that can deepen your understanding of yourself, others, and the world outside you and prepare you for a lifetime of thriving. Remember: you're not just enrolled in college; you're a full-time student in the School of Life. Stress management programs, both online[52] and on campus,[53] have proven effective in easing campus stress. Among the most effective approaches are mindfulness, an approach that focuses attention on the physical and mental sensations of the present moment[54] (discussed in detail in Chapter 13) and training in stress-reduction skills.[55]

Here are some suggestions you can put to immediate use:

- Practice the "reciprocal golden rule." Treat yourself with the kindness you may usually reserve for others. This includes accepting your flaws, letting go of regrets, and believing in the best version of yourself. (See Chapter 8 for more on self-compassion.)

- Think of not only where but also who you want to be a decade from now. The goals you set, the decisions you make, the values you adopt now will determine how you feel about yourself and your life in the future.

- Reach out to your peers. Many campuses offer support groups or peer counseling, either in person or online. Virtual peer support forums for students with problems such as symptoms of depression have proven helpful in increasing problem-solving skills, decreasing alienation and isolation, and lowering stress.[56]

- An excellent way to build your attention-paying ability is mindfulness (see Chapter 13), which involves paying close attention to what you are doing and experiencing—and improves the quality of everything you do, large or small. In studies of college students, mindfulness training helped ease the transition from high school[57] and boost resilience to inevitable setbacks.[58]

Chapter Summary

- Today's 20.2 million students attending American colleges and universities are the most diverse ever, with more women, more nontraditional-age men and women, and more minorities—and more stress, which outranks illness, sleep problems, and relationship difficulties as the number-one barrier to academic performance.

- Women consistently rate their perceived stress higher than men. Freshmen rate their stress significantly higher than seniors. Athletes and students taking more than 18 credit hours or working more than four hours a week also report greater stress.

- There are gender differences in coping with stress. Female students tend to engage in more emotionally expressive coping behaviors by seeking social support. Men handle stress through more isolated activities, such as exercise—and (less adaptively) drinking.

- Students between the ages of 18 and 25 are more likely to engage in behaviors that can increase stress and imperil health, such as eating more junk food, smoking, not exercising, and putting on weight.

- Older undergraduates often face multiple stressors but report less school-related stress compared to traditional students—perhaps a payoff of lessons acquired with age and experience and greater emotional intelligence.

- Freshman year is the most stressful, especially for first-generation students—those whose parents never experienced at least one full year of college. Often they see themselves taking on the challenging roles of being trailblazers and role models in addition to the usual academic and personal demands.

- Students who feel different from most of their peers in any way—race, ethnicity, gender identity—may see themselves as isolated and feel greater stress.

- Perceived discrimination and racism are key factors in chronic stress-related health disparities, such as increased hypertension, diabetes, cardiovascular disease, adverse birth outcomes, and mental disorders, among minority groups.

- "Minority status stress," above and beyond general stress, stems from the demands of acculturation, a complex psychosocial process in which an ethnic minority changes, both as individuals and as a group, as a consequence of contact with the ethnic majority.

- While many minority students say that overt prejudice is rare and relatively easy to deal with, subtle pressures called microaggression may undermine their academic confidence and their ability to bond with the university.

- The first step to overcoming academic stress is knowing and mastering a subject. Rather than worrying, shift your attention to the pleasure of acquiring new information and insight.

- The essential study skills include focus (ability to concentrate your attention), persistence (continuing to work even when stressed), consistency, and repetition.

- Smarter test preparation strategies include planning ahead, quizzing yourself, reviewing, and getting a good night's sleep.

- Smarter test-taking strategies include calming yourself by breathing slowly, focusing first on questions you know, writing the easier essays first, and learning from previous tests.

- Other campus stressors include lack of resources, problematic phone and Internet use, risky behaviors, illness and disability, and crime and violence.

- College stressors present opportunities to develop and hone your stress-management skills. From this perspective, every experience—good or bad, uplifting or disheartening—becomes an opportunity to learn and grow.

STRESS RELIEVERS

Change One Thought

Under the right circumstances, changing one simple thought can make a big difference. If you find yourself thinking "I'm lonely," for example, change that thought to "I am loved by someone."[59] The emotional impact can be dramatic.

Talk Back!

As you're studying, does a voice in your head keep sounding alarms: I'm never going to figure this out. I hope this isn't on the test. I can't memorize so many dates. I've always been bad at problems like these.

Send this voice a clear message: Stop!

As you study, send yourself different messages: I am getting this. I can figure this out. This is interesting!

Keep your focus on the material in front of you, not on a test. Stay in the present.

Restore Yourself

Even when dealing with pain, discomfort, and limitations, you can consciously make a place for the things that make you feel good. Here are some ideas. Add to this list with your own favorites:

- Watch a funny clip on YouTube
- Listen to your favorite song
- Call someone you like
- Hang out with a friend
- Spend time in nature

- Read for pleasure
- Do a puzzle
- Savor a chocolate
- Meditate
- Make a list of people you admire
- Take some photographs
- Sing
- Play a game
- Have a dance party—by yourself or with friends

A Do-It-Yourself Security Program

- Avoid walking alone in the evening or night. Take advantage of campus shuttle or escort services. If none is available, stick to well-lit routes.

- Train yourself to be aware of your surroundings and the people around you. Visualize potential exit routes in case of an emergency.

- Always carry your cell phone and enough money so that you can get a ride home if you find yourself in a dicey situation.

- Program the campus security number into your cell phone's speed dial numbers so you can access it with a single keystroke.

- Always lock your doors and any first- and second-floor windows at night. Don't compromise your safety for a roommate or friend who asks you to leave the door unlocked.

- Never leave your ID, wallet, checkbook, jewelry, cameras, and other valuables in open view.

- Be careful what information and which photographs you post online on social networking sites. You never know who will see them.

⊜ YOUR PERSONAL STRESS MANAGEMENT TOOLKIT

REFLECTION: Are You Showing Signs of Campus Stress?

Undergraduates describe themselves as reacting to stress in various ways. Check any that you've experienced in the last month:

- Physical
  - _____ fatigue
  - _____ sweating
  - _____ stuttering
  - _____ trembling
  - _____ no longer exercising
  - _____ eating more junk food
  - _____ developing physical symptoms
  - _____ coming down with acute infectious illnesses (cold, bronchitis, ear infection, sinus infection, strep throat)[60]

- Emotional
  - _____ anxious
  - _____ fearful
  - _____ angry
  - _____ guilty
  - _____ depressed
  - _____ less satisfied with life

- Behavioral
  - _____ poor or inadequate sleep
  - _____ crying
  - _____ eating
  - _____ smoking
  - _____ being irritable or abusive

- Cognitive
  - _____ difficulty paying attention and concentrating
  - _____ feeling distracted
  - _____ impaired memory

Count the number of checks: Your score could range from 0 to 22. Whatever your total is, mindfulness (see Chapter 13) may help. The following exercise can get you started.

TECHNIQUE: Mindful Studying

- Review the material on mindfulness in Chapter 13.

- Get into a comfortable sitting position with your spine reasonably straight. Take a moment to take five deep breaths in and out.

- Notice your surroundings—what do you see, what do you hear, what do you smell, how does your body feel?

- Continue to take deep breaths, feeling your body fill as you inhale, and imagine any stress you are experiencing being released when you exhale and release your breath.

- Visualize what you need to accomplish. Picture yourself completing your work, your mind producing great ideas, absorbing the material you are studying, or acing the exam.

- Visualize yourself after you have completed your work, feeling gratified, capable, and intelligent.

- Then begin the task at hand. If you feel your mind drifting, give yourself a study check-in and summarize in your mind what you just learned or wrote. Review material as needed. Visualize yourself focusing and completing the task, then return to your work.

- As soon as a test is scheduled, start visualizing yourself taking the exam. Feel in your body a sense of control, breathe comfortably, and smile. Fill yourself with feelings of achievement and accomplishment. Smile bigger. Breathe easily. You don't have to achieve a state of blissful calm. A little stress is actually good for performance.

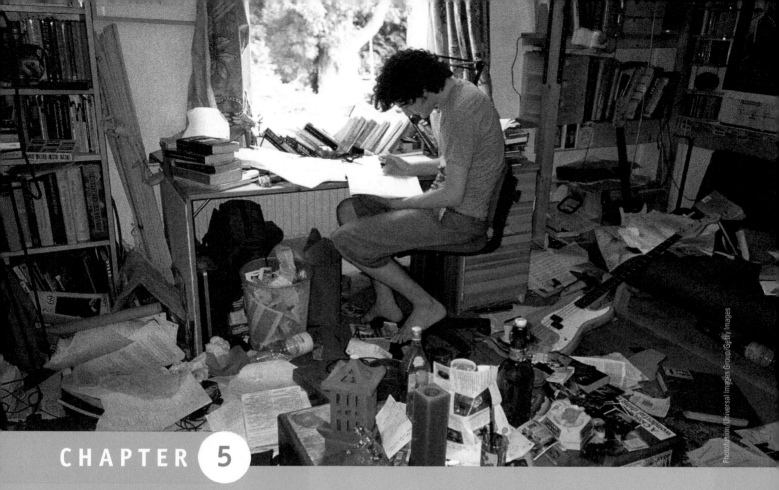

Phototusion/Universal Images Group/Getty Images

CHAPTER **5**

Your Personal Environment, Time, and Money

After reading this chapter, you should be able to:

5.1 Summarize techniques for improving your personal environment in ways that decrease stress.

5.2 Explain the importance of time management in preventing stress overload and overcoming procrastination.

5.3 Identify the key elements of financial responsibility.

5.4 List specific steps to improve your money management skills and safe-guard your financial wellbeing.

5.5 Develop a plan to take control of your daily life to decrease stress.

Use the diary in the form in Figure 5.1 or in MindTap to track how you spend your time over a three-day period. Include at least one weekend day. Set a timer on your phone, watch, or laptop to go off every half hour so you can record what you are doing in real time and how stressed you feel.

At the end of the period, analyze your diary entries. Look for patterns. How much time did you spend in class? Studying? Online? Outdoors? With friends? Are there "gaps" of lost time throughout the day? Do you see ways in which you can make better use of your time? What were you doing when your stress levels were highest? Lowest?

So far this week Josh has pulled one all-nighter, slept through his alarm two mornings in a row, missed the deadline for a sociology paper, and forgotten an appointment with his academic advisor. And it's only Wednesday.

"I don't know where the time goes," Josh complains. He tries to jot down what he's supposed to do, but then he loses the piece of paper. Some of his friends use their watches or phones to keep track of commitments, but Josh says that's not his thing. He's no better with money than he is with time. He never realizes his bank account is overdrawn until he can't get cash at an ATM. Even though it happens regularly, he's shocked—and embarrassed—when a waiter or sales clerk says his credit card has been declined.

"If I just had more time I'd get organized," Josh tells himself. But when he looks at the clothes heaped on the closet floor, the Styrofoam containers from last weekend's take-out, and the books and papers piled on his desk, he feels overwhelmed.

Where would he even begin? And even if he could beat back the chaos, wouldn't the mess return like some movie swamp monster in a week or so?

One evening a girl he invited to his room asks a question Josh can't answer: "What's that weird smell?"

Mortified, he realizes that he hasn't changed the sheets since his Mom's visit—months ago on Parents' Weekend. Josh can't count how many burrito wrappers and greasy French fries bags he must have kicked under his desk and bed. And who could guess whether his athletic shoes, socks, or jersey boxers smelled worst?

The very next day Josh buys oversized trash bags and begins excavating his room. At a discount office supply outlet just off campus, he finds some stackable plastic crates and vows to spend some time every day on clutter control. Although no one will ever consider Josh a neat freak, he no longer feels that his time and things are beyond control. And his room smells a whole lot less like a pig ranch.

Your Three-Day Activity and Stress Diary

Time	Day 1		Day 2		Day 3	
	Activity	Stress Level (1–10)	Activity	Stress Level (1–10)	Activity	Stress Level (1–10)
7:00 a.m.						
8:00 a.m.						
9:00 a.m.						
10:00 a.m.						
11:00 a.m.						
12:00 p.m.						
01:00 p.m.						
02:00 p.m.						
03:00 p.m.						
04:00 p.m.						
05:00 p.m.						
06:00 p.m.						
07:00 p.m.						
08:00 p.m.						
09:00 p.m.						
10:00 p.m.						
11:00 p.m.						
12:00 a.m.						

FIGURE 5.1 Your 3-day time diary.

Many people have at least a little "Josh" within them. What about you? Do you live in a state of order? Are you always running late? Does time seem to disappear? Do you even know when your geology project is due? What about your phone bill? Do you have enough money in the bank to cover next month's rent?

Managing your living space, time, and money doesn't require anything magical. Step-by-step techniques, like the ones described in this chapter, will enable you to choose wisely how you use basic resources. As you adopt these strategies, you will accomplish more and feel less stressed about making up for what you should have done days or weeks ago—or redoing the task you started but did not finish. You may be surprised by how your perspective changes. Rather than viewing time as thief or taskmaster, you will celebrate your skill at filling with it with things you enjoy. And rather than watching your money disappear in a blink, you may even see it grow.

Managing Your Personal Environment

....

✔ **Check-in:** Are you a neat freak with every drawer in perfect order? Do you build piles of semi-organized stuff on the floor? Are you drowning in a sea of clutter?

....

You may think of your environment in terms of air, sound, or comfort—all of which can affect your daily stress levels (see Chapter 11 for more on environmental stress). However, one underlying principle also has a significant impact: order. Living without order, rushing, and improvising all bring chaos, and chaos inevitably breeds stress. Whatever disorder you leave behind today will steal part of tomorrow from you. If you want to take control of your life, the first thing you have to do is establish in order.

Maybe part of you relishes some degree of disorder as testimony to your carefree spirit, lack of rigidity, or independence. Maybe you think that people who are tidy and punctual have less fun. Think again about how you define fun. Is frantically searching for your misplaced student I.D. card or bus pass fun? How about paying late fees on your credit cards? Or losing the reference book you need for the paper that's due tomorrow?

Every second you hunt for yet another item that's gone missing, every dollar you spend on overdue parking fines, takes away from the precious time and money you have for yourself and makes your daily life more stressful. Becoming orderly doesn't take away from fun and spontaneity. Instead it provides the structure and state of mind that enable you to avoid unnecessary stress.

Rules of Order

Disorder arises most often from putting off tasks or not completing an activity you've already begun. The deadly duo of avoidance and postponement multiply the unpleasantness of any chore or assignment. In a matter of days you face a formidable pile; in a month, you face an avalanche of routine duties you either haven't started or haven't finished.

Disorder undermines pleasure as well as efficiency because it upsets your internal well-being. You need to be in a placid physiological state to feel calm and make good choices. Notice how you feel the next time disorder disrupts your life. Say you can't find the signed medical clearance form you need to join an intramural team. As a result, you have to walk to the farthest corner of the campus and wait for who knows how long at the Student Health Service. All the while that you're searching, trudging, waiting, and raging at yourself, you're stressed out and wasting time and energy.

The alternative? Create a solution: an orderly habit that you will *always* follow, that works for *you*. For example, *always* put all your important papers in a file you *always* keep in the top right-hand corner of your desk. Or *always* back up your computer before shutting it down.

 Stress Reliever: One Simple Thing

....

Think of one thing that could make your life easier. What if you put a hook up to hold your keys so you don't spend five minutes searching for them every morning? What if you backed up your files to the Cloud every night so you'd never again lose a draft? Taking action, however small, boosts your sense of control and lowers your stress.

Your Study Space

You may tell yourself that as long as you have wi-fi, you can work anywhere—the Student Union, Starbucks, leaning against a tree on the quad, lying in bed in your underwear. You may indeed be able to check a website or send an e-mail, but work—effective, efficient, focused work—requires its own comfortable and well-designed space. You will work best in a space dedicated to a specific activity.

Now imagine how close you can come to creating this space where you live now. What would you have to do to create a place conducive to good work? Given your current budget and space, how closely can you approximate your ideal environment? When you have finished, make some notes. And then go to work on your work space.

Ideally, set aside a space for your exclusive use. It should be private, a sanctuary where others do not enter. If it's not possible to keep your workstation behind locked doors, ask the people you live with to respect this space and not touch or move the things you leave there. If you reserve one area solely for academics, every time you approach it, your mind will make unconscious associations that provide cues to help you focus on your studies.

Order demands that you have everything ready and at hand. Consider the minimum requirements. For sure, you will need a good-sized flat surface and supplies within easy reach. Think of it this way: Everything in your space should work for you and support you; nothing should work against you.

Your workspace will work all the better if it appeals to you aesthetically and beckons you to come and work. Even in a dorm room, surround yourself with your favorite colors. Over time add small touches to get as close as possible to the most ideal workspace you can imagine. An indoor plant helps purify air, and the bit of nature promotes a sense of well-being. As Chapter 15 explains, scents also make a difference. Practice a bit of aromatherapy, and buy an inexpensive diffuser to fill the air with eucalyptus, evergreen, or another pleasing scent.

As much as possible, seek good natural and artificial light so you can work without straining your eyes and adding unnecessary fatigue. In positioning your computer, keep these ergonomic points in mind:

- Set up your computer to keep glare and eyestrain to a minimum.

- Make sure you have a good, back-friendly chair and that your desk or table are the proper height.

- Place the screen at eye level (22–26 inches higher than your seat).

- Position the keyboard so that your elbows are bent at a 90-degree angle and your hands and wrists are straight.

🔧 **Stress Reliever:** Don't Hit the Sack

You've finally finished your last assignment, and you're absolutely, utterly exhausted. You look at the books stacked on the floor and the papers strewn over your desk. "Forget it," you think. All you want to do is crawl into bed.

Don't. Take 10 or 15 minutes to put your work space back in order. Gather the notes for your term paper into a file. Put your textbooks back on the shelf.

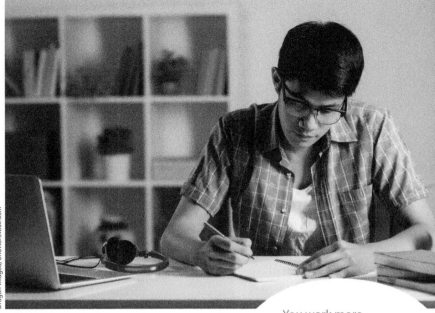

Dragon Images/Shutterstock.com

Taking the time to put your work space in order produces many benefits, including creating an inviting space to which to return. You'll love yourself for it in the morning.

You work more efficiently and effectively in an organized, uncluttered, well-lit space

Establishing Order

Don't assume that some people are just naturally neater than you or that you didn't inherit the gene for keeping track of stuff. Individuals vary in how orderly they need their environment to be so that it works for rather than against them. You don't have to become a slave of creating order. However, many college students we know are slaves of disorder. You may pride yourself on being able to roll with the punches that chaos throws at you. But why squander your time cleaning up the consequences of disorder and mismanagement?

Once your physical environment is in order—that is, when you know how and where to put your hands on what you need without delay, you will become less stressed and more serene, in other words, more in order internally. And when you are in internal order, you are empowered and your potential can truly shine.

Being orderly is a decision. If you hate spending time on meaningless tasks, create a little more order here and a little more order there in every part of your life. You do not need to make a drastic overhaul today, but choose to take small, initial steps towards a well-organized life. Make order an ongoing process. Paying attention to external order helps foster internal order.

If you don't pay regular attention to the socks piling up on the dresser or the take-out coffee cups on the floor, you'll soon find yourself surrounded once again by disarray—and feeling out of control. Inattention creates disorder. It is also how bill payments, assignment due dates, and special events are missed. Sooner or later you have to tackle the clutter. But if you let disorder become overwhelming, then clearing it becomes an all-out effort that exhausts you. So you slide immediately back into the old approach of not keeping your life in order. Some people repeat this cycle for a lifetime.

Wherever you are—at your desk, on the job, in your room, home, or car—get in the habit of leaving at least one small space more orderly than you found it. This guarantees progress because order becomes an ongoing task, rather than a once-in-a-blue-moon blitz.

 Stress Reliever: The 15-Minute Cleanup

Who has a whole day to clear out an overstuffed closet or haul months' worth of gear out of the trunk of a car? Of course, you don't. But surely you can snatch 15 minutes from the time you'd otherwise spend surfing the net or streaming videos. That's all you need to get started.

Don't wait for more disorder to accumulate. And don't fall into the trap of telling yourself that there's no point in starting until you can get it all done at once. You only create more disorder by putting off a task. Make whatever headway you can in 15 minutes every day during your regular week. On a weekend, set a timer to alert you every hour. Spend 15 minutes organizing and the other 45 minutes however you choose. Before long you will finish. And if you keep up the same pattern, you will maintain order.

Block out 15-minute slots for targeted bursts of organizational energy on your daily and weekly calendars. Why? Scheduling moves you from "someday, I've got to do this" good intentions to taking action in real time. A schedule, along with a specific commitment to always follow it strictly, will keep you focused.

Managing Your Time

Everybody gets 24 hours. No one can add a twenty-fifth hour to the day or an eighth day to the week. Although you may struggle to cram all that you need and want to do into your allotted hours, you can take control of how you use the time you have—even if you think you will always feel out of control. What you choose to do with the time you have is what matters.

Becoming conscious of time and how you use it is the crucial first step to taking control of your life. If you don't analyze where your time is going, you're likely to continue to lose it (or not use it) the same way you always have. The diary in the Pre-Chapter Check-In on page 81 can give you an objective sense of what you chose to do with time over a three-day period. Look for patterns. Calculate the number of hours you spent on various activities. Do they reflect what's most important to you?

Day Planning

Each morning, decide what you are going to do during the rest of the day and tomorrow, what your top priority will be, and how you will go about getting your work done. Write down the specific tasks you will complete by the end of the day. Some will be simple chores, like buying shampoo and toothpaste; others will be steps in an ongoing project.

Set your alarm a little earlier than usual. This does not mean you have to get up at 5:00 A.M.; you just want to rise early enough to start the day in a state of calm contemplation. Begin the day mindfully and with purpose. Don't rush out choking down a doughnut and already running ten minutes behind. People who get up a half hour to an hour earlier than they once did report amazing changes in their sense of command and their productivity.

Get to your first class or appointment a little before you have to be there. An early arrival sends a message to your brain that what you are about to do is significant and not just another throwaway experience to rush through. Just do it for a few days, and see the difference. See how this simple change helps you to feel more confident in your activities, focus better, and feel less overall day-to-day stress.

Visualize Your Time

Before you begin a task, whether it's conjugating verbs in Mandarin or making a timeline for your Ancient Civilizations class, take a few moments to visualize yourself completing the steps the process requires. This cues the mind in another way and prepares it like any other run-through or rehearsal.

Why do sports teams practice plays? In fact, why does anyone rehearse anything? Because you perform better when you rehearse. Rehearsal provides a mind map—an internal set of expectations and directions—and serves as a fundamental way of getting ready for peak performance. It also creates new connections within the brain that result in more automatic responses to task demands.

This process is also a mental focusing device. All the tugging, wiggling, spitting, and scratching that athletes engage in between pitches or tennis serves is not superstition. This chain of behaviors cues the mind and senses to a keen degree of focused readiness. If you visualize steps, you prepare yourself for action. As research demonstrates, this practice is a big aid to completing things on time.

Develop your own routine to cue yourself that it is time to work. Visualize; follow a sequence of steps; work with a sense of urgency. There is a time for leisure and a time for heightened attention and readiness. If you are working on a task, make it a matter of urgency, and you will move toward it differently. This is not about hurry, but rather about force of *in*tention and focus of *at*tention. Do things deliberately but with a concentrated sense of urgency.

If you have many tasks, do the most difficult ones early in the day. Save the easy ones for the afternoon when your circadian rhythms dip and your energy lags. Resist the notion that handling the easy ones will provide a sense of accomplishment. Your brain will read that for what it is: avoidance of the difficult things. When you come back to anything you have put off, you always resist it more. Do it first. Then notice how much better you feel—and how nice it is not to experience the stress of having a dreaded task left to complete. The rest of the day will accelerate, and your confidence will soar.

To teach yourself how to estimate time accurately, compare your predictions of how long a task will take with how much time it actually demands when you do it. Identify one assignment, such as reading a chapter or outlining a class presentation. Then just do it.

Don't take shortcuts. Work intensively and with concentration. Keep track of how much time you spend on the outline, subtracting time off for breaks or interruptions. Then see how this compares with your estimate.

Take Time for Yourself

Look back on your three-day diary and put a plus sign next to the activities that energized or excited you and a minus sign next to those that drained you. Use this information to plan ways to put more pluses on your calendar. They don't have to be major splurges. But it is important to schedule time for fun as well as coursework. Part of managing stress is living a more balanced life that has both productivity and relaxation structured into it.

Weave positive practices into your daily routine: Stream music that stirs or soothes you. Pause to watch a sunset. Positive pleasurable experiences don't have to be huge events that you anticipate for months. Small experiences can

Build "downtime" into your day so you can take a few minutes to stop, reflect, and refresh.

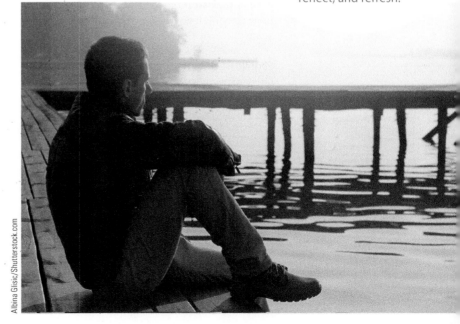

Albina Glisic/Shutterstock.com

provide just as much stress reduction. You don't have to wait for the big birthday cake of a vacation; take little bites of cupcake throughout the day every day. Catch up with a friend or family member; watch a favorite video; scroll through photos of a vacation or reunion.

When you take a break, really take one. Switch gears completely. Relax deeply. (See Chapter 12 for breathing and relaxation exercises.) Unwind in real time with no screen in front of you. Melt into a sofa. Zone out in a warm bath. Develop a routine that cues relaxation and practice it when you really need to relax deeply. Before bed, for instance, clear your mind of thoughts or read for pleasure before you repeat affirmations or review your day and the things you are grateful for.

Pre-empting Procrastination

We've all put off until tomorrow things that we would rather not face today—and come up with millions of excuses for procrastinating. But **chronic procrastination** can trip you up, slow you down, stress you out, and sabotage your best efforts. You know that. But you may not realize that procrastination isn't a character flaw. There really are only two fundamental reasons we do not complete tasks in a timely way:

- We lack smart, effective strategies and skills for making efficient use of time, or
- We fall back on inefficient, self-defeating habits that steal precious time.

In other words, either you have failed to develop good habits that you need to learn, or you have developed bad habits you need to unlearn and replace. This is particularly true of **academic procrastination**, an intentional delay in beginning or completing important and time-sensitive academic activities.[1]

Such delay, like most stress, springs from fear. People are afraid that they lack knowledge they'll need to navigate the situation they confront or that their efforts won't succeed. Hesitant to face the situation they mildly dread, they postpone a report, a phone call, or a delicate conversation, lose time, and increase their dread. When you set something aside instead of acting on it in the moment, you seldom gain an advantage unless you immediately do research on how to handle the situation more effectively. You squander time you can never regain and have made the issue at hand even larger in your own mind. The best antidotes: acquiring practical skills, such as breaking big tasks down into smaller, more doable steps, and learning to place long-term goals above short-term gratification. (See Chapter 7 on personal change.)

chronic procrastination Regular delaying of work or other activities to the extent that it interferes with your functioning and performance.

academic procrastination An intentional delay in beginning or completing important and time-sensitive academic activities.

 Stress Reliever: Begin

The single most effective antidote to procrastination is starting. Don't flog yourself to tackle the chore you hate most; just do step one. If the long-delayed job is cleaning the bathroom, tell yourself that all you are going to do now is take the basic equipment—cleaning solutions, brushes, rubber gloves, whatever—into the bathroom. Once you get there, having started the process, you will find it much easier to go ahead and complete the job.

Live in Real Time

Everyone loves a shortcut. In your hometown, do you know the best route to get from Point A to Point B, even in rush hour? Shortcuts make sense only when they enhance true efficiency rather than simply skip necessary steps. When it comes to time control, the ideal shortcut is acting in real time.

Doing things immediately skips unnecessary steps and requires less effort than doing them later. Many people fail to notice something subtler: delaying anything is procrastination on a smaller scale. Cumulatively, the consequences are the same: a serious loss of time that, if used well, could have yielded a sense of satisfaction, ease, and control. Instead, when you feel rushed and panicky, your performance is weaker than it might have been.

Say you have to lead a discussion in your political science class. You decide that in order to prepare you need to download a file and look something up in your textbook. You can take the time to jot yourself a note, and then add these items to a to-do list. Why? You're engaging in needless delay. Or you can download the file then and there, and look up the information in your textbook. This is living in real time.

The people who accomplish the most in the most efficient manner invariably handle these tasks immediately, as they arise. They manage the day-to-day part of their lives now, in real time, not later and not after a series of pointless delays. The time you spend delaying is the time in which you could have done what you delay. If you learn to respond immediately to ordinary tasks—e-mail, texts, calls you need to make—or anything else that you could finish in three minutes or less, you will learn a simple secret that will exponentially increase your efficiency. Just don't interrupt your study time to do them.

Why put your coat on the bed when you can hang it up? Why not forward the announcement of tryouts the first time your friend asks for it? Will staring several times at the button that you need to sew back on a jacket make it easier when you finally get around to doing it a month later? Will waiting to do laundry when you "have time" put a clean sweatshirt that doesn't smell funky in your closet?

If you are not going to complete an action right away, you must *in real time* take the next step required. For instance, if you cannot complete a task in three minutes, you can write it down on a to-do list and estimate how long the task will take: How much time will you need for washing and drying a load of laundry? What about folding and putting the clothes away? How long does it take to get to the grocery store, buy your items, return, and put them away?

To-do lists can help you manage and structure your day in *real time*. But if you never look at the list again or scribble little reminders on napkins from the cafeteria and stash them in your purse or pocket, writing down what you need to do only wastes time. Use a reminder or notepad app on your phone. Choose to make it a habit to write down the things you need to do and remember. There is satisfaction to be had each time you delete something from your list. There is an even greater satisfaction in making your way through the entire list and rewarding yourself for your efficiency and accomplishments.

To live in real time does not mean that you assume the "ready-fire-aim" mode. Rather, instead of setting things aside, you respond when they first come to your attention. Acting in this fashion does not rule out your considering your actions as thoroughly as warranted. And it does not rule out choosing the best time to do it later if it will take longer than three minutes. *But you must choose the specific time, and act when it arrives.* If you need to consult or consider, by all means do so; but don't put this off either. Begin it right now, carry through on it as far as possible, and then continue it at a time you choose and record. Do not set aside what you can do now.

⚒ Stress Reliever: Eavesdrop on Your Excuses

If you're a chronic procrastinator, you may not even be aware of the thoughts that run through your mind when you put something off. Every time you balk at writing the first sentence of a report, doing a literature search, making a certain phone call, or reading the first page of the assigned novel, stop and listen to what you're telling yourself. Here's what you are likely to hear:

"I'm too tired. I'll rest first, watch a little TV, and then start."

"There's no point in starting; I've got to meet my friend Navi in ten minutes."

"I've got plenty of time to do it later."

"I'll organize my desk first."

"It's too nice to stay inside."

"I don't have everything I need."

"I've been working really hard. I deserve a break."

"I'll do a better job tomorrow."

"I need a good idea to inspire me."

"I should exercise before it gets dark."

"Why do it on Friday? The instructor won't get it. It's not due until Monday."

"I can read that book in a few hours."

Think of rebuttals to yourself. For instance, you might say, "Yes, I'm tired. I'll just work for half an hour, and then I'll go to bed." Or you might tell yourself, "I'll see how much I can get done in 10 minutes." Or you could say, "I'm tired of making excuses; I choose to take time every day to focus and study because I am choosing to succeed and feel good about accomplishing something."

The Myth of Multitasking

As you read this, are you glancing at a text, listening to music, or thinking ahead to the weekend? Or maybe you're trying to multitask and do all of these at once. Stop! The brain, as neuroscientists have demonstrated, performs even simple actions one after another, in a strict linear sequence.[2] Unless they are completely mechanical ones, multitasking destroys the quality of attention given to the tasks at hand. So work when you work, play when you play. And text or snapchat when you're doing nothing more important than, say, picking laundry lint off a black T-shirt.

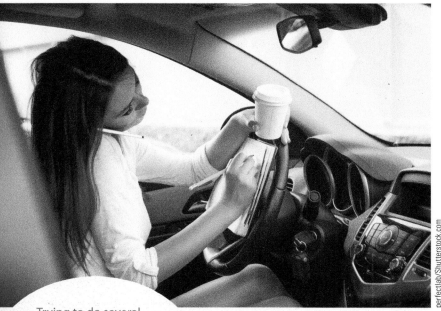

Trying to do several things at the same time can be dangerous if you're behind the wheel of a car.

perfectlab/Shutterstock.com

The Now Imperative

"Just do it," was a famous advertising slogan. We would add one more word: just do it NOW. Act in the moment a need arises. When you do, you act far more efficiently than when you delay.

The "now" part of this imperative has to do with the optimum time to act. The "imperative" part means there is no other way out. Nothing is as efficient as acting in the moment that a day-to-day need appears. When you set this standard and adhere to this imperative, you will quickly feel different about yourself and your capacities.

Whenever possible—and it is possible much of the time with a small additional amount of effort—dispatch simple things in one fell swoop. Don't pointlessly break a task down into a series of steps if they aren't necessary. Skip the list-building busy work; cut directly to the chase.

Putting off learning how to use new software is the same. You compound a problem you invested time and money to solve. All alternatives to living and acting in real time create inefficiency. These can range from a minor time loss that puts a drag on resources to (in the worst case) feeling chronically overwhelmed and unable to catch up. Don't buy gadgets and equipment you don't have time to figure out how to use. Learn to use the time saving, life-brightening devices you already have—like your brain and your attention. Don't put it off any longer; do it now. (See Part 2 of the Personal Stress Management Toolkit on page 99.)

Turn off your text message and e-mail alerts when you block out 45 minutes for reading your Econ assignment. Just do what needs doing. Become formidable in your devotion to this habit, and you will have more time for what's really important. At the time you decide to do so, go back to the text messages. They won't vanish while you are working.

To stay on track, schedule your work in 50–55 minute segments, with breaks in between. Start by taking a few moments to focus and visualize what you're about to do. Turn off anything that can ring, beep, or bother you. Stop fiddling with the screensaver on your computer. Use earplugs if necessary (not earbuds) to block noise. Build in down time, and take it according to schedule. Keep working at this pace until you complete what you set out to do. You send yourself a very empowering message when you keep your promises to yourself.

··

✔ **Check-in:** What are you doing?

··

Five minutes after you sit down to study, are you checking your text messages? Foraging for a drink or snack? Turning up your music to blot out your roommate's? Checking the score of the game? Squeezing in a quick round of your favorite computer game?

··

If so, stop everything. The external interruptions Emerson called "idle distractions" are undermining the messages you need to communicate to your brain about urgency and efficiency.

··

Time Management for Commuting and Working Students

If you commute to school, you can't roll out of bed ten minutes before class, pull on jeans, and sprint across the quad. If you work, you have to show up on time, do your job, and fit in studying where and when you can. If you don't take control of your time, you will soon feel out of control.

To beat the time crunch, begin before the term starts. Get the course catalog as early as possible so you can plan your work hours or commute around it. Try to avoid rush hour traffic or crowded subways or buses. Whenever you can, schedule classes back to back or during one part of the day (all morning or all evening, for example) so that you can concentrate academics into one block of time.

Use a calendar—either the old-fashioned paper type or one on your phone, notepad, or laptop—from the very first day of the term. This will be your most valuable time control tool. Read the syllabus for each course thoroughly the first day of class. Don't delay, or you will lose valuable time. Mark on your calendar all assignment due dates and exams. (If an assignment or task doesn't have a due date, give it one.) For any research or group assignments, make a schedule on your calendar for how you'll complete each of them. Include "begin research for sociology paper" on one day, "complete outline" a week later, and "begin first draft" on another day.

Breaking big projects up into smaller pieces and giving yourselves deadlines for each will help you stay on track. Calculate roughly how many hours you think each assignment will take. Keep in mind that most things take longer than you think, so build in extra time from the start.

Let your instructors know your work schedule, and let your boss know your class schedule. Although you cannot expect them to plan around you, they may be flexible with due dates and work hours if they know your time demands. Clear communication can help you avoid unnecessary stress.

With a schedule as tight as yours, you have to be realistic in your commitments—which means saying "no" to some of the favors asked of you. Don't feel guilty; simply explain that, even though you'd love to help a friend move or come to your cousin's dance recital, you have to work or study or commute. You also have to turn down some fun activities. Face it now: the only way to get all your assignments done will mean reading, writing, or working on projects during parts of long weekends and holidays.

Managing Your Money

✔ **Check-in:** You and your money.

How would you rate your financial management skills?

_____ Excellent

_____ Good

_____ Fair

_____ Poor

_____ Terrible

In a recent national poll, 57 percent of college students considered their money managing skills "excellent" or "good." About a third (31 percent) said theirs were "fair," while just 12 percent felt that their ability to handle money was "poor" or "terrible." However, their behaviors didn't match their self-ratings: Only 39 percent of those surveyed stuck to a monthly budget; 38 percent needed to borrow money from friends or family;

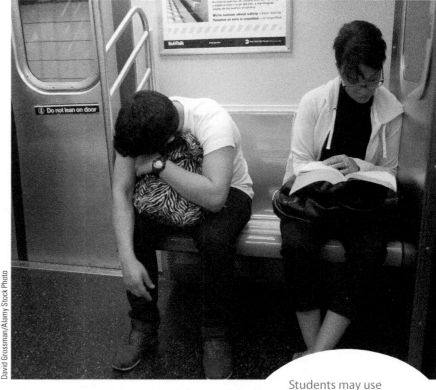

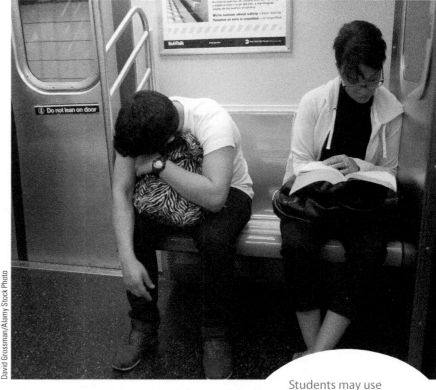David Grossman/Alamy Stock Photo

Students may use their commute time to catch up on studying or sleep.

almost half had less than $100 in their bank accounts at some point in the last 12 months.[3]

Money ranks second only to academics as a source of stress for college students.[4] In the National Student Financial Wellness Study of almost 19,000 undergraduates at 52 colleges and universities, seven in ten undergraduates felt stressed about their personal finances. Nearly six in ten worry about having enough money to pay for school; half are concerned about paying their monthly expenses.[5] (See Figure 5.2.)

People of all ages and income levels describe money as a major source of stress in their lives, but money itself isn't a stressor. It's what you do—or don't do—with it that creates stress. Not having enough may be the most common complaint about money, but even with unlimited resources, you need to know how to manage money wisely and well. College offers an ideal opportunity to learn how to handle everything from spare change to long-term loans. Once you know how to take control of your money, your money will not take control of you or your life. You will also be better prepared to pursue your goals—and have the financial resources to reach them.

College represents a huge investment for a family. If your parents are your primary source of support, talk with them about their expectations for how you handle your money. Do they expect you to get a job while taking classes? Do

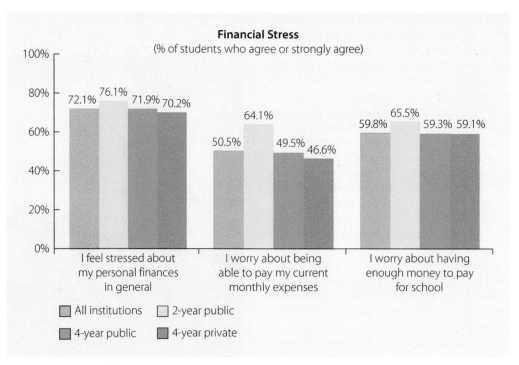

Financial Stress
(% of students who agree or strongly agree)

I feel stressed about my personal finances in general: 72.1%, 76.1%, 71.9%, 70.2%

I worry about being able to pay my current monthly expenses: 50.5%, 64.1%, 49.5%, 46.6%

I worry about having enough money to pay for school: 59.8%, 65.5%, 59.3%, 59.1%

Legend: All institutions, 2-year public, 4-year public, 4-year private

FIGURE 5.2 Most students worry about having enough money now or in the future.

Source: National Student Financial Wellness Study, Center for the Study of Student Life, Ohio State University.

they expect you to work summers rather than backpacking through Costa Rica? Be very clear on which expenses are your responsibility and your spending limits.

About two thirds of students use loans to pay for college; more than 20 percent of loan recipients expect they will have a debt of $50,000 or more by the time they graduate. The average college student graduates with $24,000 in debt, according to the Project on Student Debt. With easy access to credit cards and so many things to spend money on, many students end up owing much more.

About half of undergraduates have jobs, which helps make ends meet but can create other problems. Those working more than 10 hours a week are more likely to report academic difficulties. Students taking a fifth year or longer to complete a bachelor's degree are twice as likely to report financial stress than other undergraduates; more than two thirds say that money worries have impeded their academic performance. (See Chapter 11 for more on occupational stress.) Students stressed-out by financial pressure are more likely to reduce their courseload, withdraw from college to get full-time jobs, and take longer to graduate.[6] Like other forms of chronic stress, money worries can take a toll on students' physical and mental health.[7]

Self-efficacy (introduced in Chapter 1) can make a crucial difference. Students with greater financial self-efficacy—those who are confident and competent in handling money matters—are less likely to report financial stress.[8] The information and exercises in the following section can boost both your financial understanding and your confidence in handling money now and in the future. We also recommend participating in the money management seminars that many schools offer. Or you can visit www.cashcourse .org, a free online resource specially designed for college students sponsored by the National Endowment for Education with plenty of practical information, but no ads or agenda.

Financial Homeostasis

As with any other aspect of stress management, homeostasis or balance is key. Your income, the amount of money available to you, must cover your expenses. If you spend more, you go into debt, which generates stress as well as other problems. As a first step, you need to organize your financial records and keep track of your monthly income and expenses (See Table 5.1.).

Organizing Basics

For bills and documents, buy a simple accordion file or a portable file. Make separate folders for documents from your school, bank, and service providers. As you put things away, add reminders of any deadlines and due dates to your phone. If you know you'll be more organized with virtual files, set up a system on your computer or on cloud storage. Save electronic files to specific folders, and scan or take pictures of paper documents and upload them. You may want also to back up your files on an external hard disc.

- Bills. Set alerts on your phone and computer, or circle days on your calendar to remind your of due dates so you pay bills on time.

- Checking account. Save your canceled checks and bank statements. If they are online, save them as a PDF and print them out. You should keep three to seven years' worth of bank statements in your records for tax purposes.

- Savings and investment. File all statements from your bank savings account and any other investments such as Certificates of Deposit (CDs) or mutual funds.

- College. Keep records about your tuition payments, receipts for textbooks and supplies, courses, grades, and credits.

- Financial aid. Save applications, award letters, student loan agreements, and notes about important telephone conversations.

- Insurance. File whatever policies you have, such as car or medical coverage.

- Loan and credit-records. Keep loan agreements and payment records for car loans, credit card payments, and so on.

- Receipts and warranties. File the paperwork that comes with all major purchases, such as phones, tablets, and computers.

- Taxes. Include your tax returns, W2s, pay stubs, and so on.

- Keep records that are difficult to replace, such as your original birth certificate and Social Security card, in a bank deposit box or a fire-resistant safe.

Making a Budget

Use your money for rent, bills, and groceries first. Then look ahead to upcoming expenses to see what you need to save for. This will give you a reality check on how much you have for going out or buying new clothes. Ideally, you should be able to save as well as spend. Financial planning, starts with defining your financial goals, making plans for how to reach them, and taking action to make your goals a reality (see Table 5.2). If you write down your goals and incorporate them into your budget, you'll have a better chance of achieving them. (See Chapter 7 for more on setting goals.)

TABLE 5.1 A College Student's Budget Template

Monthly income for the month of: _____

Item	Amount
Estimated monthly income	
Financial awards	
Allowance from parents	
Other income	
Total	

Monthly expenses for the month of: _____

Item	Amount
Rent	
Utilities	
Cell phone	
Groceries	
Car expenses	
Student loans	
Insurance	
Medical expenses	
Credit card debt	
Entertainment	
Laundry	
Miscellaneous	
Total	

Semester costs for the month of: _____

Item	Amount
Tuition	
Books	
Lab fees	
Transportation	
Deposits	
Other	
Total	

How am I doing?

Item	Amount
Monthly income	
Subtract monthly expenses	
Subtract semester expenses	
Difference	

TABLE 5.2 Your Money Goals

Goal	Amount Needed	By Date	How I'll Reach My Goal
Trip home	$300	Mom's Birthday	Baby-sitting, tutoring
Car	$10,000	Next summer	Savings, bank loan, part-time job
New phone	$200	Within 3 months	Catering job, dog walking
Running shoes	$60	Two weeks	Not eating out, biking not driving
_____	_____	_____	_____
_____	_____	_____	_____
_____	_____	_____	_____

Frugal Living

When you were living with—and off—your parents, you may never have thought twice about your daily take-out cappuccino or the price of tickets for a weekend concert. That was then; this is now. You have to make choices and set priorities. If money was tight in your family, you may have already mastered ways to stretch your dollars. If you've never had to worry about money before, frugal living may be one of most useful skills you acquire in college.

Here are some tips to get started:

- Invest with your roommates in a coffee maker. Brew your own, pour it into an insulated mug, and carry it with you rather than buying a pricey coffee drink.

- Explore thrift stores when you need furniture, sports equipment, or clothing.

- Even if it's allowed, don't bring a car to campus. You can take a campus shuttle, walk, or bike to class.

- Before you make a purchase, find out if there's a student discount for it. (Search online for "student discount" and the item you want.) You can save money on everything from movie tickets to a new computer.

- If you have access to a microwave or stove and a refrigerator, prepare simple meals on your own. (You may look back fondly on your Ramen years!)

- Take advantage of free or inexpensive leisure activities: hike, play sports, go to campus-sponsored lectures and performances.

- Use apps to check prices in a store against online retailers. Read reviews before making a significant purchase. Search for online coupons and promotions.

- Know your triggers. Do you buy more than you need just because it's a "Buy two, get one free" sale? Are you a sucker for end-of-season markdowns?

- Avoid late fees on anything—library books, DVD rentals, parking tickets. They add up faster than you expect.

- Don't blow bonus money. If your grandparents send a check for your birthday, resist the temptation to splurge. Put most of it into a back-up fund for unexpected expenses or new money goals.

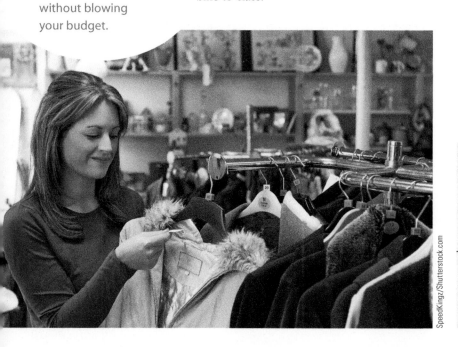

By shopping at thrift or consignment stores, you can buy items you need without blowing your budget.

🔧 **Stress Reliever:** Do I Need This? Or Do I Just Want It?

You need to buy a bus pass or gas for your car. Do you need a morning latte? A cool phone cover?

Get in the habit of distinguishing between needs and wants. After a few months on campus, track your expenses, and put a plan into action. For instance, you might

> give yourself a weekly cash allowance rather than carry a debit card, and when that week's allowance is gone, wait until next week for your "wants." Also consider using those "wants" as rewards for yourself when you accomplish tasks and meet deadlines.

Personal Finances 101

Even the smartest students can end up making dumb money mistakes. The less students know about personal finances, the greater their credit card debt—and their financial stress.

Your Credit Score

As soon as you use a credit card, take out a loan, or pay utilities, you start building your financial reputation based on your credit history, a track record of your credit use as recorded by three different credit bureaus. Your **credit score** is calculated using both positive and negative information found in your credit report, which is a summary of your credit history. The most commonly used credit score, produced by FICO, ranges from 300 to 850. (To learn which factors are considered and which have the most weight in your score, visit www.onyourown.org.)

A good credit score shows that you pay your bills in a consistent and timely manner and can be trusted to make responsible decisions and to honor commitments. Typically, one late bill or missed payment will not leave an irreparable black mark on your credit score. Several late payments, on the other hand, will. In turn, a poor credit score shows that you have a history of late or missed payments. This means you may be denied an apartment or have to pay more for a car loan, insurance, or mortgage. Prospective employers as well as landlords and service providers may check applicants' credit scores before hiring or renting to them.

To build or improve your credit score:

- Pay everything on time, from basic expenses and utilities to loan and credit card payments.

- Use only 25 percent of the total credit available to you, so it doesn't look like you're heavily relying on it to get by.

- Never max out your credit card—that's a red flag to lenders.

- Check your credit report regularly. You can request a free report by going to www.annualcreditreport.com.

- Correct any inaccuracies you see on your credit history immediately.

Banking Basics

To decide which bank is best for you, compare what different ones offer. Here are some important questions to ask:

- How much money do I need to deposit to open an account?

- Is there a transaction fee for debit card transactions?

- Is there a charge for withdrawing money from an ATM machine?

- Does it offer a student or basic checking account with low or no monthly fees?

- Does it offer online banking, mobile deposits, text alerts, and 24-hour customer service?

- Can you set up automatic transfers or bill-pay services?

- Are there penalties for monthly account use? Falling below a minimum balance? Using an ATM not owned by the bank? Overdrafts?

- Will you receive statements via mail or electronically?

Banking rules allow consumers to choose whether or not they will be charged overdraft fees for debit card and ATM transactions. By opting in, you authorize your bank to allow your transactions to go through even if you are short money in your account. This will result in the financial institution charging you fees for the overdraft. If you opt-out, your transaction will be denied.

Here are some guidelines to avoid banking penalties and problems:

- Every time you write a check, enter the amount into your checkbook register and subtract it from your balance.

- Make sure to list ATM, debit card, credit card, and online transactions in your register as well.

- Don't assume your account balance at the ATM is correct. If you made purchases that haven't been processed by your bank yet, the ATM balance will be higher than the amount of money you really have. The same is true for your online bank balance.

- When the bank mails or posts your checking account statement each month, compare the bank's figures with your own and balance your checkbook. If you have questions, ask someone at the bank to help you.

credit score A rating based on your history of paying credit card, utilities, loans, rent, and other debts.

- Keep your records safe. If you suspect someone else has gained access to your checking account, report it to your bank immediately. They can place a freeze on your account so it cannot be used.

Avoid Debit and Credit Card Stress

Using credit cards—as the majority of undergraduates do—is not only convenient but also a good way to start building credit.[9] However, it's easy for students to amass a large amount of credit debt.

Here's how to avoid this common and serious source of stress:

- Keep one or, at most, two credit or debit cards (See Table 5.3.). Resist the temptation to sign up for more simply to get a mug, flash drive, or whatever else on-campus vendors are offering.

- Shop around for a card that has no annual fee, a lower interest rate, and a 20- to 30-day grace period (the amount of time you have to pay for new purchases before interest is charged). Avoid cards that charge a one-time processing fee and cards with low introductory interest rates that shoot up in a few months. You can shop for the best credit card deals on sites such as www.bankrate.com.

- Consider getting a credit card that's secured by a bank deposit, meaning that you have enough money in a savings account to equal the credit limit on the card. A secured credit card can help you get used to handling credit while building a good credit history.

- Don't charge anything you can't pay for right away. If you have a real emergency, allow yourself three months to repay the charge in full.

- Mail the payment several days before the due date so you won't be charged a late fee.

- Stick with the card you've chosen. The longer your credit history, the more your credit score will rise.

- Subtract your credit card purchases from your checking account so you'll have enough money to pay the bill in full each month.

- Do not use a cash advance from a credit card unless you have a serious emergency. You'll probably pay a fee for the money, and you'll be charged interest immediately.

- Avoid lending your cards to anyone, even close friends. Never leave your cards in plain sight, even in your room.

At the end of your billing cycle, the card provider gives you a certain number of days (known as your grace period) to pay back what you owe, or at least a minimum payment. Paying the minimum each month is important, because you avoid a costly fee. However, if you only pay the minimum, you leave the rest of the money on your card (effectively your balance), where it will accrue interest until you pay it off. How much depends on your card.

Each credit card has a different **APR (annual percentage rate)**, the amount of interest it charges each year on your balance. A **fixed interest rate** stays the same over time. A **variable interest rate** changes over time and can be raised

APR (annual percentage rate) The amount of interest a credit card company charges each year on the unpaid balance.

fixed interest rate An interest rate that stays the same over time.

variable interest rate A rate that changes over time and can be raised at any time, or in response to your credit behavior.

TABLE 5.3 Credit Cards versus Debit Cards

Debit Card	Credit Card
Can get from bank	Can get from bank or other company
Might charge fees	Might charge fees
Can make purchases online	Can make purchases online
Money taken interest-free from checking account	Money borrowed interest-free from card provider, if paid back on time (charged interest, if paid back later)
Does not help build credit history	Helps build credit history
Free to withdraw cash from bank's ATM (charged fee if another bank's ATM)	Charged interest on cash advance from ATM or card
Does not offer rewards	Often offers rewards for use

at any time, or in response to your credit behavior. An **introductory interest rate** starts low—sometimes as low as 0 percent—but increases after a certain period of time. Many cards charge different interest rates for different types of purchases. For example, you might incur a lower interest rate on everyday purchases such as groceries and gas and a higher interest rate on a cash advance.

Digital Financial Management

Do you use Apple Pay at the bookstore? Venmo for your share of the rent or take-out bill? Affirm for a sweater on an online clothing retailer? As smartphones are replacing wallets, digital financial services are transforming consumer banking. Thanks to electronic deposits, debits, and statements, you can make financial transactions from almost anywhere, often with a single swipe.

While digital solutions may make many routine transactions faster and simpler, they don't alter the fundamentals of financial responsibility. You still need to balance income and expenses, meet payment deadlines, and monitor where your money is going. Keep track of your spending, and download records of your daily transactions. Check the balance in your accounts frequently to avoid overdrafts or spot fraudulent transactions. It may be easier than ever to buy something on impulse, but that doesn't mean you can afford to do so.

When shopping or banking online:

• Shop only on secured sites (sites with a Web address that starts with https).

• Log out of any accounts before you shut down your computer (e.g., email, bank account, student account).

• Password-protect your phone and apps. Download software updates regularly. Take advantage of security technology such as fingerprint logins.

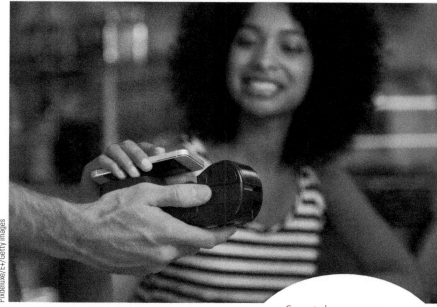

Pixdeluxe/E+/Getty Images

Debt Relief

✔ **Check-in:** Are you in over your head?

How do you know when you're in debt trouble? Check any of the statements that apply to you:

_____ You don't know how much money you owe.

_____ You use credit cards to pay for everything, even shampoo at the drugstore.

_____ You borrow from one credit card to pay another.

_____ You make only the minimum payment on your credit card bill.

_____ You miss payments.

_____ You pay your bills late.

Smartphone apps make many money transactions easier, but you need to take precautions to safeguard your accounts.

introductory interest rate A rate that starts low but increases after a certain period of time.

_____ Creditors telephone you to ask where their money is.

_____ You get a job just to pay off your credit card.

Even one checkmark is a financial stress signal. Don't wait for things to get worse. Talk to your parents, a resident advisor, or a financial aid officer. You also can seek advice from a nonprofit debt-counseling organization, such as the National Foundation for Credit Counseling (www.nfcc.org).

The sooner you can start digging out of a financial jam, the less stressed you'll feel. Put away your credit cards, but don't close down the accounts completely. You might need them at some point, and closing your accounts can have a negative impact on your credit score. Contact your creditors directly and ask them to lower your rates. Make a budget to determine how much money you can set aside to pay off debt.

Protect Your Private Information

Identity thieves often prey on college students. Avoid checking your bank balance with a public computer. If you must use one, be sure to log out of your account completely and clear the cache on the web browser. Here are some other steps to take to prevent someone else from spending your money or using your credit cards:

- Don't give anyone your Social Security, credit card, or bank account numbers unless you know why the individual or organization is requesting them. If you are unsure, ask the person to send you a request by mail instead of asking for it over the telephone. Delete e-mails requesting personal information.

- Don't just throw away papers that list important account numbers or other financial numbers. Shred anything with your name, address, credit card information, or bank account numbers before putting it in the trash or recycle bin. This includes unused credit card offers.

- Don't send your credit card number over the Internet unless you are sure the website is secure and your computer is protected by a firewall and anti-virus, anti-spyware, and other security software. Keep your security software updated.

- Keep your credit card and ATM receipts in a safe place until you've paid the credit card bill or balanced your checkbook. Then tear them up or shred them before throwing them away.

- Review your credit card statements and telephone bills for unauthorized use. If you suspect fraud, call the company immediately.

- Check your computer for malware (malicious software that affects your computer).

- If you're a victim of identity theft, report the crime to the police and your bank immediately.

- Opt out of pre-approval offers.

- Sign up for paperless billing.

- Avoid oversharing on social networks. Leave your full name, address, and birth date out of your profiles. Ignore friend requests from people you don't know.

If you suspect your identity has been stolen, act quickly. Most people who steal financial information use it within 48 hours. With a credit card, your maximum liability is $50. However, with a debit card you have to report fraud quickly to ensure you get your money back. If you report a lost or stolen debit card within 48 hours, your liability for unauthorized charges is $50. Between 49 hours and 60 days, your liability goes up to $500. After 60 days, you might be liable for all of the charges.

Alert the credit reporting agencies. Contact one of the credit reporting agencies (Equifax, TransUnion, or Experian). Ask the agency to place a fraud alert on your file to make it harder for someone to open new accounts in your name. A basic alert lasts 90 days, but you can extend it to 7 years.

Report the theft to the Federal Trade Commission. Complete its online complaint form, giving as many details as you can. Save and print out your FTC Identity Theft Affidavit. Report the theft to the police. so you have official record of the fraud. You'll need this, along with the FTC Affidavit, to prove to businesses that identity theft occurred. To remedy some of the damage, close any new accounts that have been opened in your name. Remove any unauthorized charges from your accounts. Correct any fraudulent entries on your credit report.

Taking Control

Are you squeezed for space? Running out of time? Short of cash? If so, you understandably feel stressed. How long and how severely you're stressed depends on whether you can take control and make the most of the space, time, and money available to you. What can you do today to take more control?

- Spend a few extra minutes organizing everything you need to take with you tomorrow.

Don't shut off your light and go to bed until you've cleared away the empty water bottles and stacked the papers on your desk.

- Throughout your day, capture the inevitable lulls between activities by preparing for them. Download assigned readings or apps to your phone so you have them wherever you go. If you're waiting for an appointment or a class, put the time to use.

- Work intensely. It is far better to work intensively for 45 to 50 minutes on a highly specific piece of a project and finish that piece by giving it your full attention, than to block out an hour and a half and flit in and out of concentrating.

- Keep a rainy day fund. Set aside a small amount of money every week—just so you won't be stressed by an unanticipated expense.

Chapter Summary

- Managing your space, time, and money doesn't require anything magical. Step-by-step techniques enable you to choose wisely how you use them.

- Disorder arises from putting off tasks or not completing an activity you've already begun. Disorder undermines pleasure as well as efficiency because it upsets your internal well-being.

- Wherever you are, get in the habit of leaving at least one small space more orderly than you found it. This guarantees progress because order becomes an ongoing task, rather than a once-in-a-blue-moon blitz.

- Your work space should be a private sanctuary. Everything in your space should work for you and support you. Position your computer so the screen is at eye level and the keyboard so that your elbows are bent at a 90-degree angle and your hands and wrists are straight.

- Each morning, decide what you are going to do during the rest of the day and tomorrow, what your top priority will be, and how you will go about getting your work done.

- Before you begin a task, visualize yourself completing the steps the process requires. This cues the mind and prepares it like any other run-through or rehearsal.

- If you have many tasks, do the most difficult ones early in the day. Save the easy ones for the afternoon when your circadian rhythms dip and your energy lags.

- People procrastinate because they lack smart, effective strategies and skills for making efficient use of time, or they fall back on inefficient, self-defeating habits that steal precious time.

- To-do lists can help you manage and structure your day in real time. Use a reminder or notepad app on your phone to write down the things you need to do and remember.

- The brain performs even simple actions one after another in a strict linear sequence. Unless they are completely mechanical ones, multitasking destroys the quality of attention given to the tasks at hand.

- Schedule your work in 50–55 minute segments, with breaks in-between. Whenever possible, dispatch simple things in one fell swoop.

- If you commute to campus, try to avoid rush hour traffic or crowded subways or buses. Whenever you can, schedule classes back to back or during one part of the day (all morning or all evening, for example) so that you can concentrate academics into one block of time.

- Use a calendar—either the old-fashioned paper type or one on your phone, watch, or tablet—from the very first day of the term. Mark on your calendar all assignment due dates and exams. Break big projects up into smaller pieces and give yourselves deadlines for each.

- The best way to take charge of your money is to define your financial goals, make plans for how to reach them, and take action to make your goals a reality.

- Create a set of files for all your financial information and documents so you can keep track of due dates, record payments, and identify any errors.

- Identity thieves often prey on college students. Avoid checking your bank balance with a public computer. Don't send your credit card number over the Internet unless you are sure the website is secure and your computer is protected by a firewall and anti-virus, anti-spyware, and other security software.

- Using credit cards is a good way to start building credit. Pay the whole balance. If you can't, at least pay more than the minimum due to keep interest charges down.

- The spending and saving habits that you develop in college are likely to stay with you throughout your adult life. This is one of the reasons that money management for college students is so important.

STRESS RELIEVERS

One Simple Thing

Think of one thing that could make your life easier. What if you put a hook up to hold your keys so you don't spend five minutes searching for them every morning? What if you backed up your files to the Cloud every night so you'd never again lose a draft? Taking action, however small, boosts your sense of control and lowers your stress.

Don't Hit the Sack

You've finally finished your last assignment, and you're absolutely, utterly exhausted. You look at the books stacked on the floor and the papers strewn over your desk. "Forget it," you think. All you want to do is crawl into bed.

Don't. Take 10 or 15 minutes to put your work space back in order. Gather the notes for your term paper into a file. Put your textbooks back on the shelf.

Taking the time to put your work space in order produces many benefits, including creating an inviting space to which to return. You'll love yourself for it in the morning.

The 15-minute Cleanup

Who has a whole day to clear out an overstuffed closet or haul months' worth of gear out of the trunk of a car? Of course, you don't. But surely you can snatch 15 minutes from the time you'd otherwise spend surfing the net or streaming videos. That's all you need to get started.

Don't wait for more disorder to accumulate. And don't fall into the trap of telling yourself that there's no point in starting until you can get it all done at once. You only create more disorder by putting off a task. Make whatever headway you can in 15 minutes every day during your regular week. On a weekend, set a timer to alert you every hour. Spend 15 minutes organizing and the other 45 minutes however you choose. Before long you will finish. And if you keep up the same pattern, you will maintain order.

Block out 15-minute slots for targeted bursts of organizational energy on your daily and weekly calendars. Why? Scheduling moves you from "someday, I've got to do this" good intentions to taking action in real time. A schedule, along with a specific commitment to always follow it strictly, will keep you focused.

Learn How to Tell Time

Of course, you know about the big hand and the little hand. But do you think you can knock off six calculus problems in an hour? Plow through *The Divine Comedy* in an evening? Prepare a PowerPoint presentation in 20 minutes?

Many students have a wishful-thinking view of time. They so underestimate how much time they need for their work that they overestimate how much time is available for streaming a game live on their smart phones.

To teach yourself how to estimate time accurately, compare your predictions of how long a task will take with how much time it actually demands when you do it. Identify one assignment, such as reading a chapter or outlining a class presentation. Then just do it.

Don't take shortcuts. Work intensively and with concentration. Keep track of how much time you spend on the outline, subtracting time off for breaks or interruptions. Then see how this compares with your estimate.

Begin

The single most effective antidote to procrastination is starting. Don't flog yourself to tackle the chore you hate most; just do step one. If the long-delayed job is cleaning the bathroom, tell yourself that all you are going to do now is take the basic equipment—cleaning solutions, brushes, rubber gloves, whatever—into the bathroom. Once you get there, having started the process, you will find it much easier to go ahead and complete the job.

Eavesdrop on Your Excuses

If you're a chronic procrastinator, you may not even be aware of the thoughts that run through your mind when you put something off. Every time you balk at writing the first sentence of a report, doing a literature search, making a certain phone call, or reading the first page of the assigned novel, stop and listen to what you're telling yourself. Here's what you are likely to hear:

- "I'm too tired. I'll rest first, watch a little TV, and then start."

- "There's no point in starting. I've got to meet my friend Navi in ten minutes."

- "I've got plenty of time to do it later."

- "I'll organize my desk first."

- "It's too nice to stay inside."

- "I don't have everything I need."

- "I've been working really hard. I deserve a break."

- "I'll do a better job tomorrow."

- "I need a good idea to inspire me."

- "I should exercise before it gets dark."

- "Why do it on Friday? The instructor won't get it. It's not due until Monday."

- "I can read that book in a few hours."

Think of rebuttals to yourself. For instance, you might say, "Yes, I'm tired. I'll just work for half an hour, and then I'll go to bed." Or you might tell yourself, "I'll see how much I can get done in 10 minutes." Or you could say, "I'm tired of making excuses. I choose to take time every day to focus and study because I am choosing to succeed and feel good about accomplishing something."

Do I Need This? Or do I Just Want It?

You need to buy a bus pass or gas for your car. Do you need a morning latte? A cool phone cover?

Get in the habit of distinguishing between needs and wants. After a few months on campus, track your expenses and put a plan into action. For instance, you might give yourself a weekly cash allowance rather than carry a debit card, and when that week's allowance is gone, wait until next week for your "wants." Also consider using those "wants" as rewards for yourself when you accomplish tasks and meet deadlines.

No-Stress Banking

- **Find out when your bank processes transactions.** If you make a purchase on the weekend, will it show up as a pending charge until the bank opens on Monday?

- **Make things automatic.** Set up direct deposit for your financial aid and paychecks and auto bill pay for all your routine services so you don't forget pay them.

- **Take advantage of notifications.** Many banks will email or text you if your account balance is low or something's changed on your account.

- **Password-protect everything.** Set up different passwords for your online bank account, email address (where you'll receive any statements or notifications from your bank), and smartphone and mobile banking apps.

- **Monitor your spending.** Review your online transactions and be mindful of your account balance at all times (you don't want to spend money you don't have).

- **Balance your account each month.** Verify each transaction on your statement and review your spending line by line. You want to make sure you didn't get double-charged somewhere and that your account hasn't been compromised.

⊜ YOUR PERSONAL STRESS MANAGEMENT TOOLKIT

REFLECTION: Do You Have a Procrastination Problem?

Check each of the following behaviors that apply to you:

_____ I put off studying subjects I find difficult.

_____ I put off studying subjects I'm not interested in.

_____ I put off studying subjects I find easy because I don't think they will demand much time.

_____ I put off starting papers or projects until right before the deadline.

_____ I do my grocery shopping when there is no food at all left in my fridge.

_____ I do my best work under pressure when I concentrate my energy and attention.

_____ I procrastinate in some of my subjects.

_____ I procrastinate in all of my subjects.

_____ I usually have to pull all-nighters to get my work done.

_____ I wait to have a big block of time before starting a project.

_____ I wait to do my laundry until there are no clean clothes left.

_____ I often miss deadlines because I delayed doing the work.

_____ I have missed important deadlines for filing applications, signing up for classes, and so on.

The more lines you check, the greater your problem with procrastination. Answer each of the following questions:

_____ Are you using procrastination as a smokescreen for your lack of confidence?

_____ Is it easier to delay, put off, or come up with an excuse than deal with demands and expectations? Maybe you'd rather have people conclude that you could have gotten a better grade or done better work if you hadn't procrastinated.

_____ Do you feel that no one understands how much you have to do and why you cannot meet a deadline?

_____ Do you want everyone to realize how busy and overcommitted you are?

_____ Is procrastinating your way of saying, "Don't think you can tell me what to do and when to do it"?

Consider all of these possibilities, and write a brief reflection.

TECHNIQUE: Complete the Incompletes

Every day find one thing that you began at some point but have not yet finished. It might be making the bed, replying to an email, buying a birthday card for your grandfather, replacing the bulb in your bedside lamp. Simply complete this "incomplete."

What you do doesn't matter, as long as you complete something unfinished. Do it now.

Make a daily journal entry of completed incompletes. Record what you did and how it felt to get it done. Don't let a day go by when you don't cross something off your to-do list—even if it's making a to-do list.

Your chore does not have to be something big and might take less than five minutes—folding the towels you washed last weekend, returning the charger you borrowed from a friend, paying your cell phone bill online. Most college students have such a stash of "incompletes" that they can do this exercise for a long time without running out of tasks. If you also work or have children, you may have a lifetime supply.

As you proceed, observe the surprising immediate effects. You probably feel an unexpected boost. The reason? "Incompletes" suck energy. Completing them releases the energy they monopolize. You will feel lighter and more energetic from the first completion the very first day.

When you have done this exercise daily for a week, add the following additional exercise:

- Begin one mildly unpleasant thing that stretches you a bit. Do not attempt too big a step. And select something only mildly difficult.

- Don't groan; Don't protest; Stay with us! You do not have to crawl over cut glass or endure physical challenges like a reality show contestant. But we do want you to experience what happens when you take on a mild dose of challenge instead of postponing or evading it.

- To complete this exercise, you could choose to do something practical that you find tedious, such as folding your socks or sorting old papers, or something less practical like organizing your digital photos.

- But why not kill two birds with the same stone? Why not do something practical that will simultaneously further your academic success? For instance, study for the class you find most difficult as early as possible in the day. In addition to completing one incomplete every day, faithfully add this mild stretch activity to your daily routine for three weeks, and observe the effects.

Note that choosing to do first what you might otherwise have done last creates immediate payoffs. For starters, you complete the more challenging study task when you are freshest; this alone can create a positive ripple effect. Handling tough course material early on can make it easier to comprehend. When you understand the content better, you may enjoy the work and the class more. As a bonus, your grade may improve as well.

Secondly, you send yourself powerful positive messages about your ability to handle something difficult. As you work on these tasks, the work you do works on you. By practicing simple exercises repetitively, you increase your tenacity and persistence and, in the process, make your locus of control more internal. You will be well on your way to mastering the tool of making your own luck.

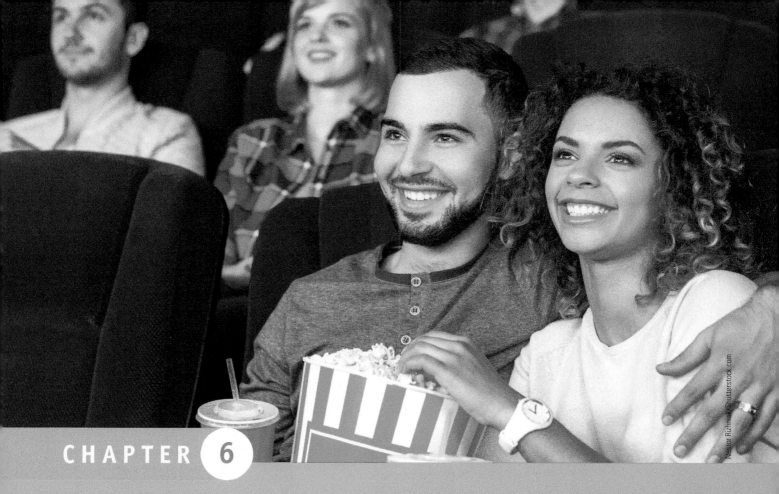

CHAPTER 6

Relationships, Social Health, and Stress

After reading this chapter, you should be able to:

6.1 Assess the influence of supportive relationships on social health.

6.2 Develop better listening and communication skills.

6.3 Discuss issues that can affect the development of healthy relationships.

6.4 Explain the ways in which social media and other forms of computer-mediated communication have changed personal relationships.

6.5 Examine the ways in which sexual and romantic relationships have changed in recent decades.

6.6 Describe the connection between a lack of close relationships and stress-related illnesses.

6.7 Identify the signs of dysfunctional relationships.

6.8 Analyze the emotional impact of breakups.

6.9 Summarize guidelines to build and maintain good relationships.

Positive Indicators

If you're currently involved with someone, read through this list of positive indicators of a healthy relationship and check all that apply.

_____ You feel at ease with your partner.

_____ You feel good about your partner when you're together and when you're not.

_____ Your partner is open with you about his or her life—past, present, and future.

_____ You can say no to each other without feeling guilty.

_____ You feel cared for, appreciated, and accepted as you are.

_____ Your partner really listens to what you have to say.

The more items you've checked, the more reasons you have to keep seeing each other.

Negative Indicators

Read through this list of negative indicators below and check those that apply. In this case, every check is a red flag warning of dangers ahead.

_____ You don't feel comfortable together.

_____ You feel angry or let down, either when you're together or apart.

_____ Your partner is very secretive about his or her life.

_____ Your partner makes you feel bad if you don't go along with what he/she wants.

_____ You don't feel cared for and appreciated.

_____ Your partner makes critical or snarky comments about the way you look, talk, dress, and so on.

Reflect on the pluses and minuses of your relationship. Are there more positives or negatives?

Tom has more than 1,000 friends—most of them virtual. Jasmine video chats daily with her high school boyfriend at another school but occasionally hooks up with someone on campus. Leena wants to come out but feels wary about approaching the girl she likes. Jessica and Nick are talking about becoming exclusive. Brad and Jason are getting married. Gretchen, divorced last year, is splitting custody of their two children with her ex.

Ask any of these undergraduates to describe their significant relationships, and you might get the same answer: complicated—as many are these days. It may be easier to interact instantaneously with people around the world, but it's as challenging as ever to communicate clearly and to forge meaningful connections.

Scientists who study relationships are just beginning to explore the brave new digital world. Will texts, tweets, and emoticons replace conversation? Can people find true love with a swipe of a finger? Does online social networking ease stress or add to it? No one knows the answers yet, but as much as technology may change our lives, one thing remains constant: We always have craved and always will crave connection.

As humans, we are wired for relationships. From our first days of life, we reach out to others, struggle to express ourselves, strive to forge bonds. The fabric of our lives becomes richer as family and friends weave through it the threads of their experiences. As individuals and as part of society, we need to care about others and to know that others care about us, to feel for others and have others feel for us, to share what we know and to learn from what others know.

Just as stress can be positive or negative, relationships can range from happy and fulfilling to draining and destructive. Healthy, mutually beneficial relationships add joy to our years and perhaps even years to our lives. Unhealthy or dysfunctional ones can be so stressful that they can undermine health as well as happiness. In the American College Health Association (ACHA) national survey, "an intimate relationship" ranked third among student stressors after academics and finances.[1]

All of us want to be acknowledged, admired, treated with respect, and rewarded—and others want the same things from us. Sooner or later we're all blindsided, disappointed, frustrated, irritated, or otherwise challenged by relationships. Sometimes you can see trouble coming and take steps to avoid it. In other cases, however hard you try, you can't run or hide from a problem. However, you can gain insight into social stress and develop skills for building stronger relationships—as this chapter will show.

Social Health and Support

Social health is the ability to:

- interact effectively with other people and with the social environment.
- develop satisfying interpersonal relationships.
- fulfill social roles.

Social health doesn't necessarily mean joining organizations or mingling in large groups, but it does involve participating in your community, living in harmony with others, communicating clearly, and forming mutually fulfilling relationships.

✔ **Check-in:** How would you assess your social health? Excellent? Average? Not as good as you'd like?

Social support refers to the ways in which we provide information or assistance, comfort, and confide in others. As large epidemiological studies have demonstrated, supportive relationships buffer us from stress, distress, and disease. People with close ties to others have stronger cardiovascular and immune systems, resist colds better, and are less vulnerable to serious illness and premature death.

Those with fewer emotional connections or in unhealthy or dysfunctional relationships are more susceptible to physical illnesses and psychological difficulties. Among college students, a sense of **belongingness**[2], feelings of connection to family, peers, and institutions, ease stress and reduce suicidal thoughts (reported by as many as half of students at some point in their lives.)

Even a hug can lessen stress and boost health. In a recent study, volunteers who hugged before being exposed to a common upper respiratory virus were much less likely to come down

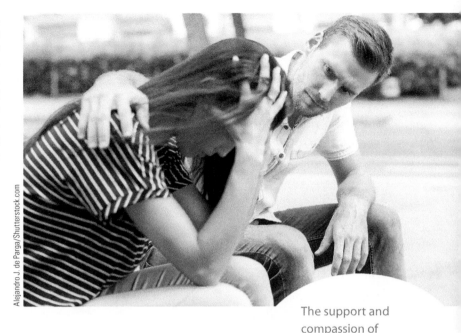

Alejandro J. de Parga/Shutterstock.com

The support and compassion of friends can buffer the harmful effects of stress.

with colds. Among those who did get sick, those who received more frequent hugs had less severe symptoms. The reason may be that hugging boosts levels of oxytocin, the bonding hormone that plays a role in the tend-and-befriend response to stress.[3]

✔ **Check-in:** Whom do you turn to when feeling stressed?

Your support network might consist of people you see almost every day; more casual acquaintances; and friends, followers, and bloggers you get to know online (social networking is covered later in this chapter). Simply staying in touch and sharing each other's lives bolster feelings of self-worth, security, and belonging. In times of stress, relationships can be a great comfort. In a national poll, three quarters of college students said that when stressed they turn to friends; nearly two thirds turn to their parents; and half turn to their siblings.

Even a relationship with a pet can soothe stress. Companion or support animals have proven beneficial in lessening psychological symptoms like anxiety and depression, easing the sting of rejection, and boosting a sense of well-being. In a recent study, students who petted or played with a dog reported less anxiety and a more positive mood.[4] The calming effects of domesticated animals has gained such wide acceptance that many colleges allow students with diagnosed mental disorders to keep support animals—dogs, cats, lizards, guinea pigs, ferrets, rats, snakes, even potbellied pigs—in

social health The ability to interact effectively with other people and with the social environment, develop satisfying interpersonal relationships, and fulfill social roles.

social support The ways in which we provide information or assistance, comfort, and confide in others.

belongingness Feelings of connection to family, peers, and institutions

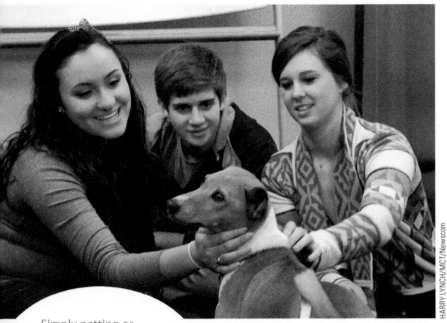

Simply petting or playing with a dog or support animal can soothe anxiety and boost spirits.

their dorms. Some bring in trained therapy dogs to interact with students during high-stress exam times. (See Chapter 15 for more on pet therapy.)

Support benefits both givers and recipients. **Altruism**—helping or giving to others—relieves physical and mental stress and protects psychological well-being. Hans Selye, the father of stress research, described cooperation with others for the self's sake as **altruistic egotism**, in which we satisfy our own needs while helping others, satisfy theirs. This concept is essentially an updated version of the golden rule: Do unto others as you would have them do unto you. The important difference is that you earn and enjoy your neighbor's love and help by offering yours. (See Chapter 10 for more on altruism.)

Getting Along with Others

More people may have come into your life since starting college than in all the years before: roommates, classmates, teammates, lab partners, teaching assistants, professors, librarians, tutors, counselors, advisors, deans, administrators, coaches, bosses, coworkers—not to mention the familiar faces on the campus shuttle or in the food court. You don't have to like them all, but learning how to get along with them can make your daily life a lot more pleasant and a lot

altruism Acts of helping or giving to others without thought of self-benefit.

altruistic egotism Offering support to others in ways that satisfy the needs of both giver and recipient.

social intelligence The skills that create relationships worth cherishing.

less stressful. That's why it's worth boosting your communications skills.

Communicating 101

Communication stems from a desire to know and a decision to tell. The first step is learning how to listen. Then you choose what information about yourself to disclose and what to keep private. In opening up to others, you increase your own self-knowledge and understanding. By mastering skills to communicate more effectively and by being responsible in your interactions with others, you can cultivate what psychologists call "**social intelligence**," the skills that create relationships worth cherishing.

A great deal of daily communication focuses on facts: the who, what, where, when, and how. Information is easy to convey and comprehend; emotions are not. Some people have great difficulty saying "I appreciate you" or "I care about you," even though they are genuinely appreciative and caring. Others find it hard to know what to say in response and how to accept such expressions of affection.

Communications often carry hidden messages about loyalty, values, morals, lifestyle choices, rivalry, compatibility jealousy, and control that play out in classrooms and workplaces. Not everyone you meet is equally as stable or trustworthy as you might wish. Keep an open mind about the people you meet, but maintain distance and discretion, particularly when it comes to sharing personal information—anything from your passwords and credit card numbers to your sexual history.

Nonverbal Communication

....

✔ **Check-in:** Body talk
....

How are you standing or sitting?
....

Are you slumping with your shoulders forward and your chin down? Or are your shoulders back and chin up?
....

How about your stomach? Is it pouching out, or are you pulling it in?
....

Try an experiment: Slouch, and then sit or stand tall. Which posture makes you feel stressed? Which boosts your confidence?

Walk around with your stomach in and your shoulders back.
....

Let your body language remind you to take charge of the way you look and feel.
....

More than 90 percent of communication may be nonverbal. While we speak with our vocal cords, we communicate with our facial expressions, tone of voice, hands, shoulders, legs, torsos, our posture. Body language is the building block upon which more advanced verbal forms of communication rest. Whether you use it to signal your interest in an attractive classmate, impress a potential employer, or soothe a child, conscious body language can make a big difference.

Here are some suggestions for sending the messages you want without being misinterpreted:

- Control your stress signals. Identify the little things you characteristically do when you're tense—whether it's fiddling with your cuticles, fidgeting with small objects, or tensing your shoulders and neck. Train yourself to become aware of what you're doing (have a friend or colleague give you a signal, if necessary), and to control them so they don't undermine the strength of what you want to say.

- Pay special attention to posture. If you sit squarely in a chair, feet on the floor and arms on the hand rests, shoulders straight, you'll

look as though you're in charge. If you slump or jiggle your foot, you'll seem disinterested, discouraged, or distressed.

- Look others straight in the eyes, especially when you're just introduced. Eye contact is the most remembered element in forming an impression of someone. When addressing a group, never look down when making an important point.

- Use gestures to add a visual dimension to your speech. According to the research findings, people who use gestures to illustrate their speech are seen as more sociable, friendly, and authoritative. But don't overdo. If you flail your arms about, you'll look overwrought and out of control.

- Avoid putting up barriers. If you cross your arms across your chest, you'll look defensive or uninterested in contact. If you keep your hand over mouth, others may assume your ideas aren't really worth hearing.

- Touch with caution. In some circumstances, a touch can be extremely effective; however, it can easily be misinterpreted. If you wouldn't want a photo of you touching the other person to appear online, don't do it.

Active Listening

Whom do you love to talk with? Your best friend, roommate, significant other, spouse, coworker, Mom, childhood pal? The guy who cuts your hair? The server at a campus cafe? Your dog? Whoever they are, we know something about them: They are good listeners (yup, even your dog). They want to hear what you have to say just as, if not more, than they want to say something to you.

Good listeners may seem lucky. They strike up conversations with total strangers. At parties everyone wants to talk to them. Their relationships tend to be rock solid. Teachers like them; bosses praise them. But luck has nothing to do with it. Listening is a skill that anyone can acquire.

Attentive, authentic listening is more than hearing words being spoken. It is hearing what's being said nonverbally as well as verbally, processing the information, being able to reflect back the content, and utilizing appropriate verbal and non-verbal responses. This is called **active or reflective listening.** It expresses real interest and makes another person feel that he or she is being understood. It also communicates to others

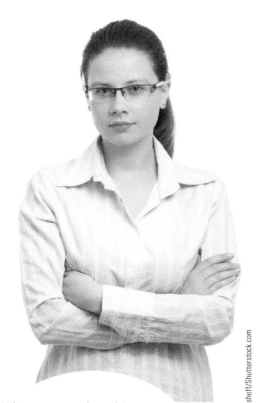

What message does this woman's expression and body language convey?

active or reflective listening Hearing what's being said nonverbally as well as verbally, processing the information, being able to reflect back the content, and utilizing appropriate verbal and non-verbal responses.

that you want to know and understand how they feel and think. This sort of sincere interest makes others feel that what they say matters simply because they are saying it.

The goal of all good listening is to seek to understand the other person before you seek to be understood. In the process you may learn more than you might imagine. If you would like to take a relationship to another level, see what happens when you listen up. And if you're shy or feel self-conscious in social settings, expect an added return on your investment. Knowing how to listen can help you—and the people around you—feel at ease. (See "Listen Up" in the Personal Stress Management Toolkit on page 123.)

How Men and Women Communicate

Gender differences in communication start early. By age 1, boys make less eye contact than girls and pay more attention to moving objects like cars than to human faces. Both mothers and fathers talk less about feelings (except anger) to sons than daughters, and boys' vocabularies include fewer "feeling" words. On the playground, if not at home, boys learn to choke back tears and show no fear. Their faces—once as openly emotional as girls'—become less expressive as they move through the elementary years.

As adults, men use fewer words and talk, at least in public, as a means of putting themselves in a one-up situation—unlike women, who engage in conversation to draw others closer. Even with friends, men mainly swap information as they talk shop, sports, cars, and computers. In studies of language, linguists have identified the differences shown in Figure 6.1, which may be based on sex or gender roles.

Agreeable but Assertive

....
✔ **Check-in:** When was the last time you asserted yourself? When was the last time you wished you had?
....

There's an old saying that "nice guys finish last," but research says shows that's not the case. Psychologists translate "niceness" into a personality trait called "agreeableness," which includes being helpful, unselfish, genuinely warm, and concerned for others. The proven benefits of agreeableness are many: less stress and conflict, strong relationships, happy marriages, better job performance, healthier eating habits and behaviors, and fewer medical complaints. But agreeable people aren't so "nice" that they are easily influenced or taken advantage of by others. In situations that call for it, they become assertive.

Assertive communication involves recognizing your feelings and making your needs and desires clear to others. It differs from:

- Passive communication, which stems from the erroneous belief that your needs don't matter. Passive communicators

Men:

- Speak more often and for longer periods in public.

- Interrupt more, breaking in on another's monologue if they aren't getting the information they need.

- Look into a woman's eyes more often when talking than they would if talking with another man.

- When writing, use more numbers, more prepositions, and more articles such as *an* and *the*.

- Write briefer, more utilitarian e-mails.

- In blogs or chat rooms, are more likely to make strong assertions, disagree with others, and use profanity and sarcasm.

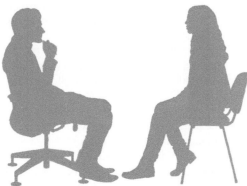

Women:

- Speak more in private, usually to build better connections with others.

- Are generally better listeners, facilitating conversation by nodding, asking questions, and signaling interest by saying "uh-huh" or "yes."

- Are more likely to wait for a speaker to finish rather than interrupt.

- Look into another woman's eyes more often than they would if talking with a man.

- When writing, use more words overall; more words related to emotion (positive and negative); more idea words; more hearing, feeling, and sensing words; more causal words (such as *because*); and more modal words (*would, should, could*).

- Write e-mails in much the same way they talk, using words to build a connection with people.

- In blogs or chat rooms, are more prone to posing questions, making suggestions, and including polite expressions.

FIGURE 6.1 He says/She says: Here are some of the gender differences in communication.

stay silent rather than speaking up, don't say what they really think, allow themselves to be bullied, give in, and try to keep the peace. Many people who cope by being passive and not expressing their feelings eventually become so irritated, frustrated, or overwhelmed that they explode in an outburst.

- Aggressive communication, which stems from the equally erroneous belief that only your needs matter. Aggressive communicators talk and interrupt others, look out only for themselves, bully others, and may shout or become violent. Aggressive people alienate others with their obnoxious behavior.

To communicate assertively, state your needs and preferences without sarcasm or hostility. Keep your ego in check, and focus on the point you are trying to make. Even at its mildest, assertiveness can make you feel better about yourself and your life. The reason: When you speak up or take action, you're in charge. And that's always much less stressful than taking a back seat and trying to hang on for dear life.

Here are some guidelines to keep in mind the next time you need to assert yourself:

- Use "I" statements to explain your feelings. For example, "I felt that . . ." or "I understood this to mean. . . ." This allows you to take ownership of your opinions and feelings without putting down others for how they feel and think.
- Listen to and acknowledge what the other person says. After you speak, find out if the other person understands your position. Ask how he or she feels about what you've said.
- Be direct and specific. Describe the problem as you see it, using neutral language rather than assigning blame. Begin statements with "When. . . ."
- Avoid generalizing or including tangential information. Focus on the exact event or situation at hand, reviewing the details.
- Address how to move forward in a productive and positive way. Suggest a specific solution, but make it clear that you'd like the lines of communication and negotiation to remain open.
- State your desired outcome, again using "I" statements, such as "I would like . . ." or "I prefer. . . ."
- Spell out the consequences. What will you do if the person's behavior or the situation

changes to your satisfaction? "If you do . . ., I will do. . . ." Be just as clear about what you intend to do if nothing changes. "If you don't . . ., I will do. . . ."

Forming Relationships

Relationships inevitably trigger stress—from the euphoric stress of shared triumphs to the dysphoric stress of conflict and loss. The way you respond determines the impact on your health and happiness.

Family Ties

Our families form the foundation of our lives. Ideally, they provide routines, traditions, clear roles and expectations, beliefs and values, and a positive emotional climate. **Family stress** is defined as a crisis that occurs in response to an event; its impact depends on its magnitude and the meaning attached to the event.[5]

For emerging adults (under age 25) who have experienced family stress during childhood or adolescence, entering college may mean breaking free from chaotic or dysfunctional relationships at home. They may gain a new perspective on family dynamics and improve their relationships with parents and siblings. For others, preoccupation with family problems can undermine their academic efforts, increase their stress, and lead to risky behaviors as a form of escape or rebellion.[6]

For students from all sorts of families, college brings new stressors, ranging from homesickness to academic pressure from parents, to providing care and assistance to relatives. Often students go through a back-and-forth process of distancing themselves from their families and seeking closeness and support. For those living at home, this balancing act may play out on a regular basis. Clear communication and genuine expressions of affection can help smooth the transition for both generations.

✔ **Check-in:** What is the most stressful relationship in your life? What steps can you take to lessen the stress?

Friendship

Friendship has been described as "the most holy bond of society." Every culture has prized the ties of respect, tolerance, and loyalty that friendship builds and nurtures. Friends can be a basic source of social support and happiness, a connection to

family stress A crisis that occurs in the response to an event; its impact depends on its magnitude and the meaning attached to the event by family members.

a larger world, and a source of solace in times of trouble. Although we have different friends throughout life, often the friendships of adolescence and young adulthood are the closest ones we ever form. They ease the normal break from parents and the transition from childhood to independence.

In our modern mobile society, we move time and again, leaving behind old friends. Social media, at the least, provide an opportunity to maintain friendships that would otherwise rapidly wither away. Everyday images of faraway friends can provide some of the same benefits as in-person friendship, including enhanced self-esteem and happiness.

Here are some of the keys to preserving and strengthening friendships:

- Don't try to fix a friend's problems. Offer support, but don't meddle—except in cases of physical danger.

- Be willing to be vulnerable. You can trust a true friend to accept you as you are—blemishes and all.

- Watch out for one-sided relationships. Is every conversation about your friend? Does your friend celebrate your good news and commiserate with your bad news?

- Know when to walk away. If you bring up a thorny issue and your friend either denies or dismisses it, turn elsewhere for a deeper relationship.

Loneliness

··

✔ **Check-in:** Have you felt very lonely at some time in the past 12 months?

··

If so, you're not alone. As many as 80 percent of those under age 18 and 40 percent of adults over age 65 report being lonely at least some of the time.[7] In the ACHA national survey, 59.2 percent of undergraduates reported feeling very lonely at some time in the past 12 months. **Loneliness**, defined as "feelings of distress and dysphoria resulting from a discrepancy between a person's desired and achieved social relations," stems from perceived, rather than actual, isolation. People may live relatively solitary lives and not feel lonely or, conversely, surround themselves with people yet feel lonely nonetheless.

Chronic loneliness, like other forms of ongoing stress, may impair the immune system and increase pain, depression, and fatigue.[8] In a review of studies involving more than 3 million people, loneliness and **social isolation**—having few or

no social contacts or activities—undermines a sense of well-being[9] and increases the risk of an earlier death for both men and women, particularly those under the age of 65.[10]

To combat loneliness, people may join groups, fling themselves into projects and activities, or surround themselves with superficial acquaintances. Others avoid the effort of trying to connect in person by mainly interacting online. The keys to overcoming loneliness are developing resources to fulfill your own potential and learning to reach out to others. In this way, loneliness can become a means to personal growth and discovery.

Shyness

··

✔ **Check-in:** Do you think of yourself as shy?

··

In some surveys, as many as 40 percent of people describe themselves as shy or uncomfortable in social situations. An estimated 10 to 15 percent of children are born with a predisposition to shyness. Other people become shy because they don't learn social skills or because they experience rejection or shame.

Some individuals are "fearfully" shy; that is, they withdraw and avoid contact with others and experience a high degree of anxiety and fear in social situations. Others are "self-consciously" shy. They enjoy the company of others but become extremely anxious in social situations.

 Stress Reliever: If You're Shy

You can overcome much of your social apprehensiveness on your own, in much the same way as you might set out to stop smoking or lose weight. For example, you can improve your social skills by pushing yourself to introduce yourself to a stranger at a party or to chat about the weather with the person next to you in a coffee shop line.

Social Anxiety

About 7 percent of the population could be diagnosed with a **social anxiety disorder** (social phobia), in which individuals fear and avoid various social situations. Because they see themselves as not handling social situations well, they worry about them in advance.

loneliness Feelings of distress and dysphoria resulting from a discrepancy between a person's desired and achieved social relations, based on perceived rather than objective isolation.

social isolation Having few or no social contacts or activities.

social anxiety disorder A fear and avoidance of social situations.

They obsess over small talk, looking foolish, getting stuck in a crowd, being awkward. To cope, they may not make eye contact, hide in a corner, go home early, or drink until they feel nothing, including anxiety. Feeling bad about the experience, they become more anxious about future social interactions. Eventually the anxiety about social situations may attach itself to everything—a condition called generalized anxiety. Childhood shyness, emotional abuse, neglect, and chronic illness increase the likelihood of this problem.[11]

The key difference between normal shyness and social anxiety is the degree of distress and impairment that individuals experience. Although people with social anxiety do not differ from others in their stress physiology, they perceive their racing hearts and sweaty palms as signs of social inadequacy. Psychotherapy can help by teaching them to recognize their stress responses as normal and manageable. Those with disabling symptoms may do best with a combination of psychotherapy and medication.

Living in a Wired World

Modern technology is changing our social DNA. Today you can use a smartphone to call, text, or video chat with almost anyone almost anywhere. You also may game with friends, blog, tweet, post on social media, upload photos and videos, and give the world (or selected citizens) front-row seats to your life.

Some experts say that with social networking, humans are only doing what comes naturally but with twenty-first-century tools—and our brains may be adapting. As neuroimaging studies have shown, the amygdala—a brain region involved in processing emotional reactions—is bigger in individuals with large, complex social networks. Thanks to **computer-mediated communication**, the conveying of written text via ever-evolving new networks, sites, and apps, these networks are getting bigger than ever.

Social Media on Campus

College-age young adults may be the most wired age group. More than nine in ten college students maintain a social networking profile, with Facebook still the most popular choice. College students aged 18 to 24 spend an average of 32.2 hours a month online; those aged 25 to 34 spend 35.8 hours.[12]

Social networks are especially appealing to college students, particularly if they leave home and move to a campus where they know few, if

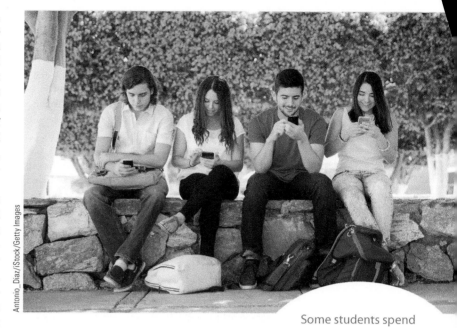
Antonio_Diaz//iStock/Getty Images

Some students spend more time on social media than in face-to-face conversations.

any, people. Many incoming students use online social networks to maintain relationships with old friends and to learn more about the new acquaintances they are making.

Facebook, the world's most popular website, was created by a college student for college students in 2004. More than 1.59 billion users around the globe have since joined and spend an average of 19 minutes a day on the site. Men and women between the ages of 18 and 25 make up about one third of all Facebook users. However, these days your parents and their friends are as likely as your peers to have Facebook pages.

The most common motivations undergraduates give for using social media are:

1. Nurturing or maintaining existing relationships
2. Seeking new relationships
3. Enhancing their reputation (being cool)
4. Avoiding loneliness
5. Keeping tabs on other people
6. Feeling better about themselves.[13]

In general, women tend to use social networking sites to compare themselves with others and search for information. Men are more likely to look at other people's profiles to find friends.

Online Eustress

Despite dire warnings about digital dangers, a recent analysis by researchers at the Pew Research Center and Rutgers University found that frequent Internet and social media users do not

computer-mediated communication The conveying of written text via ever-evolving new networks, sites, and apps.

have higher stress levels than those who use technology less. In fact, women who tweet, e-mail, and share photos score significantly lower than those who did not.[14]

Online socializing produces the same psychologically enhancing sense of community as interacting in person.[15] College students feeling stressed or down report a boost in self-esteem after viewing their Facebook profiles, perhaps because they are reminded of the personal traits and relationships that they value most.[16] Simply having a certain number of online friends and followers boosts feelings of happiness. Even more meaningful is getting support from online acquaintances—but only if it comes in response to an honest presentation of oneself.[17]

Digital Distress

The downsides of constant connection include increased awareness of stressful events, such as a job loss, accident, illness or death, in others' lives. Particularly for women, realizing that friends and acquaintances are dealing with serious difficulties adds to their own stress levels.[18] Social media sites also can make people feel inferior—if only because everyone else seems to be having a better time.[19]

Self-Disclosure and Privacy

Social networking has transformed the issues of **self-disclosure** (how much we reveal about ourselves to another person) and privacy. Rather than confide in a trusted friend, individuals may go online and reveal highly personal information to a stranger—or (if a comment or video makes its way onto a public site) to many strangers. Previously personal moments now play out in public—sometimes by choice (as in an engagement announced via a change in status), sometimes by chance (as when someone uploads a video of drunk beer-pong players).

An estimated one third to one half of teenagers and young adults with online profiles have posted photos or videos depicting what researchers call "negative health risk behaviors," such as drinking and using drugs. Their friends may view such images (of drinking more than drug use) in positive ways. Parents, friends of parents, siblings, coworkers, and potential employers often have a very different perspective.

Sexting—sending sexually explicit text messages or digital photos—is fairly common among teens and continues in college. At any age, some people tend not to consider the potential for negative fallout down the road. You may assume that a sexy selfie on Snapchat will disappear forever—but not if a screenshot makes its way to a much larger audience than you intended.

self-disclosure
Sharing personal information and experiences with another that he or she would not otherwise discover.

sexting Sending sexually explicit text messages or digital photos.

cyberbullying
Deliberate, repeated, and hostile actions that use information and communication technologies, including online web pages and text messages, with the intent of harming others by means of intimidation, control, manipulation, false accusations, or humiliation.

cyberstalking
A form of cyberbullying that uses online sites, Twitter, e-mail messages, and social media to harass victims and try to damage their reputation or turn others against them.

✔ **Check-in:** Have you ever been embarrassed by a photo, tweet, or comment posted online?

Cyberabuse

For some, the Internet has become an outlet for anger. Various "rant" websites allow anonymous users to adopt a screen name and engage in back-and-forth online flaming. Individuals who engage in virtual venting may initially feel more relaxed, but experience more anger in general and express it in maladaptive ways.[20]

Cyberbullying consists of deliberate, repeated, and hostile actions that use information and communication technologies, including tweets, texts, and messages, with the intent of harming others by means of intimidation, control, manipulation, false accusations, or humiliation. Cyberbullies may know their victims or strike randomly. Its prevalence on college campuses ranges from 8 to 21 percent.[21] Involvement in cyberbullying increases the odds of depression for both bully and victim, particularly if it includes unwanted sexual advances.[22]

Cyberstalking, a form of cyberbullying, uses social media to harass victims and to try to damage their reputation or turn others against them. Cyberstalking may include false accusations, threats, identity theft, damage to data or equipment, or the solicitation of minors for sex. Both cyberbullying and cyberstalking can be criminal offenses punishable by imprisonment. Cyberstalking occurs most often in the context of ex-partner relationships. Most of its perpetrators are male, and its victims, female. Its negative psychological impact on a victim's well-being is comparable to that caused by real-life stalking.[23]

✔ **Check-in:** Have you ever experienced cyberbullying or cyberstalking?

Sexual and Romantic Relationships

Sexual initiation is occurring earlier—at about age 16 for both genders. Men report more lifetime sex partners than women, but the difference has narrowed over time.[24] Yet even though individuals may have more sexual partners than in the past, most still value an intimate, supportive, exclusive relationship. Male and female young adults in committed relationships report greater sexual enjoyment than those engaging in hookups or casual sex.[25]

Romantic love brings eustress and distress. The "love chemicals" released within the brain when we are falling in love have effects similar to those of the hormones and neurotransmitters that intensify physiological reactions during stress. As the initial lover's high fades, other brain chemicals may come into play. The feel-good endorphins, morphine-like chemicals that help produce feelings of well-being, security, and tranquility, may increase in partners who develop a deep attachment. The hormone oxytocin, which plays a role in the "tend and befriend" stress response, as described in Chapter 1, also seems crucial in our ability to bond with others.

Gender Identity

Human beings are diverse in all ways, including sexual preferences and practices. Physiological, psychological, and social factors determine whether we are attracted to members of the same sex or the other sex. This attraction is our **sexual orientation.** **Heterosexual** is the term used for individuals whose primary orientation is toward members of the other sex. **Homosexual** refers to men and women who prefer partners of their own sex.

The **transgender** community includes individuals whose behaviors do not conform to commonly understood gender norms. These include trans youth (young people experiencing issues related to gender identity or expression), transsexuals (who identify with a gender other than the one they were given at birth), trans women (a term for male-to-female transsexuals to signify that they are female with a male history), and trans men (a term for female-to-male transsexuals to signify they are male with a female history). The terms *queer* and *genderqueer* refer to a range of sexual orientations, gender behaviors, or ideologies. LGBTQQI is an acronym for lesbian, gay, bisexual, transgendered, queer/questioning, and intersex individuals (sometimes an *A* is added for their "allies").

Lesbian, gay, bisexual, transgender, and questioning individuals may experience stress from various forms of social stigma, discrimination, and denial of human and civil rights and are at higher risk of psychiatric disorders, substance abuse, and suicide. Among lesbian, gay, and bisexual individuals, those who have not disclosed their sexual orientation may experience greater chronic stress.[26] However, coming out also can involve unique stresses.[27]

....
✔ **Check-in:** Has sexual orientation ever been a source of stress in your life?
....

Coming Out

Young people often have questions about their sexuality, but some face a stressful process of sorting out their gender identity and sexual orientation. Researchers have identified several stages:[28]

Stage One: "I Feel Different from Other Kids . . ."
Many gay, lesbian, and transgender teens say they sensed something "different" about themselves early in life, sometimes as far back as age 5. A boy may have liked to play house instead of sports, and vice versa for a girl. Patterns of social isolation from peers frequently start very young.

Stage Two: "I Think I Might Be Gay, But I'm Not Sure, and If I Am, I'm Not Sure That I Want to Be . . ."
Many homosexual youngsters may first realize that they are attracted to members of their own sex at puberty. A common response is to try to bury those feelings or to isolate themselves from other teens for fear of being exposed or "outed."

Stage Three: "I Accept the Fact That I'm Gay, But What's My Family Going to Say?"
Homosexual men and women often do not accept their sexual orientation until their late teens or their 20s. Even then they often fear their family's rejection or disapproval. As societal prejudice against gays and lesbians abates, boys and girls may arrive at this point somewhat earlier.

Stage Four: "I Finally Told My Parents I'm Gay."
In an online survey of nearly 2,000 gay and bisexual people age 25 or under, the respondents were 16 the first time they revealed their sexuality to anyone, including their parents. Many homosexual teens don't begin to date until they're on their own—possibly on a campus or in a city with a sizable gay population. Only then do they begin having the experiences that straight kids encounter earlier in their sexual development.*

Homophobia

Homosexuality threatens and upsets some people, perhaps because homosexuals are viewed as different. **Homophobia** has led to an increase in gay and "trans" bashing (attacking homosexuals and transgender individuals) in many communities, including college campuses.

Different ethnic groups respond to homosexuality in different ways. To a greater extent than white homosexuals, gays and lesbians of certain races and ethnicities tend to stay in the closet longer rather than risk alienation from their families and communities. Often they feel forced to choose between their gay and their ethnic identities.

In general, the African American community has stronger negative views of homosexuals than Caucasians do, possibly because of the influence of strong fundamentalist Christian beliefs. Stigma may contribute to a phenomenon called

_____
*American Academy of Pediatrics. "Four Stages of Coming Out." www.healthychildren.org/English /ages-stages /teen/dating-sex/Pages/Four-Stages-of -Coming-Out.aspx

sexual orientation
The direction of an individual's sexual interest, either to members of the same or the other sex.

heterosexual The term used to indicate individuals whose primary sexual orientation is toward members of the other sex.

homosexual The term used to indicate individuals whose primary sexual orientation is toward members of their own sex.

transgender The term used to indicate individuals whose behaviors do not conform to commonly understood gender norms.

homophobia
A fear of and aversion to homosexuals that can result in discrimination and gay and "trans" bashing (attacking homosexuals and transgender individuals).

"the Down Low" or DL, which refers to African American men who publicly present themselves as heterosexuals while secretly having sex with other men. This practice, which is neither new nor limited to African American men, can increase the risk of HIV infection in unsuspecting female partners.

Hispanic culture, with its emphasis on *machismo*, also takes a negative view of male homosexuality. Asian cultures, which view an individual as a representative of his or her family, tend to regard open declarations of sexual orientation as shaming the family and challenging its reputation and future.

Colleges and universities vary greatly in the resources available to gay, lesbian, bisexual, and transgender students. Most have student organizations; at about a third a paid staff member helps with the students' needs and issues. Others provide a support identification program or offer at least one course on gay, lesbian, bisexual, and transgender issues.

"Partnerships"

Although just as eager for intimacy—emotional and sexual—as older men and women, younger adults are following a different pattern than past generations as they experiment with different types of personal relationships or, as sociologists describe them, "partnerships." Among a smorgasbord of options, young adults may do the following:

- Enter into casual, short-term relationships

- Commit to a long-term monogamous relationship

- Live with a partner with or without the intent of getting married

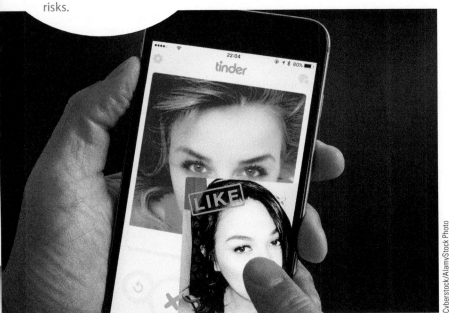

Cyberstock/AlamyStock Photo

- View marriage as the final step in a relationship that may take place after sexual involvement, shared living, childbearing, and parenting—if a couple decides to wed at all

Online Dating

Websites like match.com and eharmony.com and apps like Tinder and Plenty of Fish can connect people based on their age, appearance, location, interests, religious orientation, and ethnocultural background. Virtual flirtations may be fun, but they also entail some risks, particularly if you decide to go offline and meet in person. Finding Mr. or Ms. Right is no easier in cyberspace than anywhere else, so be realistic about where a virtual relationship might lead.

Here are some do's and don'ts of online dating:

- DO remember that you have no way of verifying if a correspondent is telling the truth about anything—sex, age, occupation, marital status, and so on. If your online partners contradict themselves or seem insincere or strange in any way, stop corresponding.

- DO be careful of what you post. Anything you put on the Internet can end up almost anywhere, including with potential employers. To avoid embarrassment, don't say anything you wouldn't want to see online or in print.

- DON'T give out your address, telephone number, or any other identifying information. The people you meet online are strangers, and you should keep your guard up.

- DON'T "date" on an office or university computer. You could end up supplying your professors, classmates, or coworkers with unintentional entertainment. Also, many organizations and institutions consider e-mail messages company property.

- DON'T rely on the Internet as your only method of meeting people. Continue to get out in the real world and meet potential dates the old-fashioned way: live and in person.

- If you do decide to meet, make your first face-to-face encounter a double or group date and make it somewhere public, like a coffee bar or a busy park.

Hooking Up

More than half of college students report engaging in some form of casual sex. A **hookup** might involve a range of physically intimate behaviors—from kissing to intercourse—characterized by a

hookup Refers to a range of physically intimate behaviors—from kissing to intercourse—with no expectation of emotional intimacy or a romantic relationship.

Dating websites and apps make virtual flirtations easy and fun—but entail some risks.

lack of any expectation of emotional intimacy or a romantic relationship. Some students have defined it more informally as "making out with no future" or "a one-time experience without any kind of responsibility to each other."[29]

Although popular media have described a pervasive "hookup culture" on campuses, researchers have challenged its prevalence. In one study, recent undergraduates did not report more sexual partners since age 19, more frequent sex, or more partners during the past year than those enrolled from 1988 to 1996. However, they were more likely to report sex with a casual date/pickup and less likely to report sex with a spouse or regular partner.[30] Other studies have documented a pattern in college hookups, which tend to peak between spring semester of the first year of college and fall semester of the second year, followed by a gradual decline over subsequent terms.[31]

A college hookup usually involves two people who have met earlier in the evening, often at a bar, fraternity house, club, or party, and agree to engage in some sexual behavior for which there is little or no expectation of future commitment. There is often minimal communication, and the hookup ends when one partner leaves, falls asleep, or passes out.

Students most likely to engage in hookups tend to be white, attractive, outgoing, and nonreligious; have higher-income and/or divorced parents, have a history of middle and high school hookups, and greater-than-typical alcohol use; are in a situation, such as spring break, that encourages hookups; and more frequently watch pornography.[32] Virtually all the students (99 percent) in one survey said they were aware of the danger of STIs in a casual sex encounter; 9 in 10 also were aware of the risks of negative emotional and mental health consequences.[33]

Students may engage in or endorse casual, commitment-free sexual encounters for various reasons, including a belief that hooking up is fun and harmless because it requires no emotional commitment, enhances their status in a peer group, and reflects sexual freedom and autonomy. Although hooking up implies no conditions and no expectations, it can and does have unanticipated and stressful consequences, including unwanted pregnancy, sexually transmitted infections, sexual violence, embarrassment, regret, and loss of self-respect.[34] (See Table 6.1.)

In a study of 483 first-year college women, half reported engaging in oral or vaginal hookup sex (compared with 62 percent who had sex with romantic partners). Hooking up was significantly correlated with depression, for several reasons that the researchers identified:

- Negative attitudes toward sex outside a committed relationship
- Risk of acquiring a bad reputation
- Failure of the hookup to lead to a romantic relationship
- Unsatisfying sex
- Pressure to go further sexually than desired[35]

Asked to identify positive aspects of hooking up, students selected "it is fun to be spontaneous," "a hookup might turn into a relationship," and "you don't have to deal with the hassle of maintaining a relationship." About one in four women reported sexual violence, including physical force, threats of harm, or incapacitation with drugs or alcohol. Hookups also increased the incidence of STIs.[36]

The motivations for a hookup may affect a participant's emotional and psychological responses. In a sample of 528 undergraduates followed for an academic year, men and women who hooked up for "autonomous," or deliberate, independently motivated reasons (such as sexual desire, pleasure, physical attraction, experimenting, exploring, novelty, excitement) did not experience depression, anxiety, lower self-esteem, or other negative impacts on their well-being. However, men and women who hooked up for "nonautonomous" reasons (low self-esteem, peer pressure, need for self-affirmation, social status, material rewards, intoxication with alcohol or drugs) were more likely to experience depression, anxiety, lower self-esteem, and lower overall well-being.[37]

Stress Reliever: Sexual Decisions

As with other behaviors, only you can and should make choices about sexual partners and activity. But to spare yourself and your partner unwanted and unneeded stress, your choices should be conscious ones rather than induced by alcohol or the heat of the moment.

When you do make a choice, reflect on it. How did the experience—whether you chose to hook-up, for instance—make you feel? Would you have done anything differently in retrospect? How did the experience affect your stress level?

TABLE 6.1 Hook-ups and Stress

Although hook-ups may seem to offer sex without stress, students report various stressful consequences, including regrets such as:

- Drinking too much and losing control
- Choosing a partner who did not meet their usual standards
- Disappointment because a hookup failed to lead to an ongoing relationship
- For men, embarrassment over their sexual performance, particularly premature ejaculation
- For women, disappointment over a lack of orgasm
- Guilt about cheating on a partner or hooking up with someone who was in a relationship
- Hurting or losing a friendship
- Worry about sexually transmitted infection (STI)
- Worry about possible pregnancy

Intimate Relationships

The term **intimacy**—the open, trusting sharing of close, confidential thoughts and feelings—comes from the Latin word for *within*. Intimacy doesn't happen at first sight, or in a day or a week or a number of weeks. Intimacy requires time and nurturing; it is a process of revealing rather than hiding, of wanting to know another and to be known by that other. Although intimacy doesn't require sex, an intimate relationship often includes a sexual relationship, be it heterosexual or homosexual.

Committed intimate relationships lessen stress and act as a buffer against its harmful effects. Simply having fewer sexual partners lowers general stress as well as the risk of sexual infections or assaults. Some research suggests that traditional-age college men receive greater emotional benefits than women from the positive aspects of romance, but are more likely than women to be emotionally harmed by the stress of a rocky patch or break-up.

Whatever their age or sex, people who lack close relationships are at high risk for a host of stress-related illnesses, including infections, heart disease, and cancer. "Love and intimacy are at the root of what makes us sick and what makes us well," says cardiologist Dean Ornish, a pioneer in mind-body-spirit medicine, "No other factor in medicine—not diet, not smoking, not exercise—has a greater impact."

Cohabitation

Although couples have always shared homes in informal relationships without any official ties, "living together," or **cohabitation**, has become more common. About one quarter of unmarried women aged 25 to 39 are currently living with a partner; an additional one quarter have lived with a partner in the past. Couples live together before more than half of all marriages, a practice that was practically unknown 50 years ago.

Cohabitation can be a prelude to marriage, an alternative to living alone, or an alternative to marriage. Personal traits, such as physical attractiveness, personality, and grooming, matter less when choosing a partner to live with than they do when selecting a prospective spouse.[38] Couples who move in together to "test" their relationship report more problems—including more negative communication, physical aggression, and symptoms of depression and anxiety—than those who are engaged or who plan to marry eventually.

Marriage

A generation ago, nearly 70 percent of Americans were married; now only about half are. The proportion of married people, especially among younger age groups, has been declining for decades. Here are the most recent statistics on Americans' unions:

- The median age for first marriage, which has gone up about a year every decade since the 1960s, has risen to 28.2 years for men and 26.1 years for women.
- Men in every age bracket through age 34 are more likely to be single than women.
- Black men and women are less likely to be married than whites, with Hispanics between the two.
- Most young adults view marriage positively, and 95 percent expect to marry in the future—except for young African Americans, who have significantly lower expectations of being wed than their white counterparts.

intimacy A state of closeness between two people, characterized by the desire and ability to share one's innermost thoughts and feelings with each other either verbally or nonverbally.

cohabitation Two people living together as a couple, without official ties such as marriage.

If you aren't already married, simply getting a college degree increases your odds of entering into matrimony in the future. College-educated women are most likely to be currently married, in part because they are more likely to stay married or remarry after divorce or widowhood. Less well-educated Americans are less likely to marry; in addition, if they do, their unions are more likely to end in divorce.

Same-sex marriages, also called gay or single-sex or gender-neutral marriages, were legally recognized as a constitutional right by the U. S. Supreme Court in 2015 and account for about 2 to 7 percent of all marriages annually. Gay and lesbian couples marry for the same reasons as heterosexuals: to affirm long-term commitment, provide emotional support, establish a family, and share life together.[39]

Because there are no social norms for same-sex unions, researchers describe these relationships as more egalitarian. Each partner tends to be more self-reliant, and homosexual men and women tend to be more willing to communicate and experiment in terms of sexual behaviors. But same-sex couples may have to deal with additional stressors such as workplace prejudice and social barriers.

Marriage and Health

Saying "I do" can do wonders for health. Compared to those who are divorced, widowed, never-married, or living with a partner, married people are healthier, live longer, recover faster from serious diseases, and have lower rates of coronary disease, cancer, back pain, headaches, mental disorders, and other common illnesses. Researchers once thought that marriage was especially beneficial to men. Married men have lower rates of alcohol and drug abuse, depression, and risk-taking behavior than divorced men. They also earn more money—possibly because they have more incentive to do so.

Married people have lower premature mortality rates, higher cancer survival rates, and fewer chronic health problems than unmarried individuals. The reason may be that marriage provides people with emotional satisfaction that buffers them against daily life stressors. In a recent study, people who felt that their spouses are always helpful in stressful times were less likely to show early signs of heart disease.[40] In terms of psychological well-being, researchers found no difference between heterosexual and homosexual spouses.[41] The same holds true for physical health benefits.[42]

While happy marriages enhance health, unhappy ones undermine it. Marital distress increases the risk of impaired immunity, cardiovascular

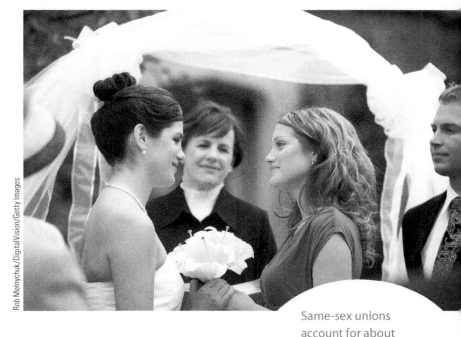

Rob Melnychuk/DigitalVision/Getty Images

Same-sex unions account for about 2 to 7 percent of all marriages.

disease, delayed healing, metabolic syndrome, and premature death. The stress triggered by negative and hostile behaviors during conflict, such as blaming or interrupting the partner, appear to be particularly detrimental to immune function, especially for women.[43]

Resolving Conflict

All couples may wish to live happily and peacefully ever after, but sooner or later, they disagree. In a five-year study of newly married couples, 36 percent sought some form of help for their relationship, most often from books on relationships and marital therapy.[44] Years of research have shown that while conflict is inevitable, the key difference between happy and unhappy couples is the way they handle disagreements.

Happier couples interject positive interactions, like a compliment or a smile, into their arguments. As long as the ratio of positive to negative interactions remains at least five to one, the relationship remains intact. By comparison, unhappy couples unfurl a barrage of negative words, gestures, criticisms, and hostility at their mates, with hardly any positive interactions.

Compared to straight couples, gay and lesbian couples use more affection and humor when they bring up a disagreement and remain more positive after a disagreement. They also display less belligerence, domineering, and fear with each other than straight couples do. When they argue, they are better able to soothe each other, so they show fewer signs of physiological arousal, such as an elevated heart rate or sweaty palms, than heterosexual couples.

same-sex marriage Governmentally, socially, or religiously recognized marriage in which two people of the same sex live together as a family.

Stress Reliever: What Not to Do in an Argument

If you want to resolve an issue, avoid these stress-aggravators:

- "You" statements, whether to criticize, tell the other person what to do, or guess what he or she is thinking or hearing.

- Listening to disparage or criticize rather than understand.

- Getting emotionally worked up.

- Staying silent about concerns for fear of provoking a fight.

- Insisting at all costs that you are right.[45,] *

---

*Heller, S. Resolution, Not Conflict. *Psychology Today*. May 30, 2013. psychologytoday.com

What can spouses do to bring out the best in their marriages? Here are some suggestions from marital therapists:

- **Focus on friendship.** If a marriage is not built on a strong friendship, it may be difficult to stay connected over time.

- **Remember what you loved and admired in your partner in the first place.** Focusing on these qualities can foster a much more positive attitude toward him or her.

- **Show respect.** Your spouse deserves the same courtesy and civility that your colleagues do. Without respect, love cannot survive.

- **Compliment what your partner does right.** Noticing the positive can change how both of you feel about each other.

- **Forgive one another.** When your partner hurts your feelings but then reaches out, don't reject his or her attempts to make things better.

Dysfunctional Relationships

Although they enrich and fulfill us in many ways, our relationships can also cause distress and sabotage our health. Mental health professionals define a **dysfunctional** relationship as one that doesn't promote healthy communication, honesty, and intimacy and that makes either person feel worthless or incompetent. Feelings of insecurity and anxiety about a dysfunctional relationship may boost stress hormones and impair the immune system.[46] Individuals with addictive behaviors or dependence on drugs or alcohol (see Chapters 12 and 13), and the children or partners of such people, are especially likely to find themselves in a dysfunctional relationship.

Physical symptoms, such as headaches, digestive troubles, tics, and inability to sleep well, can be signs of a destructive relationship. Yet, although one person may repeatedly attack, abandon, betray, badger, bully, criticize, deceive, dominate, or demean the other, the responsibility for changing the unhealthy dynamic belongs to both partners.

Emotional and Verbal Abuse

Abuse consists of any behavior that uses fear, humiliation, or verbal or physical assaults to control and subjugate another human being. Rather than being physical, emotional abuse takes many forms. (See Table 6.2 on Recognizing a Toxic Relationship.) Even if done for the sake of "teaching" or "helping," emotional abuse wears away at self-confidence, sense of self-worth, and trust and belief in oneself. Because it is more than skin deep, emotional abuse can leave longer-lasting scars.

TABLE 6.2 Recognizing a Toxic Relationship

The following behaviors are forms of abuse—verbal, emotional, or physical
• Berating
• Belittling or demeaning
• Humiliating
• Frequent criticism
• Name calling
• Blaming
• Threatening
• Accusing
• Judging
• Trivializing, minimizing, or denying what a partner says or feels
• Attempting to control various aspects of a partner's life
• Wanting to know everywhere a partner goes, with whom, etc.
• Becoming jealous of friends or family
• Threatening to harm you if you break up
• Coercion into unwanted sexual activity with statements such as "If you loved me, you would . . ."

dysfunctional Characterized by negative and destructive patterns of behavior between partners or between parents and children.

Often people who were emotionally abused in childhood find themselves in similar circumstances as adults. Dealing with an emotional abuser, regardless of how painful it is, may feel familiar or even comfortable. Individuals with low self-esteem also may pick partners who treat them as badly as they believe they deserve. Abusers also may have grown up with emotional abuse and view it as a way of coping with feelings of fear, hurt, powerlessness, or anger. They may seek partners who see themselves as helpless and who make them feel more powerful. (See Table 6.3.)

If you are in a toxic relationship, take whatever steps are necessary to ensure your safety. Find a trusted friend who can help. Don't isolate yourself from family and friends. This is a time when you need their support and often the support of a counselor, minister, or doctor as well.

Codependency and Enabling

Psychologists first identified traits of **codependency** in spouses of alcoholics, who followed a predictable pattern of behavior: While intensely trying to control the drinkers, the codependent mates would act in ways that allowed the drinkers to keep drinking. For example, if an alcoholic found it hard to get up in the morning, his wife would wake him up, pull him out of bed and into the shower, and drop him off at work. If he was late, she made excuses to his boss. The husband was the one with the substance-abuse problem, but without realizing it, his wife was **enabling** him to continue drinking. In fact, he might not have been able to keep up his habit without her unintentional cooperation.

The definition of codependency has expanded to include any maladaptive behaviors learned by family members in order to survive great emotional pain and stress, such as an addiction, chronic mental or physical illness, and abuse. Some therapists refer to codependency as a "relationship addiction" because codependent people often form or maintain relationships that are one-sided, emotionally destructive, or abusive. First identified in studies of the relationships in families of alcoholics, codependent behavior can occur in any dysfunctional family.

The characteristics of codependency include:

- An exaggerated sense of responsibility for the actions of others
- An attraction to people who need rescuing
- Always trying to do more than one's share
- Doing anything to cling to a relationship and avoid feeling abandoned
- An extreme need for approval and recognition
- A sense of guilt about asserting needs and desires
- A compelling need to control others
- Lack of trust in self and/or others
- Fear of being alone
- Difficulty identifying feelings
- Rigidity/difficulty adjusting to change
- Chronic anger
- Lying/dishonesty
- Poor communications
- Difficulty making decisions

Because the roots of codependency run so deep, people don't just "outgrow" this problem or magically find themselves in a healthy relationship. Treatment to resolve childhood hurts and deal with emotional issues may take the form of individual or group therapy, education, or programs such as Co-Dependents Anonymous (www.coda.org). The goal is to help individuals get in touch with long-buried feelings and build healthier family and relationship dynamics.

Codependency progresses just as an addiction does, and codependents excuse their own behavior with many of the same defense mechanisms used by addicts, such as rationalization ("I cut class so I could catch up on my reading, not to keep an eye on my partner") and denial ("He likes to gamble, but he never loses more than he can afford"). In time, codependents lose sight of everything but their loved one. They feel that if they can only "fix" this person, everything will be fine.

codependency An emotional and psychological behavioral pattern in which the spouses, partners, parents, children, and friends of individuals with addictive behaviors allow or enable their loved ones to continue their self-destructive habits.

enabling Unwittingly contributing to a person's addictive or abusive behavior. Components of enabling include shielding or covering up for an abuser/addict, controlling him or her, taking over responsibilities, rationalizing addictive behavior, and cooperating with him or her.

TABLE 6.3 Abusive Relationships on Campus

Types of abusive relationships reported by college students within the past 12 months	Men	Women	Average
An emotionally abusive intimate relationship	5.8	10.3	8.9
A physically abusive intimate relationship	1.6	2.2	2.0
A sexually abusive intimate relationship	0.7	2.4	1.8

Source: American College Health Association. *American College Health Association–National College Health Assessment II: Reference Group Executive Summary*, Fall 2015. Hanover, Md: American College Health Association, 2016.

Intimate Partner Violence

Intimate partner violence can occur between heterosexual, homosexual, or bisexual partners and can take different forms:

- physical violence (the threat or the use of force on one's partner to cause harm or death),

- sexual violence (the threat of or the use of force to engage a partner in sexual activity without consent, attempted or completed sexual act without consent, or abusive sexual contact), and

- psychological violence (using threats, actions, or coercive tactics which cause trauma or emotional harm to a partner.

All forms can have devastating psychological, physical, interpersonal, and occupational effects on the victim, friends and family, and society in general. Nearly half of all couples experience some form of physical aggression. In the most recent ACHA survey, about 2 percent of students had been in a physically abusive relationship in the preceding 12 months; 8 percent reported being in an emotionally abusive intimate relationship[47] (see Table 6.4).

TABLE 6.4 Risk Factors for Intimate Partner Violence

Gender. Both men and women experience acts of violence and aggression by their partners, but the violence perpetrated against women by men is likely to be much more severe and potentially injurious.

Violence in the Family of Origin: Childhood exposure to violence and abuse are risk factors for dating violence, especially for women.

Emotional States and Mental Health: Negative emotional, particularly, anger, anxiety, and depression, are associated with dating violence. Women who behave violently are more likely to be victims of partner violence and to have high levels of depression, anger, and hostility. Men show more antisocial personality characteristics and have lower educational and economic status.[49]

Substance Use and Abuse: Drugs and alcohol reduce the ability to resist unwanted physical or sexual advances and/or may prevent a victim from being able to interpret warning cues of a potential assault.[50]

Sexual Risk Taking: Hooking up with strangers and casual acquaintances.

sexual coercion Sexual activity forced upon a person by the exertion of psychological pressure by another person.

rape Sexual penetration of a female or a male by means of intimidation, force, or fraud.

College students may be at greater risk for several reasons, including alcohol use, drug use, and risky sexual behaviors. Abusive or violent partners may engage in a host of behaviors that prevent victims from fully engaging in college. This may increase the risk of depression, dropping classes, scholastic failure, and school withdrawal. which can impair their academic performance.[48]

Women attending urban commuter colleges may be at particular risk if they have partners who seek to control or limit their college experience or who feel threatened by what they may achieve by attending college.51 Minority stress (discussed in Chapter 4) may contribute to violence among lesbian, gay, bisexual, and transgender (LGBT) partners, who are much less likely than other couples to disclose what happened. In one recent study, only about a third (compared to roughly three quarters of heterosexuals) revealed a violent episode to any person, most often a friend. The reasons include a feeling that it was "not a big deal," a desire for privacy, and concern about others' reactions.52

Sexual Victimization

Sexual victimization refers to any situation in which a person is deprived of free choice and forced to comply with sexual acts. This is not only a woman's issue; men also are victimized. In recent years, researchers have come to view acts of sexual victimization along a continuum, ranging from street hassling, stalking, and obscene telephone calls to rape, battering, and incest.

Sexual coercion can take many forms, including exerting peer pressure, taking advantage of one's desire for popularity, threatening to end a relationship, getting someone intoxicated, stimulating a partner against his or her wishes, or insinuating an obligation based on the time or money one has expended. Men may feel that they need to live up to the sexual stereotype of taking advantage of every opportunity for sex. In a survey of more than 1,000 undergraduates, nearly two thirds reported knowing one or more women who have been victims of sexual assault, and over half reported knowing one or more men who have perpetrated sexual assault.[53]

Rape is defined by the Justice Department as "the penetration, no matter how slight, of the vagina or anus with any body part or object, or oral penetration by a sex organ of another person, without the consent of the victim." In *acquaintance rape,* or *date rape,* the victim knows the rapist. In *stranger rape,* the rapist is an unknown assailant. Both acquaintance and stranger rapes are serious, traumatic crimes that can have a devastating impact on their victims. "Date" rapes on campus are typically less violent and involve less force by the assailant, less resistance by (and less injury to) the victim, but nonetheless cause serious psychological consequences, including traumatic stress.[54]

When Love Ends

As the old song says, breaking up is indeed hard to do. Sometimes two people grow apart gradually, and both of them realize that they must go their separate ways. Many do not end their relationships because love disappears. Rather, a sense of dissatisfaction or unhappiness develops, which may then cause love to stop growing. The fact that love does not dissipate completely may be why breakups are so painful. It hurts to be rejected; it also hurts to inflict pain on someone who once meant a great deal to you.

Breaking Up and Rejection

✔ **Check-in:** Do you think it's more difficult to initiate a breakup or to be rejected?

In surveys, college students generally say that it's harder to break up with someone you once cared about. Those who decided to end a relationship report greater feelings of guilt, uncertainty, discomfort, and awkwardness than their girlfriends or boyfriends. Psychological research suggests otherwise.

While the pain does ease over time, it can help both parties if they end their relationship in a way that shows kindness and respect. Your basic guideline should be to think of how you would like to be treated if someone were breaking up with you:

- Would it hurt more to find out from someone else?

- Would it be more painful if the person you cared for lied to you or deceived you, rather than admitting the truth?

- What can you say?

- "I don't feel the way I once did about you."

- "I've realized that you and I want different things in life."

- "I don't want to continue our relationship"

Rejection hits with a double whammy: Physiologically, it increases the inflammatory responses that contribute to asthma, cardiovascular disease, rheumatoid arthritis, and other chronic illnesses[55]; Psychologically, it elicits a flood of self-derogatory thoughts such as "I'm undesirable" or "I'm unlovable" and wrenching emotions such as shame and humiliation. No other stressor increases the risk of depression more. Individuals who break up with a partner are ten times more likely to develop depression than others. For the person who was dumped, the likelihood of depression doubles.[56]

> 🔧 **Stress Reliever:** How to Deal with Rejection
>
> Remind yourself of your own worth. You are no less attractive, intelligent, interesting, or lovable because someone ends a relationship with you.
>
> Accept the rejection as a statement of the other person's preference rather than trying to debate or defend yourself.
>
> Think of other people who value or have valued you, who accept and even see as appealing the same characteristics the rejecting person viewed as undesirable.
>
> Don't withdraw from others. Although you may not want to risk further rejection, it's worth the gamble to get involved again. The only individuals who've never been rejected are those who've never reached out to connect with another.

Divorce

According to the most recent estimates, 40 to 50 percent of first marriages end in divorce, affecting about 2.5 million adults a year. Divorce rates have been leveling off among persons born since 1980, especially among college-educated women.[57] This may reflect a delay in getting married, increasing selectivity when choosing partners, or a preference for cohabitation rather than marriage.[58]

Many marriages dissolve simply because one partner's commitment to maintaining the relationship declines. Even couples who are initially very happy can go on to divorce if they begin to engage in more negative communication and emotion and provide less mutual support.

Divorce, one of the most powerful stressful life events, can have long-term consequences for mental and physical health, including these:

- Long-term decreases in life satisfaction
- Heightened risk for a range of illnesses
- Poor prognosis for those already ill
- Increased risk of early death[59]
- Higher chance of heart attack[60]

Good relationships grow stronger and closer through years of living and loving together.

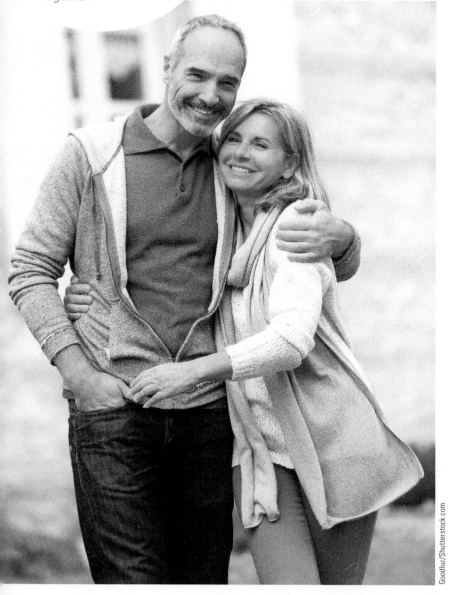

Goodluz/Shutterstock.com

Building Better Relationships

As with other significant endeavors, good relationships require work—through hard times, despite conflicts, over months and years and decades. Here are some guidelines for nurturing a healthy, happy relationship:

- Recognize that both people in the relationship have the right to be accepted as they are, to be treated with respect, to feel safe, to ask for what they want, to say no without feeling guilty, to express themselves, to give and receive affection, and to make some mistakes and be forgiven.

- Remember that no one in a relationship has the right to force the other to do anything, to tell the other where or when to speak up or go out, to humiliate the other in public or private, to isolate the other from friends and family, to read personal material without permission, to pressure the other to give up goals or interests, or to abuse the other person verbally or physically.

- Be willing to open up. The more you share, the deeper the bond between you and your friend will become.

- Be sensitive to your friend's or partner's feelings. Keep in mind that, like you, he or she has unique needs, desires, and dreams.

- Express appreciation. Be generous with your compliments. Let your friends and family know you recognize their kindnesses.

- Know that people will disappoint you from time to time. We are only human. Accept your loved ones as they are. Admitting their faults need not reduce your respect for them.

- Listen respectfully to your partner's point of view even when you disagree. If you argue, stick to the topic; don't attack the person. Never use the vulnerabilities only you know about as weapons.

- If you're in the wrong, say you're sorry, even if only for something small. It feels good to own your actions and take responsibility. You never know how much it may mean to someone to hear it.

- Healthy, mutually beneficial relationships add joy to our years and perhaps even years to our lives. Unhealthy or dysfunctional ones can be so stressful that they can undermine health as well as happiness.

- Social health is the ability to interact effectively with other people, develop satisfying interpersonal relationships, and fulfill social roles.

- Social support refers to the ways in which we provide information or assistance, comfort, and confide in others. People with close ties to others have stronger cardiovascular and immune systems, resist colds better, and are less vulnerable to serious illness and premature death.

- By mastering skills to communicate more effectively and by being responsible in your interactions with others, you can cultivate what psychologists call "social intelligence," the skills that create relationships worth cherishing.

- More than 90 percent of communication may be nonverbal. Body language is the building block upon which more advanced verbal forms of communication rest.

- Attentive, authentic listening means hearing what's being said nonverbally as well as verbally, processing the information, being able to reflect back the content, and utilizing appropriate verbal and non-verbal responses.

- Assertiveness doesn't mean being aggressive or telling someone off. To communicate negative feelings and thoughts in a non-provocative way, focus on specifics, avoid verbal jabs, and make sure you're talking with the person who is directly responsible for a problem.

- Loneliness, defined as "feelings of distress and dysphoria resulting from a discrepancy between a person's desired and achieved social relations," is a common stressor that increases the risk of depression and poor psychological and physical health.

- As many as 40 percent of people describe themselves as shy or uncomfortable in social situations. Some shy people are born with a predisposition to shyness. Others become shy because they don't learn social skills or because they experience rejection or shame.

- About 7 percent of the population could be diagnosed with a social anxiety disorder (social phobia), in which individuals fear and avoid various social situations. The key difference between normal shyness and social anxiety is the degree of distress and impairment that individuals experience.

- College-age young adults may be the most wired age group. In general, women tend to use social networking sites to compare themselves with others and search for information. Men are more likely to look at other people's profiles to find friends. The sexes even differ in their profile photos: Women usually add portraits, while men prefer full-body shots.

- Frequent Internet and social media users do not have higher stress levels than those who use technology less. Socializing online can produce the same psychologically enhancing sense of community as interacting in person.

- The downsides of constant connection include increased awareness of stressful events, such as a job loss, accident, illness or death, in others' lives. Social media sites also can make people feel inferior.

- Social networking has transformed the issues of self-disclosure (how much we reveal about ourselves to another person) and privacy. Sexting—sending sexually explicit text messages or digital photos—is fairly common among teens and continues in college.

- A minority of Internet users—from 1 to 10 percent in various studies—report symptoms associated with addictive behavior. Like other addictions, "problematic" Internet use may lead to preoccupation, withdrawal, difficulty with control, disregard for harmful consequences, loss of other interests, desire for escape, hiding the behavior, and harmful effects on relationships or work- or school-related performance.

- Cyberbullying consists of deliberate, repeated, and hostile actions that use information and communication technologies with the intent of harming others by means of intimidation, control, manipulation, false accusations, or humiliation. Cyberstalking uses social media to harass victims and try to damage their reputation or turn others against them.

- Physiological, psychological, and social factors determine whether we are attracted to members of the same or the other sex. Homosexual is the term used for individuals whose primary orientation is toward members of their own sex; heterosexual, for those who prefer partners of the other sex.

- Lesbian, gay, bisexual, transgender, and questioning individuals, who may experience stress from various forms of social stigma, discrimination, and denial of human and civil rights, are at higher risk of psychiatric disorders, substance abuse, and suicide.

- Younger adults may enter into casual, short-term relationships, commit to a long-term monogamous relationship, live with a partner with or without the intent of getting married, or view marriage as the final step in a relationship that may take place after sexual involvement, shared living, childbearing, and parenting—if a couple decides to wed at all.

- Websites like match.com and eharmony.com and apps like Tinder and Plenty of Fish can connect people based on their age, appearance, location interests, religious orientation, and ethnocultural background. Virtual flirtations entail risks, particularly if you decide to go offline and meet in person.

- A hookup might involve a range of physically intimate behaviors—from kissing to intercourse—characterized by a lack of any expectation of emotional intimacy or a romantic relationship.

- Although hooking up implies no conditions and no expectations, it can and does have unanticipated consequences, including unwanted pregnancy, sexually transmitted infections, sexual violence, embarrassment, regret, and loss of self-respect.

- College students in committed relationships experience fewer mental health problems, are less likely to be overweight/obese, or to engage in fewer risky behaviors (such as binge drinking). The reason may be that a loving relationship lessens stress and acts as a buffer against its harmful effects.

- About one quarter of unmarried women aged 25 to 39 are currently living with a partner; an additional one quarter have lived with a partner in the past. Couples live together before more than half of all marriages, a practice that was practically unknown 50 years ago.

- The proportion of married people, especially among younger age groups, has been declining for decades. Same-sex marriages, also called gay or single-sex or gender-neutral marriages, account for about 2 to 7 percent of all marriages contracted in a single year.

- Compared to those who are divorced, widowed, never married, or living with a partner, married people are healthier, live longer, recover faster from serious diseases, and have lower rates of coronary disease, cancer, back pain, headaches, mental disorders, and other common illnesses.

- Marital distress undermines immunity at a cellular level and increases the risk of cardiovascular disease, delayed healing, metabolic syndrome, and premature death.

- A dysfunctional relationship is one that doesn't promote healthy communication, honesty, and intimacy and where either person is made to feel worthless or incompetent.

- Abuse consists of any behavior that uses fear, humiliation, or verbal or physical assaults to control and subjugate another human being. Rather than being physical, emotional abuse takes many forms and wears away at self-confidence, sense of self-worth, and trust and belief in oneself.

- Codependency describes any maladaptive behaviors acquired by family members in order to survive great emotional pain and stress, such as an addiction, chronic mental or physical illness, and abuse.

- Intimate partner violence can include physical violence, sexual violence, and psychological violence.

- Physiologically, breakups increase the inflammatory responses that contribute to chronic illnesses. Psychologically, they elicit a flood of self-derogatory thoughts and increase the risk of depression.

- Divorce, one of the most stressful life events, can have long-term consequences for mental and physical health, including heightened risk for a range of illnesses and an increased risk of early death.

 ## STRESS RELIEVERS

If You're Shy
You can overcome much of your social apprehensiveness on your own, in much the same way as you might set out to stop smoking or lose weight. For example, you can improve your social skills by pushing yourself to introduce yourself to a stranger at a party or to chat about the weather with the person next to you in a coffee shop line.

Sexual Decisions
As with other behaviors, only you can and should make choices about sexual partners and activity. But to spare yourself and your partner unwanted and unneeded stress, your choices should be conscious ones rather than induced by alcohol or the heat of the moment.

When you do make a choice, reflect on it. How did the experience—whether you chose to hook up, for instance—make you feel? Would you have done anything differently in retrospect? How did the experience affect your stress level?

What Not to Do in an Argument
If you want to resolve an issue, avoid these stress-aggravators:

- "You" statements, whether to criticize, tell the other person what to do, or guess what he or she is thinking or hearing.

- Listening to disparage or criticize rather than to understand.
- Getting emotionally worked up.
- Staying silent about concerns for fear of provoking a fight.
- Insisting at all costs that you are right.

How to Deal with Rejection

- Remind yourself of your own worth. You are no less attractive, intelligent, interesting, or lovable because someone ends a relationship with you.

- Accept the rejection as a statement of the other person's preference rather than trying to debate or defend yourself.
- Think of other people who value or have valued you, who accept and even see as appealing the same characteristics the rejecting person viewed as undesirable.
- Don't withdraw from others. Although you may not want to risk further rejection, it's worth the gamble to get involved again. The only individuals who've never been rejected are those who've never reached out to connect with another.

⊜ YOUR PERSONAL STRESS MANAGEMENT TOOLKIT

REFLECTION: Building Blocks of a Good Relationship

As with other significant endeavors, good relationships require work—through hard times, despite conflicts, over months and years and decades. As you strive to improve the ties that bind you to others, keep in mind the characteristics of a good relationship. Check the ones that are most important to you.

_____ Trust. Partners are able to confide in each other openly, knowing their confidences will be respected.

_____ Togetherness. In a healthy relationship, two people create a sense of both intimacy and autonomy. They not only enjoy each other's company but also pursue solitary interests.

_____ Expressiveness. Partners in healthy relationships say what they feel, need, and desire.

_____ Staying power. People in committed relationships keep their bond strong through tough times by proving that they will be there for each other.

_____ Security. Because a good relationship is strong enough to absorb conflict and anger, partners know they can express their feelings honestly. They also are willing to risk vulnerability for the sake of becoming closer.

_____ Laughter. Humor keeps things in perspective—always crucial in any sort of ongoing relationship or enterprise.

_____ Support. Partners in good relationships continually offer each other encouragement, comfort, and acceptance.

_____ Physical affection. Sexual desire may fluctuate or diminish over the years, but partners in loving, long-term relationships usually retain some physical connection.

_____ Personal growth. In the best relationships, partners are committed to bringing out the best in each other and have the other's best interests at heart.

_____ Respect. Caring partners are aware of each other's boundaries, need for personal space, and vulnerabilities. They do not take each other or their relationship for granted.

Read through the items you've checked, and reflect on how they play out in your relationships. What would you like to experience more of? What steps would you take to achieve this? If you are in an intimate relationship, consider sharing this self-survey and your responses with your partner.

TECHNIQUE: Listen Up!

Replay three conversations you've had in the last 24 hours with three different people. Relive them in your mind. In your Journal, answer the following questions:

- What was the purpose of the conversation? Killing time? Flirting? Trying to get information you needed for a class or assignment?
- Who initiated the conversation?
- Who talked more?
- What questions did you ask, if any?
- How much did you really listen?
- How well did you listen?
- What do you remember?
- What did you hear?
- How interested were you in knowing the other person, as opposed to merely scoring points or getting information you needed?

- What did you come to learn or understand about the other person?

- How well did you put yourself in the other person's shoes, if at all?

On the basis of your answers, rate your listening skills on a scale of 1 (you talkin' to me?) to 10 (Dr. Phil). Here are some suggestions if you want to raise your listening skills to a higher level:

- Make eye contact. You don't have to stare intently, but make sure you feel a visual connection.

- Let the other person know you are listening. It is okay to nod your head or throw in an occasional "Mmhmm" or "I see." Don't interrupt, though.

- Validate what people are sharing with you. Acknowledge when something significant is said.

- Only ask questions that will expand or clarify what the person is saying.

- If you're not clear on a point, say something like, "So what you're saying is . . ." Occasionally you can briefly summarize what you have heard.

- Do not leap ahead and start thinking about what you're going to say. Keep your focus on the other person.

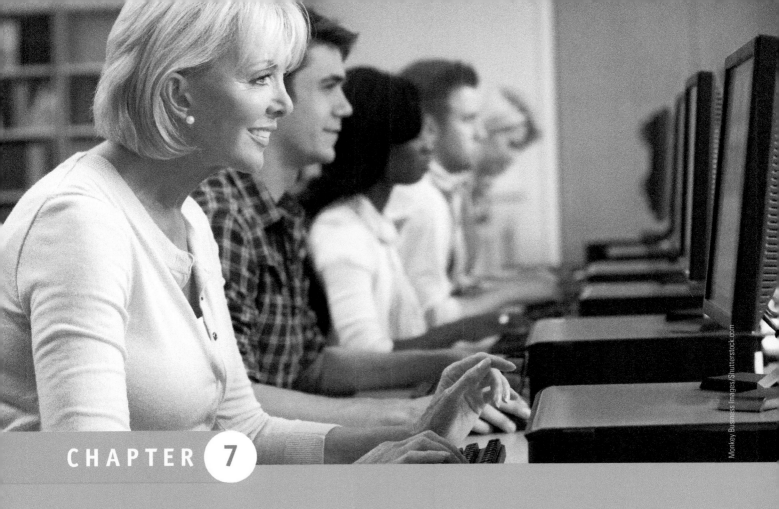

CHAPTER 7

Personal Change

After reading this chapter, you should be able to:

7.1 Identify factors that influence our view of change.

7.2 DIfferentiate individual behaviors and characteristics according to Prochaska's Stages of Change model.

7.3 Elaborate on steps to take to develop goals for successful personal change.

7.4 Discuss language that characterizes change.

7.5 Utlilize available resources to support change.

7.6 Summarize factors to consider when faced with a decision.

7.7 Recognize components necessary to sustain behavior change.

Ask yourself the following questions:

_____ What am I doing now that I want to stop doing?
_____ What am I not doing now that I want to do?
_____ What am I doing now that I would like to increase?
_____ What am I doing now that I would like to decrease?

Write down your answers, although you don't have to share them with anyone. Roll them around in your mind. Add, subtract, or edit as you read through this chapter.

Not yet thirty, Ana has seen a lifetime of changes. With her father in the military, she moved again and again as a little girl to a new home in a new neighborhood. Every time she enrolled in a new school—half a dozen in all—she had to once again try to fit in and make new friends. When one or the other of her parents was deployed overseas, her role in the household changed as she took on more responsibility for her little brothers.

When Ana started college, the changes accelerated. Her father retired early with a service-related disability; her mother took on extra shifts to bring in more income. Ana transferred from her state university several hours away to a local community college so she could live at home and help out. Unable to keep up with academics as well as her family obligations, she dropped out.

Several years later, her father's health has improved. One of Ana's brothers enlisted in the Army; another got a scholarship to her old university. And now she's enrolled in a community college, wondering how she's ever going to keep up with her young, energetic classmates.

Ana keeps scrambling to do everything the best she can, yet there's a knot in her stomach that never quite goes away. She can't shake the nagging sense that she could and should be coping better. "Step it up," she tells herself, but Ana doesn't know even where to begin. Sometimes she simply wishes the world would stop changing and stand still so she could catch up.

For all of us, each day ushers in all kinds of changes, great and small. People come in and go out of our lives; businesses boom and bust; politicians win and lose; seasons pass. These external changes occur whether or not you want or welcome them. Though not all of these changes affect you, some do affect you directly and require adaptation, which, by definition, can induce stress.

Some changes occur without any conscious effort on your part. Every day your body manufactures new cells; your muscles break down and build up new tissue; your brain fires neurons that establish new connections. But change is not something that just happens to you; you can choose to initiate changes that can prevent, reduce, or buffer stress and its potentially harmful impact. When you deliberately change a nonproductive thought, feeling, or behavior, you are choosing to take control—of your time, your health, your relationships, your achievements, and your future. Making changes to manage stress better carries an even greater benefit: it increases your chances of success in changing health behaviors.[1]

Just think of how college students lived and learned thirty years ago: They wrote papers with typewriters, listened to music on audiocassettes, and mailed letters home. Yes, technology has changed, but the people who learned to use computers, smartphones, and e-mail had to make changes too. This chapter provides a primer on how to make positive changes and adaptations in your life.

Choosing Change

Because of your past experiences, you may find anything outside your comfort zone—which may be a rather small chunk of psychological real estate—stressful. This is understandable: All you know is how you have done things so far. Like blinders, your past experiences limit your vision. You look at life through the lens of your preexisting ideas, biases, and fears. If you had a serious illness as a child, every visit to a doctor may be terrifying; if you once stuttered or lisped, you may remain self-conscious every time you open your mouth. To change your perception of stress, you have to set aside such preconceptions and expand your sense of how far you've come and how capable you've become.

Of course, you cannot control every aspect of your life. All of us enter the world with certain givens, and there is an element of unpredictability to what happens around us. But you decide what to eat; whether to drink or smoke; when to study, sleep, and exercise; how to express your sexuality; if you want to repair or end a friendship. You may not notice the consequences of your choices for months or even years, but their ultimate impact is undeniable.

Every time you learn something new, whether it's rock climbing or rocket science, you expand your possibilities and enhance your ability to cope. Whenever you stretch yourself to understand another point of view, you change your range of knowledge. When you tackle a challenging task and dare to fail, you change your capacity to grow. Without such changes you would remain a smaller, paler, narrower shadow of who and what you can become. And your world would seem smaller and more stressful.

Thanks to decades of research, we now know what sets the stage for change, the way change progresses, and the keys to lasting change. We also know that personal change is neither mysterious nor magical but a methodical process that anyone can master.

✔ **Check-in:** What is the biggest change you've experienced in your life?

Why Change Seems Stressful

Perhaps the greatest misconception about—and barrier to—personal change is the notion that you have to change who you *are*. You don't. The problem never is and never will be who you are. The problem—and what you may need to change—is what you *do*.

The idea of who you are resides at the center of your sense of reality. It is part of the glue that holds your reality together. You believe that if you know anything, you know yourself. And you feel that you *know* what is possible for you.

What you *actually* know is what you have habitually believed and how you have consistently behaved. You have what police call an "m.o.," or *modus operandi*, a way of doing things and a way of thinking about things that seldom varies in significant ways unless you consciously decide otherwise. You tie your shoes the same way, part your hair on the same side, lead with the same foot as you step into the shower, rerun the same habitual thoughts and feelings through your brain.

When asked to attempt something different or new, you may think you can't do it on the basis of your past history. You mistake what you have never habitually done for something you cannot do. If you've never been punctual, you can't see yourself suddenly being on time. If you've always been disorganized, you can't imagine a clutter-free workspace. If you've gorged on junk food for years, you don't think a salad could ever satisfy you. If you fly off the handle at every slight, your temper seems untamable.

But all of life consists of doing things you never did before and beginning to do them before you are sure you can. No rehearsal completely prepares you for the first day at a new school, or a championship game, a driving test, or an interview. Preparation helps, but there is a moment—often not entirely at your discretion—when you must deliver. The experience can be scary, but it is the key to growing and moving forward with your life.

Remember that you, with all your talents and quirks, your passions and preferences, are more than the sum of your habits. You can change your behaviors and still feel, not just like yourself, but also like the best possible and most complete version of yourself.

What You Need to Know about Change

You don't decide to change one evening and wake up a changed person in the morning. There is no on-off toggle switch, no all-or-nothing experience that clearly divides your life into what was and what will be. You are changing as you read these words because new ideas are entering your brain. Will they ultimately lead to lasting change? That depends, again, on your choice, but if you are open, the process of change is already underway. (We will explain more about the stages of this process later in this chapter.)

Don't worry about being ready to make changes. You have the capacity and the strength you need; you have only to decide to use them. As you do, keep in mind the following fundamentals:[2]

- **Personal change demands no prerequisites.** You don't have to wait for a burst of insight or a jolt of inspiration. You don't need a guru, coach, or therapist. Change starts with something extremely commonplace: observing what you do *now* and thinking through different satisfying. Once you create this vision, you can prepare your change plan.

- **Personal change occurs in steps.** Unless you have been blessed with extraordinary natural talent, you don't sit down at a piano for the first time and play a Beethoven concerto. Instead you start with the classic five easy pieces. Slowly, steadily, you make progress until one day something seems to click. Suddenly you're making music rather than playing notes. But you've also learned all kinds of other things: how to position your body, use your fingers and hands, recognize rhythm, read notes—so much! When you take small, methodical steps toward a goal, you acquire more than one new competence: If you pay attention, you teach yourself how to make a change.

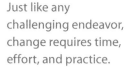

Just like any challenging endeavor, change requires time, effort, and practice.

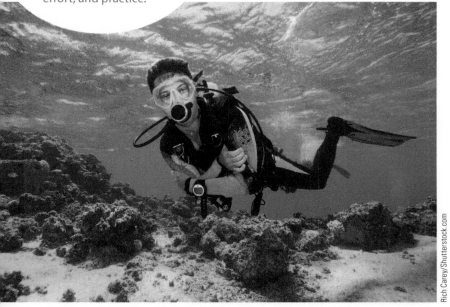

Rich Carey/Shutterstock.com

- **Personal change proceeds better with scientifically tested tools.** Many people change by trial and error. If they want to lose weight, for instance, they try the latest trendy diet—then the next and the next. Unfortunately, the diet yo-yo may leave them heavier than ever. But there are powerful research-based tools that dramatically increase the chance of successful change. In fact, if you use them consciously and consistently, they make change nearly inevitable. Some are as simple as focusing your attention with laser-like intensity or changing the language you use when talking to yourself. These tools, applied conscientiously, will spare you a lot of wasted time and needless frustration.

- **Personal change replaces old habits with new skills.** You couldn't get through the day without habits. Your daily routine consists of habitual behaviors like combing your hair, getting dressed, taking notes, texting friends, and a variety of other things. But if you take the time to step back and observe yourself, you may identify some habits that get in your way and slow you down.[3] Maybe you're always running behind; maybe you've never gotten a grip on managing money; maybe you drink or gamble more than you want. You can replace these negative behaviors with positive new *skills* (the word people use for habits they like and want to keep) that empower and energize your life.

- **Personal change requires time as well as effort.** To change you must adopt an appropriate long-range perspective. Instead of planning a quick fix, the emotional equivalent of a crash diet, think in terms of revising forever the specific, decisive aspects of your life that will make a difference. People who lose weight and keep it off don't go on—and inevitably off—a diet. They permanently change the way they eat and exercise. The key word is "permanently." Lasting revisions take time and diligence, although not as much as you might suppose—and certainly not more than you can muster.

✔ **Check-in:** What is one habit or behavior that you would like to change?

What You Can and Can't Change

Some people change very little in life. Sure, over time they may get fatter and flabbier, gather lines, and go gray. But they wear their hair the same way, buy the same brand of shoes, eat the same breakfast, and cling to routines for no reason other than the ease of staying within their comfort zone. Yet as both research and real life show, many others do make important changes. Individuals of every type train for marathons, quit smoking, switch fields, write screenplays, take up the saxophone, or learn to tango even if they never danced before in their lives.

What is the difference between these two groups? The way they think. People who change do not question whether change is possible or look for reasons why they cannot change. They simply decide on a change they want and do whatever is necessary to accomplish it. Changing, which always stems from a resolute decision, becomes job one. When people do not change, the reason is not that change isn't possible, but that they put the brakes on change or limit their possibilities.

Of course, there are things you can't change. You can't alter when and where you were born. You can't do anything but complain about the weather. You cannot fly like a bird regardless of how furiously you flap your arms. But often you think you cannot do something simply because you have never done it before.

To make a change—whether it's to eliminate a bad habit or to create a good one—you have to do two things:

- Repeat new actions in order to forge new connections in the brain.
- Resist the natural tendency to follow the well-trod path of least resistance.

For highly elaborate changes such as learning to write with your non-dominant hand, this process can be long and arduous. But if you observe yourself closely, you will see that you are already adept at creating simpler habits. In a large lecture hall, you may return to the same seat every day. If you attend church regularly, you may head for the same pew. You don't stop to consider alternatives. Changing forces you to do so. It requires both new neural pathways and repetition over time to overcome the inclination to return to older, more familiar patterns.

Although venturing into new territory can feel stressful, the discomfort is temporary. Every time you repeat your new behavior, you strengthen the new connections in your brain. If you have ever worked with weights, you remember how sore your biceps felt in the beginning. But if you persisted, your muscles grew bigger and stronger. The original weight became easier to lift, and soon you could hoist heavier loads.

A similar process occurs as you make a change in your behavior. The first steps feel awkward and uncertain, but they become fluid with time and practice. It is important to remind yourself that just because something may feel strange or uncomfortable, the feeling will pass. The next time will feel more comfortable, and may become something you deeply enjoy.

> **Stress Reliever:** Own the Future
>
> Make a list of some positive attributes you plan to acquire. Write a series of statements describing the new improved you—all in the present tense. Why? Using the present tense creates a hypnotic-like demand that your behavior match the description. Some examples:
>
> _____ I am organized.
>
> _____ I am psyched.
>
> _____ I am ready for this test.
>
> _____ I can do this.

The Stages of Change

Psychologists have developed many theories about why we do the things we do. Some theories emphasize the role of the unconscious; others focus on the dynamics of our relationships or our thoughts and habits. Psychologist James Prochaska and his colleagues, by tracking what they considered to be universal stages in the successful recovery of drug addicts and alcoholics, developed a way of thinking about change that cuts across psychological theories. Their "transtheoretical" model focuses on universal aspects of an individual's decision-making process rather than on social or biological influences on behavior.[4]

Instead of conceptualizing change as an exertion of effort or will, Prochaska identified various stages that people move through as they progress from being clueless, to conscious, to committed to making a change. This process begins slowly before you make a deliberate decision to change. Rather than marching in linear fashion from one stage to the next, most people spiral through the following stages: (See Figure 7.1.)

Precontemplation

You are at the **precontemplation** stage if you, as yet, have no intention of making a change. Even though you feel stressed or sense that something is not quite right or not quite the way you want it to be, you haven't identified exactly what's wrong, let alone thought about looking for solutions. You are vaguely uncomfortable, but this is where your grasp of what is going on ends.

precontemplation
The time when a person has no intention of making a change.

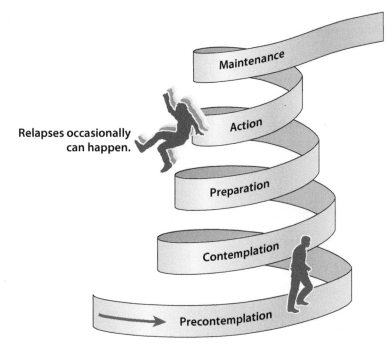

Relapses occasionally can happen.

Maintenance

Action

Preparation

Contemplation

Precontemplation

FIGURE 7.1 The stages of change form a dynamic spiral.

contemplation The stage of change in which, although you'd prefer not to change, you realize that you must.

During the contemplation stage of change, you think about the way things are and the way you'd like them to be.

If you feel healthy and are busy with your classes and activities, for instance, you may never think about exercise. Then you notice you get winded walking up stairs. Still you don't quite register the need to do anything about it.

During precontemplation, change remains hypothetical, distant, and vague and seems unlikely. Yet you may speak of something bugging you and wish that things were somehow different. If you ignore or override this discomfort or find sufficient distractions,

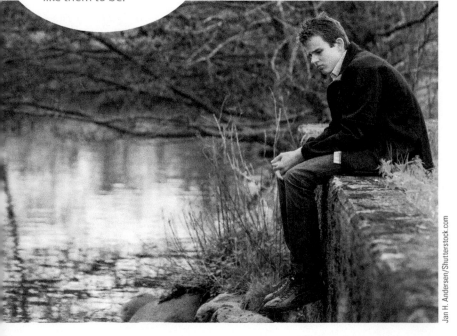

Jan H. Andersen/Shutterstock.com

precontemplation can last indefinitely, and you won't change.

Contemplation

In the **contemplation** stage, you begin to get it. You acknowledge that something is amiss and begin to consider what is and whether you can do anything about it. You still prefer not to have to change, but you start to realize that you can't avoid reality. Maybe your grades have plummeted, and you're facing academic probation. Maybe you're been putting in such long hours at work that you doze off during lectures. As you begin to weigh the trade-offs of standing pat versus acting, you may alternate between wanting to take action and resisting it. You may question your ability to change and feel moody and irritable, reflections of the ambivalence and indecisiveness you feel.

✔ **Check-in:** Are you contemplating a change?

The way you talk to yourself expresses your feeling that change is necessary but demonstrates your lack of commitment to taking action. Here are some examples of how the contemplation stage sounds:

_____ "I've got to do something about this."

_____ "I can't go on this way."

_____ "I hate that I keep . . ."

_____ "I should . . ."

_____ "Maybe I'll do it someday—not tomorrow, but one day."

_____ "I'm fed up."

Preparation

At some point you stop flip-flopping, make a clear decision, and feel a burst of energy. This decision heralds the **preparation** stage. You gather information, make phone calls, do research online, and look into exercise classes at the gym. You begin to think and act with change specifically in mind, even if you hold something back.

Part of preparation is getting internally accustomed to the idea of change and the impact it will make on you. This takes the form of mental rehearsal as you imagine what life will be like when you change. Trying things on for size in your mind helps you ready yourself to deal with higher expectations and new demands. In this phase you face your fears openly.

If you eavesdrop on what you're saying to yourself, you would hear statements such as, "I am going to do this," and you set a date, such as, "I will begin on New Year's Day." Yet you may not share your plans with others. Despite all the internal progress you've made, you aren't necessarily ready to go public and commit to change.

Action

The **action** stage is the stage of actively modifying your behavior according to your plan. Your resolve is strong, and you know you're on your way to a better you. You no longer keep your plan under wraps—not that you could. Change produces signs that are visible to others. You may not join your old friends for poker games, or midweek beer pong tournaments. You may talk to your adviser about dropping a course or signing up for a free tutorial.

In the action stage, things you mulled over and incubated for years unfold quickly. The more attention you devote to nurturing and solidifying your new habits, the faster they fall into place. In a relatively short time, you acquire a sense of comfort and ease with the change in your life.

Maintenance

Maintenance is about locking in and consolidating gains. This stabilizing stage, which follows the flurry of specific steps taken in the action stage, is absolutely necessary to retain what you've worked for and to make change permanent. Although it may sound as dull as changing oil and rotating tires, maintenance is an active, vital phase of the change process that provides the final ingredient needed for permanently reshaping your life.

In this stage, you strengthen, enhance, and extend the changes you've initiated. You bring the rest of what you do into line with the change to support it. By securing the progress you've made, even if you hit a plateau or slip backward, you can regain your footing and keep moving forward. It may even be helpful to have a slip up with your new change. Perhaps after a long day of classes, followed by your new habit of spending an hour in the library to immediately begin homework and reading, you get home and feel drained. Instead of preparing that healthy dinner for yourself you'd planned on, you pick up a burger and fries instead. This could be a helpful learning experience. For days you know you are likely to be especially tired at the end of the day, you can prepare food in advance that will last for a few meals. Now you've learned how to tweak your new change to make it work best for you.

Relapse

Some therapists add another stage: **relapse**, or reverting to old behaviors, which is often part of the process of change. Behavioral change is a process rather than a one-time event. People often spiral through the various stages several times before the desired change becomes stable.[5]

Even with considerable inner reserves and advance planning, you may lose your footing. Whatever you do, do not consider any stumble a failure. The only failure will be failing to mine the situation to discover as much information as you can. Mistakes and setbacks teach exactly what you need to move forward—especially if you think you have hit the wall or crashed and burned.

Do a post-mortem on this little episode. Seek the support of a counselor or wise friend at this time, someone who can help you identify the factors which led to your relapse and help you find the motivation to try again. Then regroup, reload, and launch Plan B. Avoid drama. Consider all of this as nothing more than a mid-course correction. When you drive, you make hundreds of tiny course corrections in order to travel in a straight line. It is the same with change. Sometimes when you're driving, you come to a detour. The same happens with change.

....

✔ **Check-in:** Read through the descriptions of the stages of change again, and ask yourself: Where am I?

....

Is This the Best Time to Make a Change?

Yes. Trust us on this. If you wait for change to happen spontaneously or for circumstances to change, you will keep waiting. Hoping fortune will come and smile upon you is not a method for change. Fortune has already smiled and given you the present moment. If you create a weekly study schedule for yourself right now, we doubt that you'll regret it come finals week.

Postponing change is not simply postponing; it is a failure to act. Any apparent advantage usually turns out to be imaginary. If you wait until you have more money or more time, or until you're comfortable with what the future holds, you may end up waiting forever. If you wait to be in the right mood to change, you inevitably will wait longer than

preparation The stage of change in which you begin to think and act with change specifically in mind, even if you're not quite ready to start.

action The stage of change in which you actively modify your behavior according to your plan.

maintenance The ongoing stage of change that involves locking in and consolidating gains to make change permanent.

relapse Reverting to old behaviors.

necessary. In order to change, you need something other than time, money, or a certain mood. You need the skills we describe later in this chapter.

On the other hand, rather than waiting for the perfect time to come, you may fear that your ideal moment has passed. Think again. There is no one single moment, no one single choice, that defines a life. Believing that you missed your chance, believing that the time is not right or ripe for change, is a way to justify not changing. All of us have passed on important opportunities. If you keep looking back, you get trapped in regret and ignore the opportunities that exist now. You cannot relive or undo the past, but you have this moment in time. You decide what you want to do with it.

What if you're too busy right now? Who isn't? Using excuses to resist change is only hurting you and your potential. Start small—in fact, it is best to start small, but do start. Do not fall into the "if I can't exercise for an hour, I won't exercise at all" trap. If something is worth doing, it is worth doing for whatever amount of time you can give it. And it is worth starting now. You deserve it.

> **Stress Reliever:** Are You Ready to Cross the Line in the Sand?
>
> Imagine that you are standing in front of an imaginary line in the sand. One side represents life as you have lived it in the past; the other, your new life. Crossing the line represents a complete, final, no-turning-back decision to make a change of series of changes that will help you create the life you want.
>
> This exercise is even more powerful if you act it out and physically cross from one side of a room or a space to the other as a symbolic commitment to change.

Athletes visualize every movement they must make to perform at their best.

See the Steps of Change

If you imagine a hypothetical event, such as winning an award or being selected to represent your school at a national conference, you are more likely to consider it possible and to make it happen. In studies of world-class athletes, those who practiced positive visualization performed better than those who exercised just as much but did not use this psychological technique.

However, it's important to visualize not just the final moment of triumph, but the actual steps and activities that lead up to it. As social psychology research has shown, if you visualize yourself completing the various steps of a project just before sitting down to it, you will be much more likely to complete your work in the allotted time.

An Olympic gold-medal 400-meter hurdler named Edwin Moses, who set four world records in his event, used to visualize an entire race, imagining every single stride he would take, seeing himself crossing each hurdle and then sprinting to the finish line. Sports psychologists contend that his visualization of the entire race was more effective than just imagining the moment when the gold medal slipped over his head. Visualizing the steps of any process creates a readiness to complete the process just as you've imagined it. It also reduces anxiety around taking those steps towards change.

Practice your positive visualization at least twice a day, once in the morning and once in the evening. Even better, stop just before you begin any task to visualize briefly how you want to conduct yourself during the activity.

Let's say it's time to devote a block of time to studying for that difficult class. Before you begin, visualize yourself taking notes or underlining passages. See yourself reading your textbook and doing online practice quizzes with interest, enthusiasm, and comprehension. Inject a mild note of urgency; add a great deal of attention.

The more detailed your vision of your positive behaviors, the more benefits you'll derive from the exercise. End each visualization with your personal equivalent of an Olympic gold medal—whether that's stepping on the scale with a smile, crossing the finish line of a charity fun run, or acing a test.

Motivating Change: Go for Your Goals

As you've already learned, stress is (to a great extent) in the eye of the beholder. When your eyes are focused on a dream, on something big that you want out of life, or on smaller dreams of relationships you wish to develop, skills you wish to master, self-understanding you wish to cultivate, or adventures you want to pursue, you see purposeful action and challenge not as stresses, but as steps to take on your way to your goal.

Goals carry us from dreaming to doing by giving us purpose and direction. They also provide a rationale and a set of priorities to guide us in selecting which changes we want to make and when. As road maps that lead to destinations, action plans provide us with a way to reach our goals by suggesting an itinerary for getting us there. People who set goals, write them down, and review them reach them faster. They also report less stress, greater happiness, and more life satisfaction.[6]

Once you decide that you want to make a personal change in your life, setting goals is the best way of getting from Point A to Point B—and eventually all the way to Point Z. Setting goals means setting a course for your life. Without goals, you remain stuck. With goals, you learn, you grow, and you become what you wish. Here are some specific steps to take:

- See it, say it, write it. Create an image of your goal. Maybe you see yourself performing on stage, hanging your paintings for an exhibit, or anchoring the local news. Describe and define your goal in your mind. Then put it in words and commit it to paper. Until you write down what you want, it's only a wish. Feel free to amend, modify, refine, expand and extend your goals—and then check off each one as you reach it.

- Identify your resources. Do you have what you need—knowledge, skills, time—to succeed?

- Systematically analyze barriers. Think through, in very concrete and specific terms, what is likely to get in your way. For each obstacle, list solutions.

- Set goals that focus on changing behavior and make them as specific as possible. If your goal is to study abroad for a semester, this is what you might write:

- Today's goal: I will go online and identify the program and location that most interests me.
- This week's goal: I will meet with my advisor and a financial aid advisor to make sure studying abroad won't interfere with my required courses or my scholarship.
- This month's goal: I will download and complete the application.

Your Big Dream

Big ideas and big dreams energize and motivate us by making the work of change worthwhile. Only when we allow and encourage big-picture thinking in ourselves do we begin to stretch and extend beyond what we consider our limits. By directing all of your potential toward something that gets your juices flowing, a dream or a compelling big-picture vision helps you engage fully and melts away irritations, obstacles, and inconveniences. Sure, the road may be rocky at times, but remember that you are writing your story along the way to your goals. Remind yourself, "I am choosing to follow my dreams and take every chance to problem solve as a learning experience."

Give yourself this advantage: Begin to think in terms of dreams and constructing a life that is the stuff of dreams. This won't just happen without your conscious, active involvement; you have to make it happen through your choices and your actions. Choices create the specific itinerary for converting your big picture from blue-sky fantasy to the bedrock upon which you build. By having a dream, you will know which changes to make and actions to take. (See the Personal Stress Management Toolkit on page 143.)

Your Destination Goal

You wouldn't board a bus without knowing where you want to go, but it's easy to drift through our days with only a vague sense of where we're heading. Unfortunately, goals that don't lead somewhere—like wanting to be happy or rich—tend to go nowhere. A specific, focused, realistic goal, such as selling your designs for phone and tablet cases online or learning a new language, provides a solid destination that can fast-forward you into the future.

A long-term goal transforms your brain into a satellite dish picking up the signals that are most relevant to your quest. Rather than staying in the "wouldn't it be nice if . . ." mode, a destination goal instructs your mind to focus on an objective. Then while you get to work on the short-term goals and action steps, your unconscious mind searches for additional possibilities and creative solutions.

Setting Long-Term Goals

- Review your descriptions of your dreams and visions, and translate them into one overarching dream and a handful of specific, long-term goals. If your dream is to live and work in Paris, one obvious long-term goal would be to become fluent in French.

- Write no more than five or six long-term goals in this fashion.

- Do not set a time limit for these goals. The reason? If you set a deadline for a long-term goal, you may slow your progress by eliminating opportunities for your unconscious mind to find truly creative and efficient solutions that could come more quickly. You don't want to direct your mind to wait until some stated time if it can come up with results sooner.

- To ensure that your unconscious mind pays attention to your goals, repeat each goal five times in the morning and five times in the night until you reach it. This exercise makes your long-term goal function as a command directing you to make efforts toward meeting it.

Your Short-Term Goals

Short-term goals are tools for reaching immediate objectives in brief time frames, such as one week. An example of short-term goal planning might be to meet with a financial aid officer, check certain websites about summer internships, or read a certain book within a week. A short-term goal has specific objectives and an unambiguous deadline for meeting it.

Here are some guidelines:

- Decide on specific objectives you want to accomplish within a brief time period and write them down. For instance, you may want to discover and evaluate any and all Chinese-language groups or activities on campus.

- Schedule time to accomplish your goal. You might set aside time between classes to meet with a Chinese language professor. Mark in your calendar when you are going to complete a task.

- Announce your goals to one other person. Agree to check in with him or her at a specific time every week to report on your progress and to set new goals to reach by your next meeting.

- Schedule time to look at your list of short-term goals every day, and take the actions

necessary to reach them. Make this a non-negotiable imperative.

- Whenever you achieve a goal, check it off, tell a friend, or just raise your hands above your head like an athlete who's just clinched a championship. This builds your sense of "I can do it. I am doing it. Look how far I've come!"

 Stress Reliever: Own Your Goals

Are you thinking of becoming a pre-med because your mother never had the chance to fulfill her dream of becoming a doctor? Are you going out for soccer because of your grandfather's passion for the game? Are you trying one major after another because you would really rather train to be a paramedic than get a degree in liberal arts? Are you taking evening courses because your supervisor suggested them or because you want to move into management?

Whenever you're setting goals—whether long-term or short-term—these guidelines are critical:

- Set only your own goals. Don't allow others to set them for you, and don't set goals for others.

- Always write your goals down, and look at them often. Putting a goal in writing moves you from wishing to doing, from contemplation to preparation and action. When you write goals down, you become more committed to making your words come true.

- Give each goal a rating from 0 to 10 for the degree to which the goal is one you embrace as your own, using 0 for one that you do not embrace at all and 10 for a goal fully embraced by you. Make a second rating to express the importance of accomplishing each goal, using 0 for a goal completely unimportant to you and 10 for one as important as you could imagine.

The Language of Change

You've already learned how words affect your perceptions and responses to stress. Change has a vocabulary all of its own. Even tiny little words like "try" take on new meanings. Are you, for instance, "trying" to get organized? If so, you've just tripped over your own feet. "Try," as in "try to do it if you can" is a sorry, sickly little word that insinuates itself regularly into otherwise reasonable requests and kills their power. In fact, "I'll try" in response to a request is usually a polite form of refusal. If your professor gives you a date and time to discuss your final grade, would you "try" to make it? This use of "try" differs completely from the "try" that means to "test or examine."

The word "try," meaning "to attempt," is a weasel word that contains a built-in implicit directive to stop short of succeeding. When someone says, "just try your best," isn't he or she suggesting that you mount some kind of effort but not expect to be successful? In fact, to comply fully with the directive "just try your best," you *have* to stop short of bringing something to a full, successful conclusion. The "just" tells you how far to go. "Try your best" is the same as saying, "Don't worry. I don't expect you to make it."

Soft language with its built-in slack gives you and others permission to accept less than your best. When you talk to yourself this way, you listen to, and follow, the implied directives.

....
✔ **Check-in:** Think for a moment.
....

Would you say "try your best" to a heart surgeon before going under the knife?
....
Then why say it to yourself?
....

Loophole Language

Language that expresses unequivocal intention sounds different and makes entirely different demands on the listener. With it, you create an internal environment of clear objectives and directives. For example, if you say about your zoology final, "I'm gonna try to study hard for it," the word "try" sends a message to your brain that cancels out the "study hard for it." But if you say "I am going to focus and study thoroughly for my final," the language *requires* a different kind of commitment. That's what we're talking about.

People also sabotage themselves by saying "if" or "if only." You probably have used phrases like, "If I could get organized," or "If only I could stick with my exercise plan." Such statements reinforce the notion that you're never going to change.

Instead of another "if," say to yourself, "When I get organized," or "When I start working out." This simple switch sets the stage for believing what is actually true—that you already can and will be able to change your lifestyle.

Another way to prevent dodging change is to use the word *how* rather than *why* to explain your actions. For example, if you ask yourself *why* you sometimes drink too much, you might answer, "Things aren't going well in my life," or "I get bored in the evening." If you ask yourself *how* you drink too much, you might answer, "I start playing drinking games with my friends," or "I don't keep track of how many beers I have."

Give yourself new operating instructions and insist that you always follow them. Tell yourself that whenever you reach for another drink, you will always consider *how* you are choosing or deciding to drink more rather than answering the why question with another excuse for doing so. When you ask how, be sure to know that you do have a basis for how you choose to drink more.

> **Stress Reliever:** Don't Try. Do.
> ....
> For one week, forbid yourself to use the word "try" in relation to actions you are going to take. Observe the effect. You will quickly discover how often you use the word—and perhaps why you use it too. You will also feel how different it is to shed this linguistic hideout. You may feel that you are eavesdropping on your own unconscious. Also note how different it is to forbid yourself to use the word than it is to try not to use it.

Real Talk

If your instructor asked if you'd like to get an A in this course, would you say, "sort of" or "kind of"? We hope not. Vague language invites you to hold back, especially when you're talking about what you want to do. Add "really" to the mix, and you dilute what you're saying even more.

What does it mean to say, "I sort of really want to do it" or "I mean I kind of could be into that"? This kind of speech carries an ambivalence virus that infects your thinking and your ability to move on things. When you speak of goals, use definitive, unequivocal language to describe what you want and how you intend to get it. Say, "I will do it"—with no kind of, sort of vagueness attached or implied. Notice the difference from the wishy-washy conditional tense and passive voice of, "I would like it to get done today." These statements sound different because they are different. Speaking with purpose will change the way you and others perceive you. It is important to remember that goals are not met by being "kind of interested" or "sort of trying."

When you start a sentence with "it" or use the passive voice, you suggest that things happen independent of your will or because of external events not under your direction. Compare the differences between the following:

- "It needs to get done."
- "I need to do it."
- "I am doing it today."

All three express differences in locus of control and intention to complete the action. While you are not in control of everything, the first statement suggests that there is no point in exercising the power you do have and thus excuses you from responsibility. The second statement talks about a need. There is no stated intention and no directive to complete. The difference between the first and third is night and day in terms or urgency and intention to complete the task at hand.

Ducking responsibility, however appealing at the moment, always costs you heavily. When you linguistically evade responsibility, you reduce personal power and control and invite the passivity that the passive voice implies. Although we're not teaching a grammar lesson, we hope you get the message. By taking greater responsibility *for* your language and *with* your language, you demand that you take greater responsibility for your actions and with your life.

Look for ways to embrace and increase responsibility when you talk. Using the active voice—I am, I do, I will—frees you to seek ways in which you can exert a directing force upon your life. When you use the active voice and embrace as much responsibility for your actions as you can, you will notice a greater sense of mastery and personal efficacy.

Say "I am writing the essay this afternoon." Then do it. Do not say. "I'm going to take a stab at that essay today or tonight—whenever I can get to it." Deconstruct the second sentence, and you will easily recognize how vague your operating instructions are. The odds of your finishing it this afternoon by saying it the second way are next to nothing. Why? Because you didn't say anything that remotely expresses this specific intention and the instructions to your brain are vague. To follow those vague instructions your brain actually has to take vague actions and not complete the task. In plain language, you aren't planning to, so you won't.

Boosting Your Power to Change

Remember the story of Robinson Crusoe? Shipwrecked on a desert island, he had to change in order to survive. His original destination and goals no longer mattered. He had to deal with a completely new reality. He did so by using the island and the boat wreckage to provide everything he needed to survive. Instead of mourning what he lost, he played the hand he was dealt to its maximum advantage. If he had done otherwise and spent his time grieving for what should or might have been, he would have perished.

When you're facing a challenge or a change (or the challenge of change), think like Robinson Crusoe: Use what you've got. Take advantage of every opportunity. Don't mope and whine. Don't pine for something you lack, like more money or a supportive partner. Become the master of what you have and what is available to you.

Exploit the advantages of what seem to be disadvantages. If you feel that you don't have enough money, for example, become expert at stretching your resources. Use your student ID to get into museums and movies at a lower price. Investigate all the free classes, craft studios, movies, music and dance facilities, recreational

When facing a challenge or making a change, you have to draw on every resources within and around you.

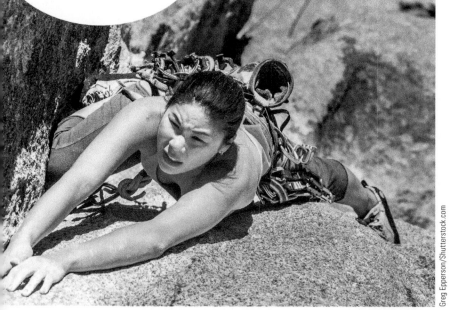

Greg Epperson/Shutterstock.com

programs, and other opportunities available on and off campus. Enjoy local free concerts. Sign up for deal-offering websites, such as Groupon, LivingSocial, ScoutMob, Google Offers, Amazon Local, or Savvy Circle. You don't need an extravagant budget. Pay attention and you will be awash in great opportunities for special experiences. And remember: Every sunset is free, and there's no charge for walking in the moonlight.

If you're thinking ahead to your career (and you should be), you may worry about how to go about getting job experience. Rather than hustling for whatever low-paying job you can scrounge, volunteer to work for free doing something you find meaningful or in a field of interest. Once you get that opportunity, become as useful and productive as you can. Do not fall victim to conventional thinking—your own or someone else's—about what you must achieve on what timetable.

Act on what you *have* now and where you *are* now. You may become so valuable to the organization for which you volunteer that when you say you can't afford to stay longer, they offer you a paying position because they don't want to lose you. Whether they do or not you will have had an experience in the environment you were seeking and had the chance to learn.

Although most Olympic athletes are born with natural talent, all must work hard to develop their agility, strength, skills and mental toughness. The best, the strongest, the swiftest, and the most skilled would never make it to the Olympics, let alone to the medal stand, if they did not make the most of what they have. You do the same when you do everything you can with whatever is at your disposal and exploit every opportunity to achieve your goals.

⚙ Stress Reliever: Do You Give Up Too Soon?
···

Despite good intentions and considerable progress, many people give up their goals just before reaching their rainbow's end— and congratulate themselves for getting that far. Would you ever board a plane for Chicago and say, "Well, we got three-quarters of the way there!" as if that were good?
···
Persist, persevere and don't settle for "almost there." If you stall on the final stretch, do a quick reality check. Maybe you need to break down some steps into

smaller bits or add a few more to reach your goals. Don't hesitate to seek more support, or simply allow yourself more time. Not only be gentle with yourself, but also be firm. Keep working towards your goals.

Beyond Willpower

Do you know people with a will of steel? If they're on a diet, they can resist the most delectable pastries; if they're getting into shape, they rise at dawn to get in a three-mile run; if they're on deadline, they focus with laser-like intensity. Psychologists say such individuals have high trait self-control, which means they do better at avoiding temptation, resisting impulses, and blocking out distractions.

However, researchers have discovered a secret behind their seemingly superhuman self-discipline: They don't simply resist temptations; they avoid them. Successful dieters, for instance, don't buy candy—let alone keep a stash in the closet. They put their running shoes by their bedside to remind them to get moving first thing in the morning. And when they're crashing on a project, they turn off phones and alerts, close the door, and get the job done. As we put our 2016 resolutions into practice, then, we should take a page from their book and try to avoid tempting situations instead of just relying on willpower. "If you can avoid temptation," the researchers concluded, it will not even occur to you: success without effort."[7]

You can also use the opposite approach: Display reminders of what you're trying to achieve. Hang your bathing suit in plain sight to inspire your weight loss plan; download a photo of an Olympic athlete to motivate yourself to work out; if you're saving to study or travel abroad, turn an image of your desired destination into your screen saver.

Making Personal Change Inevitable

When you were little, change was a completely normal, everyday event. You amazed your parents with how quickly you changed—and you amazed yourself as you added remarkable feats like walking and talking to your repertoire. Children caught up in the magic of daily discoveries change without considering alternative ways of being. They try new things, fail where they will, pick themselves up, and try again.

At some point in life, for whatever reason, we start saying about some ingrained habit, "It's just the way I am." That's not true; it's the way you *have been until now.* Declaring that you can't change wastes time you could be using to make change inevitable. And change is inevitable—if you do the work.

The first step on the way to successful change is to commit quietly but fully and vow not to stop before reaching your goal. If you don't decide to change, your old habits win out; the moment you decide, you become formidable, like some hungry animal that will hunt relentlessly until it finds food. Things become clear; life becomes simpler because when you decide, you simplify it; one priority rises to the top. Making an unequivocal choice for change unleashes a nearly unstoppable force, especially if you tune into the pleasure.

A decision to move from where you are requires a concrete plan. This may sound daunting, but you already have a grasp of how to go about it. If you ever plotted ahead of time how to tell your parents about your plan to backpack in Europe or how to get the attention of the cute classmate across the aisle, you have experience in setting out a plan. Making a plan concrete simply requires taking that kind of strategizing and elaborating on it.

No matter how complex a desired change may be, you can break it down into finite steps. Once you develop a step-by-step plan and consistently follow it, you can replace any habit, however tenacious. However, for a while the new habit will have to compete with the old ingrained one. You will have to exert effort until you have locked in the new behavior.[8]

Just as when you learned to swim, when you begin your first efforts to change, you may cling to the side or rely on artificial supports like water wings far longer than you need to. Both are ways of cheating yourself. At some point you have to give up what makes you feel secure in order to make the next step. You have to let go of the edge.

Change becomes inevitable if you persist even when you fear that you're in over your head and when your efforts seem to have no apparent effect other than hassling and irritating you. Change takes time, but usually only the early results are disconcerting. Change tinkers with deeply entrenched habits and patterns of thinking that exist beyond your consciousness. You will have some temporary hell to pay for this disruption. But if you understand that new routines feel upsetting only until you become accustomed to them, you will persist in the face of challenges that otherwise might discourage you.

Any habit can be changed. Change is no mystery. You do the work, and you make the change. But you have to keep choosing to change until you get there.

> ### 🔧 Stress Reliever: "Shaping" Change
>
> "Shaping" is a behavior modification technique that uses rewards and incentives to motivate change and reinforce progress. Whenever you meet one of your goals, reward yourself with a positive reinforcer. Here are some examples:
>
> _____ A long walk
>
> _____ Sitting on a bench by a pond outside and watching the sky or sunset
>
> _____ Twenty uninterrupted minutes of reading for pleasure
>
> _____ Listening to your favorite music
>
> _____ Looking through old photos in digital storage
>
> _____ Watching a favorite classic movie
>
> _____ Sleeping in on Sunday
>
> _____ _____
>
> _____ _____
>
> _____ _____

Are You Getting in Your Own Way?

You may not even be aware of any tendency to trip over your own feet until you start to change. Because you consider whatever you habitually do as normal, you may have accepted self-defeating behavior, not as a choice, but as simply the way you are. In fact, you made many choices in the process of becoming who you "naturally" are. Everything that feels normal and natural now was once a matter of choice and felt awkward and new in the beginning. When you can recognize this element of choice, you have the opportunity to make a new one.

Try the following simple exercise: If you wear a wristwatch, take it off, and place it on the other wrist. Leave it there for a day. Notice whether it feels unnatural or odd, and whether this feeling changes.

Of course, there isn't anything "natural" about wearing your watch on one wrist or the other. It's simply a matter of choice—like the way you shave or apply moisturizer. You always do these things the same way. Change them, and notice how you feel. The point isn't to throw yourself off, but to show that you can continue unhelpful or pointless habits because they feel "normal" and balk at very useful changes because they feel strange at first.

If even simple changes can unsettle you, how will you fulfill your potential or accomplish a life choice or a dream? Small patterns migrate from specific situations and grow into big, generalized patterns until you come to view a simple habit as who you fundamentally are. If you see that you haven't persisted, for instance, you may conclude that you lack persistence and that you can't finish things you start. If you see that you avoid things, you come to think that you are a coward.

Say you are putting off filing the final part of your application for study abroad. Avoiding the paperwork may seem a small thing. But focus on the following: What is it you fear about reaching your goal? What is holding you back? New demands to live up to? New expectations from others? The unknown challenges of spending time in a foreign country? Disappointment if you aren't accepted? Figure it out because if you delay, you create a new stress—avoiding. Then, by not solving the tendency to avoid, you make the stakes higher still.

As you analyze ways in which you may be tripping yourself up, keep another thing in mind: If you have not reached a change goal as rapidly as you wanted, do not try to save face by quitting. Otherwise after all your hard work, you will pull away from the struggle before you reap the rewards.

Achieving any important, satisfying goal takes time and work. If you sign on only for what is immediately fun and easy, your shrink your life down to a limited range of shallow activities and interests and block yourself from making changes that would set you free. And you never find out what it's like to spend a semester in Rio studying Portuguese.

Changing for Good

Every day you face choices, including the choice of change. Maybe you're still in the precontemplation or contemplation stages—the two longest phases in the process of change. Or you may be ready to begin the third stage of preparation and to take concrete steps toward your goal.

Wherever you are, you need not remain frozen in this moment, looking over your shoulder, your gaze fixed on the past, always just about to make the choice that will change your life but never quite making it. You have only to turn, face the present moment, and begin to work from your current position. Until you do, you remain

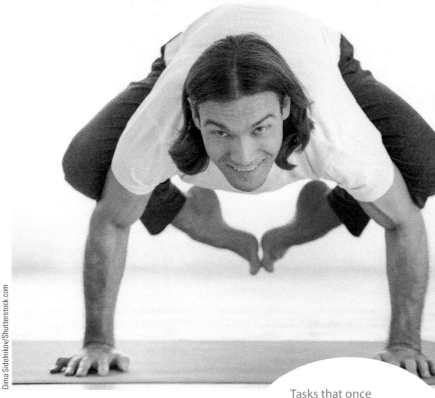

Tasks that once seemed impossible can be mastered with persistence.

mired in what you already know rather than moving ahead to what you have yet to learn. The pain you want to avoid is knowing what to do but not doing it.

Every day you choose whether and how to express love, creativity, and excellence. Regardless of what you choose, your choices have consequences. Ask yourself: What am I doing with my time? What do I need to do to express who I am? Pick one new thing to do each day that can raise your "standard of living." What is the center point of your life? How do you nurture and nourish your body and your spirit? Are you so busy doing everything that you enjoy nothing?

If you read a few pages from a good book every evening and spend a bit of time thinking about how you want to make tomorrow satisfying, you will begin something you will not want to set aside. If you turn off your car radio and drive everywhere in silence, you create a noise-free zone where you can hear yourself think. Better yet, get out of your car and walk or bike.

You can make better choices. The small decisions of everyday life—what to eat, where to go, when to study—are straightforward. Larger issues—which major to choose, what to do about a dead-end relationship, how to handle an awkward work-study situation—are more challenging. However, if you think of decision-making as a process, like change, you can break down even the

Dima Sidelnikov/Shutterstock.com

most difficult choices into manageable steps. The following can help whenever you face a decision:

- Set priorities. Rather than getting bogged down in details, step back and look at the big picture. What matters most to you? What would you like to accomplish in the next week, month, year? Look at the decisions you're about to make in the context of your values and goals.

- Inform yourself. The more you know—about a person, a position, a place, a project—the better you will be able to evaluate it. Gathering information may involve formal research, such as an online search for relevant data, or informal conversations with teachers, counselors, advisers, family members, and friends.

- Consider all your options. Most complex decisions don't involve simple either/or alternatives. List as many options as you can, along with the advantages and disadvantages of each. Talk to a friend or family member about your options to feel out what feels seems right for you; they could suggest alternatives that haven't crossed your mind.

- Tune in to your gut feelings. After you've gotten the facts and analyzed them, listen to your intuition. While it's not infallible, your sixth sense can provide valuable feedback. If something just doesn't feel right, try to figure out why. Are there any fears you haven't yet confronted? Do you have doubts about taking a certain path? "Going with your gut" is not just a pat expression. Researchers have learned that the gut contains neural tissue that is effectively the same as brain cells.

- Consider a worst-case scenario. When you're close to a final decision, imagine what will happen if everything goes wrong—the workload becomes overwhelming, your partner betrays your trust, your expectations turn out to be unrealistic. If you can live with the worst consequences of a decision, you're probably making the right choice.

Managing Your Behaviors

Every new electronic device—computer, phone, tablet, television, gaming console—comes with operating instructions. Maybe you read them carefully and follow every step; maybe you toss them aside and wing it. Human beings don't come with a helpful owner's manual. Yes, responsible adults—parents, grandparents, teachers, mentors, coaches—teach you the basics. But sooner or later you have to wing it—at times not as successfully as you might wish. However, the behaviors you've tried in the past aren't encoded on a hard drive. You always have the option of rewriting your operating instructions so you behave in ways that can reduce day-to-day stress.

Take an everyday situation that many people find stressful: waiting, which can feel like torture for folks who hate wasting time. Perhaps whenever the line to drop in during a professor's office hours is too long or all the dryers in the laundry room are busy, you bolt, losing the time you already devoted to your mission and failing to complete what you have to do. Here's how to turn things around:

- Imagine a situation in which you have to wait, see yourself in it, and then, at the point at which your impatience formerly overwhelmed you, find a new behavior to substitute for leaving. Consider as many possibilities as you want before coming up with a new alternative. You might decide to open an app of Spanish verbs you need to memorize or to start a visualization exercise like the one described on page 143.

- When you choose, develop an internal instruction to tie a new, adaptive behavior to a specific triggering event. A trigger can be either the event that prompted the old behavior or the event you want to associate with the new behavior—for example, standing in a slow-moving line. With time, your operating system will learn to look at previously tedious or stressful situations as opportunities to accomplish something and reduce stress.

- Put your new specific operating instruction in the following form: "Whenever I stand in any line, I will *always* . . ." Then insert the behavior you decide will work best for you. If you choose the Spanish verbs, the sentence would end "click on the app of Spanish verbs and begin to memorize them." Note the use of the word *always* in the instructions. Always use *always* in your specific operating instructions.

- Practice. Nothing increases the speed at which you adopt new behaviors like rehearsal in real life. Each day create as many opportunities as possible to use your new instructions. For the best results, rehearse a new behavior consistently when you are cool and unflustered. This will help you internalize the instructions and become mentally accustomed to the new choice.

- Continue your new specific operating instructions whether you encounter success or failure in the actual situation. Your goal is to make the new behavior become your automatic response, and you need *many* repetitions to overlearn any new behavior enough to make it automatic.

Chapter Summary

- When you deliberately change a nonproductive thought, feeling, or behavior, you are choosing to take control—of your time, your health, your relationships, your achievements, and your future.

- Change starts with observing what you do now and thinking through different choices that might make your life easier, more efficient, less stressful, or infinitely more satisfying. Once you create this vision, you can prepare your change plan.

- When you take small, methodical steps toward a goal, you acquire more than one new competence: If you pay attention, you teach yourself how to make a change.

- Personal change replaces negative behaviors with positive new skills (the word people use for habits they like and want to keep) that empower and energize your life.

- To change, you must adopt an appropriate long-range perspective. Instead of planning a quick fix, the emotional equivalent of a crash diet, think in terms of revising forever the specific, decisive aspects of your life that will make a difference.

- To make a change—whether it's to eliminate a bad habit or to create a good one—you have to do two things: repeat new actions in order to forge new connections in the brain and resist the natural tendency to follow the well-trod path of least resistance.

- The "transtheoretical" model of change focuses on various stages that people move through as they progress from being clueless, to conscious, to committed to making a change.

- During the precontemplation stage, you may speak of something bugging you and wish that things were somehow different. If you ignore or override this discomfort, precontemplation can last indefinitely, and you won't change.

- In the contemplation stage, you acknowledge that something is amiss and begin to consider what it is and whether you can do anything about it.

- In the preparation stage, you begin to think and act with change specifically in mind. Part of preparation is getting internally accustomed to the idea of change and its impact on you.

- Action is the stage of actively modifying your behavior according to your plan. In a relatively short time, you acquire a sense of comfort and ease with the change in your life.

- The maintenance stage is about locking in and consolidating gains. This stabilizing stage, which follows the flurry of specific steps taken in the action stage, is absolutely necessary to make change permanent.

- Visualizing the steps of any process creates a readiness to complete the process just as you've imagined it. It also reduces anxiety around taking those steps towards change.

- Goals carry us from dreaming to doing by giving us purpose and direction. They also provide a rationale and a set of priorities to guide us in selecting which changes to make.

- A long-term goal transforms your brain into a satellite dish picking up the signals that are most relevant to your quest. Rather than staying in the "wouldn't it be nice if . . ." mode, a destination goal instructs your mind to focus on an objective.

- Short-term goals are tools for reaching immediate objectives in brief time frames, such as one week. A short-term goal has specific objectives and an unambiguous deadline for meeting it.

- Change has a vocabulary all of its own. Using the active voice—I am, I do, I will—frees you to seek ways in which you can exert a directing force upon your life.

- When you're facing a challenge or change, take advantage of every opportunity. Exploit the advantages of what seem to be disadvantages.

- The decision to move from where you are requires a concrete plan. No matter how complex a desired change may be, you can break it down into finite steps.

- Change becomes inevitable if you persist even when you fear that you're in over your head and when your efforts seem to have no apparent effect. Change takes time, but usually only the early results are disconcerting.

🌐 STRESS RELIEVERS

Own the Future

Make a list of some positive attributes you plan to acquire. Write a series of statements describing the new improved you—all in the present tense. Why? Using the present tense creates a hypnotic-like demand that your behavior match the description. Some examples:

_____ I am organized.
_____ I am psyched.
_____ I am ready for this test.
_____ I can do this.

Are You Ready to Cross the Line in the Sand?

Imagine that you are standing in front of an imaginary line in the sand. One side represents life as you have lived it in the past; the other, your new life. Crossing the line represents a complete, final, no-turning-back decision to make a change of series of changes that will help you create the life you want.

This exercise is even more powerful if you act it out and physically cross from one side of a room or a space to the other as a symbolic commitment to change.

Own Your Goals

Are you thinking of becoming a pre-med because your mother never had the chance to fulfill her dream of becoming a doctor? Are you going out for soccer because of your grandfather's passion for the game? Are you trying one major after another because you would really rather train to be a paramedic than get a degree in liberal arts? Are you taking evening courses because your supervisor suggested them or because you want to move into management?

Whenever you're setting goals—whether long-term or short-term—these guidelines are critical:

- Set only your own goals. Don't allow others to set them for you, and don't set goals for others.

- Always write your goals down, and look at them often. Putting a goal in writing moves you from wishing to doing, from contemplation to preparation and action. When you write goals down, you become more committed to making your words come true.

- Give each goal a rating from 0 to 10 for the degree to which the goal is one you embrace as your own, using 0 for one that you do not embrace at all and 10 for a goal fully embraced by you. Make a second rating to express the importance of accomplishing each goal, using 0 for a goal completely unimportant to you and 10 for one as important as you could imagine.

Don't Try. Do

For one week, forbid yourself to use the word "try" in relation to actions you are going to take. Observe the effect. You will quickly discover how often you use the word—and perhaps why you use it too. You will also feel how different it is to shed this linguistic hideout. You may feel that you are eavesdropping on your own unconscious. Also note how different it is to forbid yourself to use the word than it is to try not to use it.

Do You Give Up Too Soon?

Despite good intentions and considerable progress, many people give up their goals just before reaching their rainbow's end—and congratulate themselves for getting that far. Would you ever board a plane for Chicago and say, "Well, we got three quarters of the way there!" as if that were good?

Persist, persevere and don't settle for "almost there." If you stall on the final stretch, do a quick reality check. Maybe you need to break down some steps into smaller bits or add a few more to reach your goals. Don't hesitate to seek more support, or simply allow yourself more time. Be gentle with yourself, but also be firm. Keep working towards your goals.

"Shaping" Change

"Shaping" is a behavior modification technique that uses rewards and incentives to motivate change and reinforce progress. Whenever you meet one of your goals, reward yourself with a positive reinforcer. Here are some examples:

_____ A long walk
_____ Sitting on a bench by a pond outside and watching the sky or sunset
_____ Twenty uninterrupted minutes of reading for pleasure
_____ Listening to your favorite music
_____ Looking through old photos in digital storage
_____ Watching a favorite classic movie
_____ Sleeping in on Sunday
_____ _____
_____ _____
_____ _____

REFLECTION: Dream Big

If you already know your dream, write it here:

_____

_____

_____

_____

_____

If you do not have a specific dream or vision yet, the following exercise will help you create one. As quickly as you can, write down your vision, your big picture dream, and your wildest, most outrageous, even your most far-fetched hopes and goals. (Yes, you can include becoming a rock star, professional athlete, CEO, or President.) Do not judge or edit—just keep writing until you have written everything you can think of.

Now answer the following questions. Write quickly, allowing no more than 60 to 90 seconds for every answer.

- What do you want your life to be like?

- What draws your attention and taps into your enthusiasm? What fascinates you, intrigues you, tickles your curiosity?

- What would you do if you were guaranteed 100 percent success?

- If you had all the self-esteem necessary to be unstoppable, what would you do differently?

- As a child, what did you first seriously imagine you would do when you grew up? What was your first true ambition?

- What qualities continue to inspire respect and awe in you? What qualities would you develop in yourself if you knew how?

- What would you plan to do in the future if you didn't have to earn money to make a living?

Take a look at these questions daily until you hit paydirt or run out of new things to say. If you can answer all of them the first day, great. If you draw a blank on one or more of them, take another look the next day and see what comes to you. Don't worry about not answering right away. Whether the questions remain consciously on your mind or not, they continue to work outside your conscious awareness.

TECHNIQUE: Create a Timeline

You live in time, and you need a clear sense of time in order to succeed. If you are still in the process of identifying your goals and dreams, a timeline may seem premature. Don't worry; you can fill in some parts later. A timeline is part blueprint and part itinerary. As you gather information and formulate your goals, you can make revisions as you see fit.

Think of the timeline at this point as at best a rough draft. Use a pencil so it feels less scary or binding. Remember that the timeline is a guide meant for your benefit alone.

Get a large, poster-sized sheet of paper. On the top half, construct a timeline of your life with an arbitrary life span of 90 years. Mark the events of your life up to the present moment, noting major milestones.

Don't get bogged down. You can approximate dates and include no more than ten or twelve major life events (entering kindergarten, your soccer team's regional championship, graduating from high school, and so on).

If you have already had a wider range of life experiences than traditional-age college students, you might include your first job, serving in the military, getting married, or having a child. Use words, pictures, photographs…whatever works best for you.

Mark the spot on your timeline that represents today.

Based on your self-appraisal and the change you have in mind, mark the date by which you think you will be ready to make your desired change. This is not the same as making a deadline for change, but a measure of your current sense of when you will be ready to change.

Look at your timeline and pencil in the major steps you need to take each day, week, or month to make your desired change.

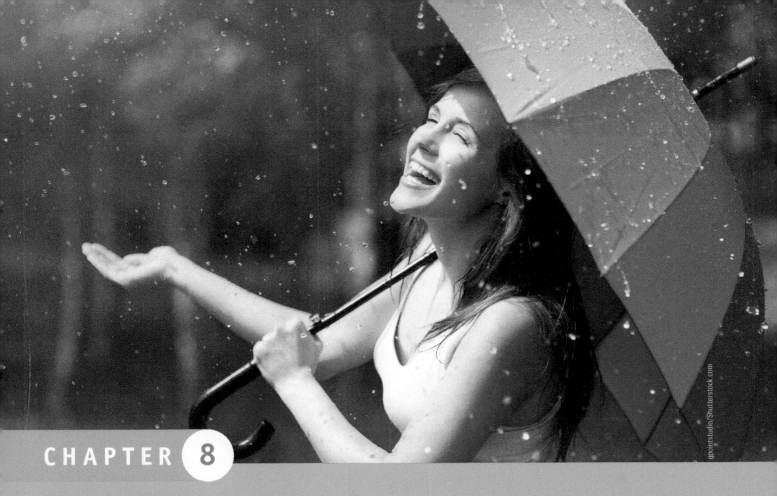

CHAPTER **8**

Psychological Approaches

After reading this chapter, you should be able to:

8.1 Summarize the characteristics of psychologically and emotionally healthy individuals.

8.2 Explain emotional intelligence and the qualities of people with a high emotional quotient.

8.3 Describe how strategies to develop positive strengths and virtues help in finding meaning and purpose in life.

8.4 Outline common negative emotions experienced by college students.

8.5 Discuss some types of risky behaviors among college students.

8.6 Develop fundamental skills to manage stress successfully.

Below are 8 statements with which you may agree or disagree. Using the 1–7 scale below, indicate your agreement with each item by indicating your response for each statement.

7—Strongly agree
6—Agree
5—Slightly agree
4—Neither agree nor disagree
3—Slightly disagree
2—Disagree
1—Strongly disagree

_____ I lead a purposeful and meaningful life
_____ My social relationships are supportive and rewarding
_____ I am engaged and interested in my daily activities
_____ I actively contribute to the happiness and well-being of others
_____ I am competent and capable in the activities that are important to me
_____ I am a good person and live a good life
_____ I am optimistic about my future
_____ People respect me

Scoring: Add the responses, varying from 1 to 7, for all eight items. The possible range of scores is from 8 (lowest possible) to 56 (highest possible). A high score represents a person with many psychological resources and strengths.

Source: Diener, E et al (2009). New measures of well-being: Flourishing and positive and negative feelings. Social Indicators Research, 39, 247–266.

Nate considers himself a nice guy—until someone pushes his buttons. It doesn't matter if it's a jerk who cuts in front of him in line or a clumsy waiter who splashes him with water. Nate doesn't just fly off the handle; he rockets into full-throttle rage. His face reddens; his muscles tense; his voice grows louder. It takes every ounce of self-control in his body to keep from throwing a punch.

One night as he was driving with his girlfriend, a car swung into his lane without signaling. Nate furiously honked his horn. When the driver slowed down, he cut off the vehicle and charged out of his car to confront the idiot behind the wheel. The driver turned out to be a terrified older woman who had been trying to calm her grandchild. When the boy began to cry, Nate felt like the idiot.

"You've got real anger issues," his girlfriend said. "Until you deal with them, I don't want to be around you."

Nate wasn't just living in a state of constant stress; he was pulling others into the same noxious place. But until his girlfriend emailed him links to anger management workshops, he never thought he could take control of his temper. Anger, he learned, was just a feeling like any other that he could choose to act on, ignore, or learn to control.

Like stress, emotions can be positive or negative, healthy or unhealthy. Positive emotions such as love and hope lighten our spirits and fill our hearts. Negative emotions can trigger and prolong the stress response, eventually endangering psychological and physical well-being. Letting our feelings run our lives inevitably leads to stress—for ourselves and everyone around us. Yet although emotions can be extremely intense, we are more than what we feel, and we can develop the insights and skills essential for psychological and emotional well-being.

Psychological and Emotional Health

mental health The ability to perceive reality as it is, respond to its challenges, and develop rational strategies for living.

emotional health The ability to express and acknowledge one's feelings and moods and exhibit adaptability and compassion for others.

emotional intelligence A set of skills that contribute to the accurate appraisal, expression, and regulation of emotion in oneself and in others and the use of feelings to motivate, plan, and achieve in one's life."

EQ (emotional quotient) The ability to monitor and use emotions to guide thinking and actions.

Emotionally healthy individuals face challenges with confidence and optimism.

Unlike physical health, psychological well-being cannot be measured, tested, X-rayed, or dissected. Yet psychologically healthy men and women generally share certain characteristics:

- They can cope with the stressors of everyday living.
- They value themselves and strive toward happiness and fulfillment.
- They establish and maintain close relationships with others.
- They accept the limitations as well as the possibilities that life has to offer.
- They feel a sense of meaning and purpose that makes the gestures of living worth the effort required.

✔ **Check-in:** How many of these characteristics do you have?

Psychological health encompasses both our emotional and mental states—that is, our feelings and our thoughts. As discussed in Chapter 3, **mental health** refers to our ability to perceive reality as it is, to respond to its challenges, and to develop rational strategies for living. A mentally healthy person doesn't try to avoid conflicts and distress, but can cope with life's transitions, traumas, and losses in a way that allows for emotional stability and growth.

Emotional health includes feelings and moods, both of which are discussed later in this chapter. Characteristics of emotionally healthy persons include the following:

- Determination and effort to be healthy.
- Flexibility and adaptability to a variety of circumstances.
- Development of a sense of meaning and affirmation of life.
- An understanding that they are not the center of the universe.
- Compassion for others.
- The ability to be unselfish in serving or relating to others.
- Depth and satisfaction in intimate relationships.
- A sense of control over mind and body that enables them to make health-enhancing choices and decisions.

Emotional Intelligence

What matters more than what we feel is how we handle our feelings. Psychologists refer to this form of internal self-management as **emotional intelligence**, defined as "a set of skills hypothesized to contribute to the accurate appraisal and expression of emotion in oneself and in others, the effective regulation of emotion in self and others, and the use of feelings to motivate, plan, and achieve in one's life."[*] **EQ (emotional quotient)** refers to the ability to monitor and use emotions to guide thinking and actions. (See Table 8.1.)

Emotional intelligence consists of several dimensions, including:

- Accurate recognition and expression of emotions while feeling them.
- Ability to create and maintain healthy interpersonal relationships.
- Ability to control and marshal emotions in order to remain focused and reach goals.
- Recognition and understanding of what others are feeling and empathy with them.
- Ability to manage emotions, regulate moods, handle stress, and rebound from emotional setbacks.

The brain regions involved in emotional intelligence overlap significantly with those involved

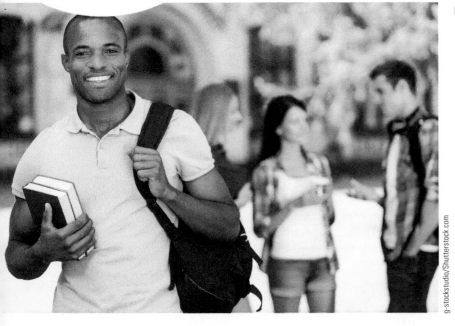

g-stockstudio/Shutterstock.com

TABLE 8.1 What's Your Emotional IQ?

	Disagree	Sometimes	Agree
1. It's easy for me to describe how and why I feel different emotions.			
2. I have a good grasp on nonverbal cues and communication.			
3. My thoughts are influenced by my feelings.			
4. I am good at reading other people's emotions.			
5. I can usually identify exactly what I am feeling.			
6. I accept when I need to pay attention to uncomfortable feelings.			
7. I am open with my feelings and emotions.			
8. I am good at reading people's facial expressions.			
9. I am aware of changes in my mood.			
10. I typically can understand what causes my emotions.			
11. I consider myself to be empathetic.			
12. I don't refocus my thoughts on information over emotions.			
13. I have a good understanding of my emotional reactions.			
14. I know how to manage my emotions.			
15. I usually can understand the reasons for other people's emotions.			
16. I can evaluate the effects my emotions have on me and my actions.			
17. I don't let my emotions take full control over me and my actions.			
18. I am good at picking up on when people are being fake.			
19. In an average week, I experience a range of emotions.			
20. I share my feelings with family and friends.			
21. I don't try to ignore or bottle up my feelings.			
22. It's easy for me to describe what and why I feel things.			
23. What people around me are feeling has an affect on me.			
24. I can handle strong emotions.			
25. I can understand how feelings and emotions change.			

Use this quiz to identify aspects of your emotional intelligence that you could strengthen or improve. Explore which emotions or emotional experiences may be challenging for you and why. Also reflect on your emotional strengths. Think about why some of these statements ring true for you and what impact this has on your thoughts, feelings, and behaviors.

Score 1 point for each "Disagree," 2 points for each "Sometimes," and 3 points for each "Agree." Add up all of your points. If you scored between:

- 25–40 = low emotional IQ
- 40–60 = average emotional IQ
- 60–75 = high emotional IQ

Source: Salovey, P., & Mayer, J. D. (1989). Emotional intelligence. Imagination, cognition and personality, 9(3), 185-211.

in general intelligence—and in effective stress management.[2] Women generally score slightly higher in emotional intelligence than men, but in both sexes, individuals who are outgoing, dependable, and independent-minded tend to have higher EQ scores. However, everyone is capable of cultivating greater emotional intelligence, which grows as we learn from life experiences—including stressful ones.

Individuals with a high EQ are less prone to depression and anxiety and more productive at work. They bounce back more quickly from serious setbacks and illnesses and report better ties with friends and family, more satisfying romantic relationships, more emotional support, more intimacy, and more affection as well as greater life satisfaction and psychological well-being. Among the aspects of emotional intelligence that most benefit students, particularly when under stress, are focusing on clear, manageable goals and identifying and understanding emotions rather than relying on gut feelings.[3]

---

positive psychology
The scientific study of ordinary human strengths and virtues.

positive psychiatry
Promotes positive psychosocial development in those with or at high risk of mental or physical illness.

downward spiral
A progression of negative thoughts and feelings that can lead to depression or self-destructive behaviors.

positive spiral
A progression of positive thoughts and feelings that leads to fulfilling events and experiences.

> ### Stress Reliever: The XYZ Technique
>
> How do you put difficult emotions into words? Think "X-Y-Z":
>
> - I felt X (frustrated, hurt, disappointed)
> - when you did Y (didn't follow through, made fun of me, didn't call)
> - in situation Z (at the meeting, when you promised, in front of my parents).

The Power of Positivity

Positive psychology and **positive psychiatry** focus on the aspects of human experience that lead to happiness and fulfillment—in other words, on what makes life worthwhile.[3] The goal of these approaches is not simply to feel good momentarily or to avoid bad experiences, but to build positive strengths and traits that enable us to find meaning and purpose in life.[4]

Emotional Spirals

We rarely feel just one emotion. A certain feeling leads to another and then another. Psychologists describe this cascade as a self-perpetuating spiral that includes thoughts, emotions, and behaviors. In a **downward spiral**, sadness, for instance, spins into rumination on a loss, which leads to social withdrawal, which generates deeper sadness, more negative thoughts, and greater isolation, pulling individuals downward into depression or self-destructive behaviors. Downward spirals tend to narrow an individual's perspective and increase susceptibility to stress.

Positive emotions give rise to **positive spirals** in which feelings of gratitude, for instance, feed a sense of optimism, which increases sociability, which fuels a desire for more pleasurable experiences. Upward spirals increase openness to other people, new ideas, and new activities and expand an individual's social ties. As positive experiences accumulate, they deepen and expand positive feelings, build resilience to temporary setbacks, and counter the negative effects of stress.[5]

> ### Stress Reliever: Accentuate the Positive
>
> Do's:
>
> - Smile. A happy face makes for a happy spirit.
> - Focus. By being fully present in the moment, you'll experience it more intensely.
> - Share your joy. Talking about and celebrating good experiences extends positive feelings.
> - Travel through time. Vividly remembering or anticipating positive events—a technique called "positive mental time travel"—boosts levels of happiness and life satisfaction.
>
> Don'ts:
>
> - Don't hide your feelings. Suppressing positive feelings—because of shyness or a sense of modesty, for instance—diminishes them.
> - Don't get distracted. Unrelated worries and thoughts detract from the here-and-now of a positive experience.

- Don't find fault. Paying attention to negative aspects of otherwise positive experiences sabotages levels of happiness, optimism, self-esteem, and life satisfaction.

- Don't go there. "Negative mental time travel"—reflecting on what went wrong or what may go wrong—can lower self-esteem and foster depressive symptoms.

"Undoing" Stress

In difficult situations, positive feelings alter the processing of emotions in ways that "undo" some of stress's harmful effects, including the following:[6]

- **Restore and Cleanse** Positive emotions shorten the after-effects of the stress response by relieving tension and cleansing your body of stress hormones. Unlike panic and fear, which narrow focus and attention, positive emotions enable us to be more flexible and open in our thinking.[7]

- **Broaden and Build** As more than a decade of research has shown, "broadening and building" approaches such as cultivating gratitude and acceptance can help buffer against stress, promote resilience, lower the risk of mental disorders, and enhance physical well-being.

Positive psychology interventions that have proven effective in undoing or lessening stress include:

- Counting one's blessings
- Savoring experiences
- Practicing kindness
- Pursuing meaning
- Setting personal goals
- Building compassion for oneself and others
- Identifying and using one's strengths (which may include traits such as kindness or perseverance).

Boost Self-Esteem

Each of us wants and needs to feel significant as a human being, with unique talents, abilities, and roles in life. A sense of **self-esteem**, of belief and pride in ourselves, gives us confidence to attempt to achieve at school or work and to reach out to others to form friendships and close relationships. Self-esteem is the little voice within that whispers, "You're worth it. You can do it. You're okay."

Self-esteem is based not on external factors like wealth or beauty, but on what you believe about yourself. It's not something you're born with; it develops over time. It's also not something that anyone else can give to you, although those around you can either enhance or diminish your self-esteem.

When we face stress, a healthy sense of self-esteem can do much more than simply boost confidence. It endows us with a layer of emotional resilience when we encounter rejection and failure (See Chapter 10 for more on resilience). Low self-esteem renders us more vulnerable to many of the psychological injuries of daily life, while high self-esteem strengthens our emotional immune system.[8]

The seeds of self-esteem are planted in childhood when parents provide the assurance and appreciation youngsters need to push themselves toward new accomplishments: crawling, walking, forming words and sentences, learning control over their bladder and bowels. Adults, too, must consider themselves worthy of love, friendship, and success if they are to be loved, to make friends, and to achieve their goals. Low self-esteem is more common in people who have been abused as children and in those with psychiatric disorders, including depression, anxiety, alcoholism, and drug dependence.

One of the most useful techniques for bolstering self-esteem is developing the habit of positive thinking and talking. Negative observations,

self-esteem Confidence and satisfaction in oneself.

A child builds self-esteem with every new accomplishment—one step at a time.

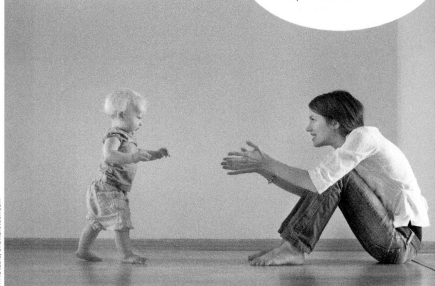

MNStudio/Shutterstock.com

such as constant criticisms or reminders of minor faults, undermine self-image. Positive affirmations—compliments, kudos, encouraging words—have the opposite effect.

---

conscientiousness
Striving for competence and achievement, self-discipline, orderliness, reliability, deliberativeness.

extraversion
A personality trait correlated with being active, talkative, assertive, social, stimulation-seeking.

self-compassion
A healthy form of self-acceptance in the face of perceived inadequacy or failure.

How do you practice self-compassion?

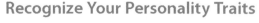

> **🔧 Stress Reliever:** Reframe
>
> ┈┈┈┈┈┈┈┈┈┈┈┈┈┈┈┈┈┈┈┈┈┈
>
> Think of something that is stressing you out. Can you look at it in a more positive way? Try incorporating some of the following attitude-adjusting strategies:
>
> ┈┈┈┈┈┈┈┈┈┈┈┈┈┈┈┈┈┈┈┈┈┈
>
> • Accept that some things are out of your control.
>
> ┈┈┈┈┈┈┈┈┈┈┈┈┈┈┈┈┈┈┈┈┈┈
>
> • Challenge your negative thoughts.
>
> ┈┈┈┈┈┈┈┈┈┈┈┈┈┈┈┈┈┈┈┈┈┈
>
> • Be compassionate and forgiving, both to yourself and to those around you.
>
> ┈┈┈┈┈┈┈┈┈┈┈┈┈┈┈┈┈┈┈┈┈┈
>
> • Keep it real. Don't let your expectations become unreasonable or catastrophic.
>
> ┈┈┈┈┈┈┈┈┈┈┈┈┈┈┈┈┈┈┈┈┈┈
>
> • Avoid extremes. Thinking in absolute terms such as "always" or "never" is bound to bring you down.

Recognize Your Personality Traits

Why do some students consistently take steps to minimize stress while others seem to be stress magnets who repeatedly put their well-being at risk? The answers may lie within their personalities. Two personality traits in particular—conscientiousness (striving for competence and achievement, self-discipline, orderliness, reliability, deliberativeness) and **extraversion** (being active, talkative, assertive, social, stimulation-seeking)—correlate with very different health behaviors and responses to stress.[9]

College students who rate high in conscientiousness tend to wear seat belts, get enough sleep, drive safely, use safer sex practices, exercise, not smoke, drink less, and eat healthful foods—all helpful for managing stress. They carefully weigh the risks and benefits of their behaviors and delay immediate gratification for the sake of long-term benefits, such as preventing cardiovascular disease or sexually transmitted infections.

Students who score high in extraversion are more likely to put their health at risk. They drink more alcohol, smoke, engage in risky sexual behaviors, and don't get enough sleep. The reasons may involve brain chemistry. Individuals with low levels of certain neurochemicals may pursue highly stimulating (though stressful) behaviors that trigger an adrenaline rush that makes them feel more alert and excited.

Personality is not destiny. If you see yourself as low in conscientiousness or high in extraversion, you can take deliberate steps that will lower your stress and safeguard your health. For instance, you might fulfill your need for stimulation and excitement with less risky alternatives, such as rock climbing or volunteering with student-led emergency response services.

Practice Self-Compassion

Self-compassion is a healthy form of self-acceptance that some psychologists describe as being kind to yourself in the face of suffering. By practicing a "reciprocal golden rule," you treat yourself with the kindness usually reserved for others. This includes accepting your flaws; letting go of regrets, illusions, and disappointments; and taking responsibility for actions that may have harmed others without feeling a need to punish yourself. In contrast, individuals low in self-compassion are extremely critical of themselves and obsessively fixate on their mistakes. Compassion for others seems to breed compassion for yourself, and vice versa.[10]

Individuals high in self-compassion tend to:

• Be understanding toward themselves when they make mistakes.

• Recognize that all humans are imperfect.

• Not ruminate about their errors in judgment or behavior.

• When feeling inadequate, engage in soothing and positive self-talk.

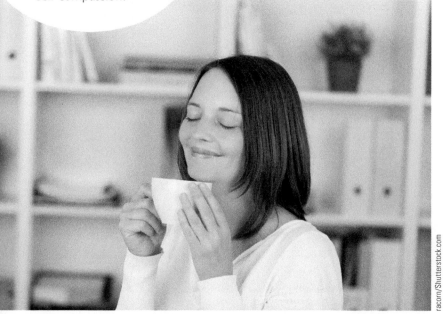

racorn/Shutterstock.com

- Recognize that failure is an unavoidable part of the human experience.
- Feel a greater sense of connection to others, even in the face of disappointment.
- Not exaggerate the significance of painful thoughts (though they're mindful of them).
- Manage frustration and stress by quelling self-pity and melodrama.

After a traumatic life event, self-compassion may help individuals recognize the need to care for themselves, reach out for social support, engage in less self-blame and self-criticism, and look back on the time as an emotionally difficult event rather than an experience that defines or changes them.[11] It also motivates people to learn from their mistakes and improve themselves after an initial failure.[12]

Meet Your Needs

Newborns are unable to survive on their own. They depend on others for the satisfaction of their physical needs for food, shelter, warmth, and protection, as well as their less tangible emotional needs. In growing to maturity, children take on more responsibility and become more independent. No one, however, becomes totally self-sufficient. As adults, we easily recognize our basic physical needs, but we often fail to acknowledge our emotional needs. Yet they, too, must be met if we are to be as fulfilled as possible.

The humanist theorist Abraham Maslow believed that human needs are the motivating factors in personality development. According to his theory, we first must satisfy basic physiological needs, such as those for food, shelter, and sleep. Only then can we pursue fulfillment of our higher needs—for safety and security, love and affection, and self-esteem. The goal is to reach a state of **self-actualization**, in which we function at the highest possible level and derive the greatest possible satisfaction from life (see Figure 8.1).

Among the characteristics of self-actualized individuals is **autonomy**, or independence. Autonomous individuals are true to themselves. As they weigh the pros and cons of any decision, whether it's using or refusing drugs or choosing a major or career, they base their judgment on their own **values**, not those of others. Their ability to draw on internal resources and cope with stress has a positive impact on both their psychological well-being and their physical health. Those who've achieved autonomy may seek the opinions of others, but they do not allow their decisions to be dictated by external influences. In autonomous individuals, their locus of control—that is,

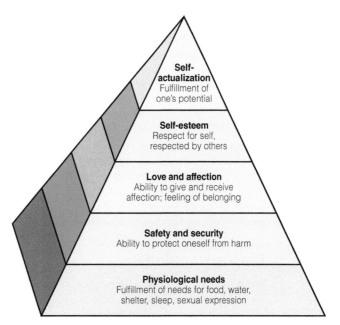

FIGURE 8.1 Check-in: Where do you see yourself on Maslow's pyramid of needs?

where they view control as originating—is *internal* (from within themselves) rather than *external* (from others). (See Chapter 1.)

Cultivate Gratitude

✔ **Check-in:** What three things are you thankful for today?

A grateful spirit brightens **mood**, boosts energy, and infuses daily living with a sense of glad abundance. Although giving thanks is an ancient virtue, gratitude refers to appreciation, not just for a special gift, but for everything that makes life a bit better: other people, nature, positive circumstances, kind gestures, direct help. Gratitude affirms the goodness in the world and acknowledges other people—or higher powers, from a spiritual perspective—as their source.

Grateful people feel more frequent and intense positive emotions, have more positive views of their social environment, use more productive coping strategies, sleep better, and appreciate their lives and possessions more. By acknowledging how others support and affirm us, gratitude strengthens relationships and encourages us to go beyond the gifts we and repay them or "pay them forward."

A "lifestyle orientation" of feeling grateful has been shown to reduce stress levels over time. College students who keep gratitude journals report higher levels of happiness, feel better about their

self-actualization A state of wellness and fulfillment that can be achieved once certain human needs are satisfied; living to one's full potential.

autonomy Ability to draw on internal resources; independence from familial and societal influences.

values The criteria by which one makes choices about one's thoughts, actions, goals, and ideals.

mood Sustained emotional state that colors one's view of the world for hours or days.

The Power of Positivity 151

lives as a whole, are more likely to have made progress toward important personal goals, exercise more regularly, and report fewer negative health symptoms.[9] (See the Personal Stress Management Toolkit on page 164.)

Gratitude changes your life in striking ways. As you enhance appreciation in your daily life, you see things from a larger perspective. Your relationships improve, and you will more aware of what you have. Being deeply grateful can increase your reverence for life and make you a champion of the betterment of others. Gratitude leads the way to maturity and awareness and also bestows contentment and profound life satisfaction.

Pursue Happiness

Happiness is not the absence of stress, but an abundance of eustress. Education, gender, and race don't determine how happy you are. Asked if they were "feeling good and functioning well," men and women with different backgrounds and varying levels of education have similar odds of achieving high levels of emotional well-being.[13]

As long as you have enough money to cover basic needs, you don't need more wealth or more possessions for greater joy. Even people who win a fortune in a lottery return to their baseline of happiness within months. Health both affects and is affected by happiness. As long-term studies show, happiness enhances immunity, speeds healing, and may even reduce the risk of dying—both in healthy people and in those with diagnosed diseases.

Many people assume that they can't be happy unless they get into a certain school, earn a certain grade, win a certain job, make a certain income, fall in love with a certain person, or look a certain way. But according to psychologist Sonja Lyubomirsky, author of *The Myths of Happiness*, such notions are false. "People find a way to be happy in spite of unwanted life circumstances," she notes, "and many people who are blessed by wealth and good fortune aren't any happier than those who lack these fortunes."[14]

While possessions bring temporary delight, the thrill invariably fades. The joy we feel when we get something we desire—whether it's a new phone or a sports trophy—doesn't last because of "habituation," the capacity to become accustomed to life changes and take them for granted. The bliss of acquiring the latest smartphone or game console generally fades in six to twelve weeks. The bliss of making a new friend, which is more dynamic and engaging, lasts longer. Children, despite all the challenges they bring, yield more joy than many possessions, according to studies of parents.[15]

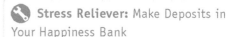

Stress Reliever: Make Deposits in Your Happiness Bank

At the end of each day, think of one thing that made you happy and describe it in words (written or recorded). When you're feeling down, tap into this happiness fund to lift your spirits.

The Types of Happiness

Researchers distinguish between two types of happiness:

- **hedonic,** which involves accumulating material things and enjoying pleasurable activities, and
- **eudaemonic,** which is based on a sense of higher purpose and service to others.

Hedonic happiness has been linked with high levels of the stress-related biological markers that promote inflammation throughout the body and low levels of markers of antibodies to fight infection. In contrast, eudaemonic happiness fosters expression of genes that produce protective antibodies and suppresses genes that promote inflammation.

One of the most effective ways of increasing eudaemonic happiness is performing small acts of kindness. While there is no set formula for their variety and frequency, Lyubomirsky advises a minimum of a good deed once a week, which provides as much of an emotional boost as a thrice-weekly activity. She also recommends variety—taking out the trash when it's your roommate's turn one time, for instance, and buying a hot chocolate for a homeless person the next—because simple repetitions lose their ability to boost happiness.[16]

Don't Worry, Be Happy

Some skeptics dismiss "happichondria" as the latest feel-good fad. However, happiness researchers, cite mounting evidence suggesting that happiness is, to a significant degree, a learned behavior. Among 5,000 students in 280 countries who completed a massive online open course (MOOC) on happiness, positive feelings such as affection, amusement, and enthusiasm kept going up as the course progressed while sadness, anger, and fear declined.[17]

You too can worry less and smile more. Here are some suggestions:

- **Spend time with happy, upbeat individuals.** In surveys of college students,

hedonic Happiness derived from accumulating material things and enjoying pleasurable activities.

eudaemonic Happiness based on a sense of higher purpose and service to others.

the happiest generally spent the least time alone and shared one distinctive characteristic: a rich and fulfilling social life, including a romantic relationship as well as rewarding friendships.

- **Up your appreciation quotient.** Regularly take stock of all the things for which you are grateful. (See "Reflection" in the Personal Stress Management Toolkit on page 164.) To deepen the impact, write a letter of gratitude to someone who's helped you along the way.

- **Watch videos of kittens, puppies, and other adorable creatures.** Japanese researchers have shown that looking at pictures of appealing animals—from pets to pandas to grumpy cats—not only improves mood but also focuses attention to enhance performance on various tasks.[18]

- **Create your own imaginary video.** Visualize several of your happiest memories in as much detail as possible. Smell the air. Feel the sun. Hear the sea. Play this video in your mind when your spirits slump.

- **Immerse yourself.** Find activities that delight and engage you so much that you lose track of time in a state that psychologists call "flow." Experiment with creative outlets. Look for ways to build these activities into your life.

- **Seize the moment.** Rather than wait to celebrate big birthday-cake moments, savor a bite of cupcake every day. Delight in a child's cuddle, a lively conversation. Cry at the movies. Cheer at football games. This life is your gift to yourself. Enjoy it!

Become Optimistic and Hopeful

✔ **Check-in:** Do you usually anticipate the best or the worst possible outcome?

Mental health professionals define **optimism** as the "extent to which individuals expect favorable outcomes to occur." They view it as "an active priority of the person, not merely a reflex that prompts us to look on the sunny side."[19] The different ways in which optimists and pessimists cope with stress can affect their well-being. Studies have established "significant relationships" between optimism and cardiovascular health, stroke risk, immune function, cancer prognoses, physical symptoms, pain, and mortality rates. The more optimistic the person, the more pronounced the favorable effect on immunity.[20]

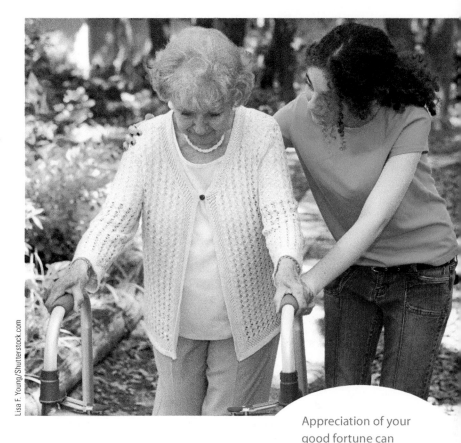

Lisa F. Young/Shutterstock.com

Appreciation of your good fortune can inspire you to reach out to those who need help.

For various reasons—because they believe in themselves, because they trust in a higher power, because they feel lucky—optimists expect positive experiences from life. When bad things happen, they tend to see setbacks or losses as specific, temporary incidents. In their eyes, a disappointment is "one of those things" that happens every once in a while rather than the latest in a long string of disasters. In terms of health, optimists not only expect good outcomes—for instance, that a surgery will be successful—but also take steps to increase this likelihood. Pessimists, expecting the worst, are more likely to deny or avoid a problem, sometimes through drinking or other destructive behaviors. Even when perceived stress is high, optimism lowers stress and stabilizes levels of the stress hormone cortisol.[21]

Individuals aren't born optimistic or pessimistic, hopeful or despairing. Researchers have documented changes over time in the ways that individuals view the world and what they expect to experience in the future.[12] Optimism breeds hope, another life-affirming positive emotion. College students who score high in hope solve problems more effectively, avoid self-criticism and negative self-talk, and are less likely to report symptoms of depression. Among the strategies that enhance hope are identifying goals, imagining success, identifying potential ways to overcome barrier, and interpreting failures positively.[22]

optimism Tendency to seek out, remember, and expect pleasurable experiences.

Detoxifying Negative Feelings

✔ **Check-in:** Track your moods.

Every day, rate how much each emoji matches how you have been feeling on a scale of 1 to 10. At the end of the week, average your daily ratings into a collective score. Track how your feelings change throughout the term.

Fear

Enthusiasm

Anger

Affection

Sadness

Amusement

We experience three to four times more negative emotions than positive—perhaps because alertness to potential dangers helped our early ancestors survive. However, just as you can learn to enhance positive emotions, you can learn to detoxify negative ones. (See Table 8.2.)

Fear

✔ **Check-in:** What do you fear most? Are your fears based in reality? What single step might you take to lessen your fears?

If you peel away all the layers of emotions involved in stress, at its innermost core you'll find the same thing: fear. Faced with stress, people hunker down and hold to their current position even if it is not an ideal or healthy one. They are afraid of the unknown, afraid of failing, afraid of embarrassing themselves, afraid of disappointing, afraid of discovering they do not have what it takes, or afraid that if they make it through one stressful challenge, people will expect even more of them in the future. And fear engenders even more fear—and stress.

You may assume that people who boldly take on stressful challenges do so because they aren't afraid. This isn't true. Those who push the envelope and venture beyond their comfort zones take fear seriously for what it is: a signal to use caution. If you feel fear, it's wise to investigate its source. It's far better to perceive danger than ignore it and act recklessly. But fear or the possibility of danger shouldn't stop you in your tracks. Instead of running for cover, realize that where there is danger, you must be appropriately cautious. Driving a car or striking a match carries a risk of danger, but you don't avoid either. Instead you heighten your attention so you do them safely.

If you work with fear correctly, fear will become your ally in managing stress. Let your inner alarm guide you to assess a situation accurately without going overboard. Don't leap before looking, but don't retreat before finding out what to expect. Get information. Doing so is the only way to determine whether a danger is real and what specific threat it presents.

Giving in to fear leads to mindlessly freezing in your tracks. If you let that happen, your life will be safe and predictable—and barren. A certain level of fear, like a certain level of stress, can inform and motivate you and can alert you to authentic hazards. Then you can evaluate and decide what level of daring makes sense.

The downside of fear is that, if not handled appropriately, it has a way of making your worst, most stressful nightmares come true. When you are afraid of something, you try to avoid it—and whenever you do so, you are more likely to experience what you fear most.

TABLE 8.2 Negative Feelings on Campus

Negative Feelings Reported by Students at Any Time Within the Last 12 Months:	Percent
Feeling overwhelmed by all they had to do	85.1
Feeling exhausted (not from physical activity)	81.6
Feeling very sad	63.5
Feeling overwhelming anxiety	57.7
Feeling that things were hopeless	47.8
Feeling so depressed that it was difficult to function	35.3

Source: American College Health Association. *American College Health Association–National College Health Assessment II: Reference Group Executive Summary.* Fall 2015 Hanover, MD: American College Health Association, 2016.

Picture yourself standing on the free-throw line to shoot two foul shots. Your team is one point behind with one second left on the clock. If you shoot hoping not to blow it, you are more likely to miss than if you say to yourself, "These guys are going down!" The reason: When you worry about failure rather than going on the offensive, your fear creates muscular tension that disrupts the fluidity of your shot.

The same thing happens whenever you have to do something you find exceptionally stressful, such as speaking in public. If you have to make a presentation in class, focusing on not making a fool of yourself is the kiss of death. Even if you do a great deal of research, you are far less likely to give a good talk if you are trying to avoid giving a bad one. Concentrate instead on what you want to say and what you want people to understand. Tell yourself that you have something fantastic to share with your audience and that everyone is going to enjoy and learn from this time together.

Fear also can stem from faulty assumptions about what the future will bring. People often anticipate that things will turn out badly and feel convinced that their prediction is a fact. Do you ever assume that you can foresee exactly what is going to happen in your life—that you're going to fail a test, blow an interview, or say or do something embarrassing at a public event? If so, the following exercise can help you tune up your internal "predict-o-meter" (see Figure 8.2).

Anger

....

✔ **Check-in:** Are you a hothead? Do you frequently lose it, blow up, explode, go ballistic, have a fit?

....

The terms we use for getting angry reveal its dangers. Anger is a bomb, and if you have a short fuse, you and everyone around you are in harm's way. In-your-face eruptions of anger may seem funny on television. In real life, they are tedious and tiring. They also can damage your family, your friendships, your career, and your ambitions. If you don't learn to tame it, your temper can get you thrown off a team or a job, out of a class, and even into jail.

Mild irritation or moderate and controlled anger is one thing. Tantrums, outbursts. and chronic rage are another. Whatever its trigger, anger unleashes the stress response, which revs the body into a state of combat readiness, multiplying the risk for bodily harm, stroke, and heart attack—even in healthy young individuals. Full-blown anger bypasses the rational parts of the brain so you lose the opportunity to take control of what you feel, say, and do. You let somebody else take

Sometimes we believe that we can predict exactly what is going to happen in our lives. Has your inner predict-o-meter ever told you: "I'm going to bomb this test," "I won't fit in," or "I can't do it"? But how often has your predict-o-meter been spot on? Science has proven that we cannot predict the future, yet we often find ourselves convinced our predict-o-meter is right. And often, this leads to great stress and anxiety

For this activity, think of a time when your predict-o-meter told you something negative was going to happen in a situation or event. Then, write down what happened in real life. Often, what actually happens is never as bad as our anxiety tells us it will be.

What my inner predict-o-meter said was going to happen….	What really happened….

FIGURE 8.2 Is your crystal ball accurate?

Steve Pepple/Shutterstock.com

charge of you because clearly you are not in control. This is neither inevitable nor unavoidable.

Taming a toxic temper, like other behavioral changes, requires skillpower, not willpower. The first step is recognizing the earliest signs of anger when you still have time to engage the rational parts of your brain. Be mindful of your heart rate, breathing, and muscle tension if your anger begins to brew. Make a reasoned choice about what to do, rather than merely going nuclear. Analyze the situations that trigger a rage attack

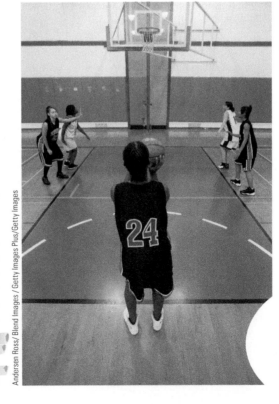

Andersen Ross/ Blend Images / Getty Images Plus/Getty Images

Telling yourself you can do it boosts your chance of succeeding under pressure.

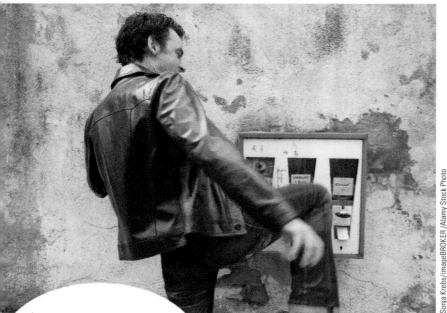

 Do you ever respond to frustration with an outburst of rage?

Sonja Krebs/imageBROKER/Alamy Stock Photo

letting the light of heaven shine through. Breathe deeply and fully inhabit the moment. Let your anger blow away in the breeze. If you can't go outdoors, visualize a soothing or inspiring natural scene.

Mood Control

Feelings come and go within minutes. A mood is a more sustained emotional state that colors our view of the world for longer periods. According to psychological surveys, bad moods descend upon us an average of three out of every ten days. The most effective way to banish them is by changing what caused them in the first place—if you can figure out what made you upset and why. Ask yourself what you can do to fix what went wrong or to remedy a loss. If there is, take action and solve it. Rewrite the report. Ask to take a makeup exam. Apologize to the friend whose feelings you hurt. Tell your parents you feel bad about the argument you had.

If there's nothing you can do, accept what happened and focus on doing things differently next time. Resolving to try harder in the future has proven as effective in improving mood as taking action in the present. You also can try to think about what happened in a different way and put a positive spin on it. This technique, known as *cognitive restructuring or reframing*, helps you look at a setback in a new light:

so you can anticipate them, change the ways in which you respond, and keep in mind the consequences of an anger outburst. Most importantly, these skills can keep you, not your temper, in control of your life.

Some people think of anger as the psychological equivalent of the steam in a pressure cooker that has to be released or else it will explode. That's not the case. "Venting"—in person or online—only makes anger more dangerous by prolonging intense emotions and stress. To deal with anger, you have to figure out what's really making you mad.

Usually the jammed snack machine is the final straw that unleashes bottled-up rage over a more difficult issue, such as a domineering parent or boss. Monitor yourself for early signs of exhaustion and overload. While stress alone doesn't cause a blowup, it makes you more likely to overreact. (See the Personal Stress Management Toolkit on page 164.)

 Stress Reliever: Step Outside

Being outside puts the irritations of daily living into perspective. Let your gaze linger on silvery ice glazing a branch or an azalea bush in wild bloom. Follow the flight of a bird; watch clouds float overhead. Gaze into the night sky and think of the stars as holes in the darkness

Stress Reliever: Reappraise

Ask:

• What lessons did this teach me?

• What would I have done differently?

• Could there be a silver lining or hidden benefit?

If you can't identify or resolve the problem responsible for your emotional funk, the next best solution is to concentrate on altering your negative feelings. For example, try setting a quick, achievable goal that can boost your spirits with a small success. Clean out a drawer; sort through the piles of paper on your desk; send an e-mail or text message to an old friend. Or try some of the stress-reducing techniques described in Part IV of this book.

Taking Charge of Risky Behaviors

Addictive behaviors and substances may seem like quick escapes from stress, but ultimately they turn into dead ends. Gaming or gambling can start off as enjoyable diversions but consume ever-increasing amounts of your time, energy, and money. Drugs—street drugs as well as improperly used medications—and tobacco are dangerous, even life-threatening. The same is true of alcohol in more than moderate amounts. The entire range of risky behaviors can intensify the stress in your daily life and create unforeseen and unpredictable new stresses.

Gambling

Gambling has become a more serious and widespread problem. College students who gamble say they do so for fun or excitement, to socialize, to win money, or to "just have something to do." Simply having access to casino machines, ongoing card games, or Internet gambling sites increases the likelihood of gambling. About half of students who gamble at least once a month experience significant problems related to their gambling, including poor academic performance, heavy alcohol consumption, illicit drug use, unprotected sex, and other risky behaviors.

✔ **Check-in:** Are you at risk for problem gambling?

Among young people (ages 16 to 25), the following behaviors indicate increased risk of problem gambling. Check any that apply to you.

_____ Being male.

_____ Gambling at an early age (as young as age 8).

_____ Having a big win early in one's gambling career.

_____ Consistently chasing losses (betting more to recover money already lost).

_____ Gambling alone.

_____ Feeling depressed before gambling.

_____ Feeling excited and aroused during gambling.

_____ Behaving irrationally during gambling.

_____ Having poor grades at school.

_____ Engaging in other addictive behaviors (smoking, drinking alcohol, illegal drug use).

_____ Being in a lower socioeconomic class.

_____ Having parents with a gambling or other addiction problem.

_____ Having a history of delinquency or stealing money to fund gambling.

_____ Skipping class to go gambling.

The more items that you've checked, the more you should be aware of your potential risk. Try taking a complete break from gambling for 30 days. If you can't, seek professional counseling.

Alcohol

About two-thirds of college students drink alcohol. The most common reason is to relax. Because it depresses the central nervous system, alcohol can make people feel less tense and stressed—even though it does nothing to relieve the cause of the stress and may make some stressors worse. The biggest dangers come from drinking without thinking. When you drink without thinking, you give up control and turn your life over to alcohol. And when you lose control, you lose—and you pay the price in stress. You can end up a hapless spectator or a victim of consequences you never intended. (See Table 8.3.)

Although the percentage of college students who drink alcohol has remained the same over recent decades, what has changed is the percentage of students who engage in mindless, dangerous drinking. More students today binge, drink to get drunk, participate in drinking games, or drink to excess at athletic rallies, celebrations, and spring breaks. As a result, more students are being injured, assaulted, or raped in alcohol-related crimes—and are dying as a result of alcohol poisoning or alcohol-related accidents.

TABLE 8.3 Consequences of Drinking

College students who drank alcohol reported experiencing the following in the last 12 months when drinking alcohol:*

Percent (%)	Male	Female	Average
Did something you later regretted	29.9	29.0	29.2
Forgot where you were or what you did	27.1	24.4	25.2
Got in trouble with the police	2.9	1.7	2.1
Someone had sex with me without my consent	0.9	2.4	1.9
Had sex with someone without their consent	0.4	0.2	0.3
Had unprotected sex	21.6	20.0	20.4
Physically injured yourself	12.7	11.1	11.7
Physically injured another person	2.6	0.7	1.3
Seriously considered suicide	2.9	2.7	2.9
Reported one or more of the above	49.4	45.6	46.7

*Students responding "N/A, don't drink." were excluded from this analysis.

Source: American College Health Association. *American College Health Association–National College Health Assessment II: Reference Group Executive Summary.* Fall 2015 Hanover, MD: American College Health Association, 2016.

According to the American College Health Association's National College Health Assessment, about three in ten students report doing something they later regretted as a result of their drinking.[23] If just thinking about your alcohol use makes you feel stressed, this is a red flag. Take the following self-survey to get an accurate sense of your alcohol consumption.

✔ **Check-in:** Your alcohol audit

If you drink, answer the following questions to get an honest assessment of your alcohol use.

_____ When did you last have a drink?

_____ How many drinks did you have?

_____ Why did you choose to drink?

_____ How often do you drink?

_____ When do you drink? Where?

_____ Why do you usually drink?

_____ What is the most you have ever drunk in a single episode? Who were you with? How did you feel afterward?

_____ How many times have you gone on a binge (more than four drinks if you're male or more than three drinks if you're female in a single episode)? When and where did these heavy drinking episodes occur? How did you feel afterward?

_____ Did you ever find that you were not able to stop drinking once you started? How often has this happened?

_____ Have you ever failed to do what was expected of you because of drinking? How often?

_____ Have you ever felt guilt or remorse after drinking? How often?

_____ Has a relative, friend, doctor, or other health worker ever expressed concern about your drinking or suggested you cut down?

_____ Have you ever passed out from drinking? Do you not remember things that happened while you were drinking?

_____ Have you ever felt that you needed more alcohol than you used to in order to get the same effect?

_____ Have you ever tried to cut down or stop drinking but couldn't?

Review your answers carefully, and think about your drinking. On a scale of 1 (no reason for concern) to 10 (I have a drinking problem), how do you rate your concern about the role of alcohol in your life? Write down this number and the date.

If drinking problems run in your family, you need to think about drinking even more carefully than other students. In both women and men, genetics accounts for about 50 percent of a person's vulnerability to serious drinking problems. Do research on alcoholism in your family, going back to your grandparents and including uncles, aunts, and cousins. Gather as much information as you can about the risks for children of alcoholics. We suggest that you discuss your vulnerability with your doctor, a mental health professional, or a counselor at your school.

Binge Drinking

According to the National Institute of Alcohol Abuse and Alcoholism, a **binge** is a pattern of drinking alcohol that brings blood-alcohol concentration (BAC) to 0.08 gram-percent or above. For a typical adult man, this pattern corresponds to consuming five or more drinks in about two hours; for a woman, four or more drinks.

An estimated 4 in 10 college students drink at binge levels or greater. They consume 91 percent of all alcohol that undergraduates report drinking. Binge drinkers are more likely to be under age 24 and to be male than female, although more women report binge drinking than in the past.[24] Binge drinkers are more likely to use other substances, including nicotine, marijuana, cocaine, and LSD, to be injured or hurt, to engage in unplanned or unprotected sexual activity, and to get in trouble with campus police.

Students tend to binge-drink at the beginning of the school year and then cut back as the semester progresses and academic demands increase. Binge drinking also peaks after stressful times, such as after midterms or finals, and during letting-off-steam occasions, such as football weekends and Spring break.[25]

> 🔧 **Stress Reliever:** Set a Drinking Quota and Write it Down
>
> ....
>
> "My limit is ___ drink(s) whenever I drink."
>
> ....
>
> Sign and date the entry.

Defensive Drinking

If you are of legal age and don't want to abstain from alcohol, make a list of strategies you can use to limit your drinking. Here are ones commonly reported by other students:

_____ Eating before, while, and after drinking.

_____ Assigning a designated driver.

_____ Keeping track of how many drinks you are having.

_____ Avoiding drinking games.

_____ Planning in advance not to exceed a set number of drinks.

_____ Alternating alcoholic and nonalcoholic drinks.

_____ Pacing drinks to one or fewer per hour.

_____ Asking a friend to let them know when they had enough.

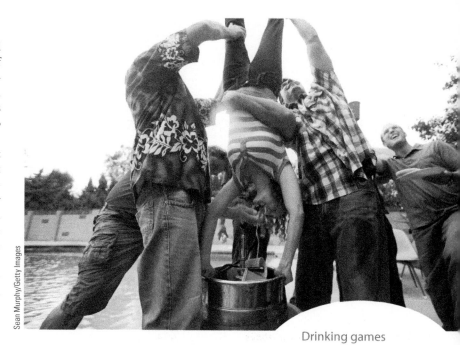

Sean Murphy/Getty Images

Drinking games can lead to extreme intoxication, alcohol-related injuries, and alcohol poisoning.

_____ Choosing not to drink alcohol.

_____ Choosing a non-alcoholic look-alike, like alcohol-free beer or plain soda.

_____ Drinking at least one glass of water for every alcoholic beverage you consume.

Before leaving for a party or a bar, put a check next to the strategies you plan to use. The next day check the ones you actually did use. If your drinking strategies didn't work well, come up with new ideas to try in the future.

Drugs

As a kid you may have played with matches even though your parents warned you about the dangers. Did you get burned? Let's hope not, but you could have been. Certainly your judgment was immature. Or maybe you rode your bike down steep hills to see how fast you could go or whirled round and round until you were dizzy. Seeking thrills and slightly altered states is a part of growing up. In fact, the lust for them makes a lot of money for amusement parks. Because our **culture** is awash in drugs, you may also have become curious about them. Maybe you experimented. Or maybe you just said no. Either way you have survived so far and made it to college.

Now you are in another time of experimentation and discovery. As a student, you can stretch yourself intellectually, expand yourself socially, challenge yourself physically, and experience a different kind of excitement. Students who report higher stress levels are more likely to become heavy drug users.[26] A minority of students—far fewer than you think—begin or continue to use

binge Pattern of drinking alcohol that brings blood-alcohol concentration (BAC) to 0.08 gram-percent or above—typically consuming five or more drinks in about two hours for a man and four or more drinks for a woman.

culture The set of shared attitudes, values, goals, and practices of a group that are internalized by an individual within the group.

Being with people who are drinking doesn't mean you have to drink as much as they are. Here are some effective ways to get your message across. Visualize situations in which you might use them. Rehearse before you go out:

_____ "Just have one beer."	"I have a bet with someone (no need to say it's you) to see how long I can go without drinking."
	"I can't stop at one, and I'm not going there tonight."
_____ "How about a round of tequila shooters for everyone?"	"No, the last time I tried tequila I swore I'd never do it again."
_____ "Why aren't you drinking?"	"I don't drink."
	"I've got practice/work/a job interview/whatever/first thing tomorrow"
_____ "Can I buy you a drink?"	"Not tonight, thanks. Maybe next time."

drugs. They may argue that parents, teachers, and other authorities exaggerate their dangers. At times they do, but this does not mean that drugs are safe.

All drugs—prescription medicines and street drugs—are dangerous. The only way to be absolutely sure of avoiding the stress caused by drugs is not to use them. This choice—the one more than six in ten college students make—is more than safe: it's smart. Drugs interfere with learning and education by making it more difficult to pay attention, concentrate, and remember. They create problems with people who love you. The use of illegal drugs can, as you know, lead to terrible, life-changing consequences for you and your family.

Legal drugs, when used for reasons other than that for which they were prescribed, can be even stronger and more deadly. Drugs produce short- and long-term side effects that can range from mood changes to potentially fatal abnormalities in your breathing and heart rate. Most importantly, drugs can steal control of your life and your future—or steal your very life.

There are other less obvious reasons not to go down the path of drug use. For one thing, there is no need to. As Table 8.4 shows, you can experience all the sensations drugs can offer in other ways.

Tobacco

Stained teeth; bad breath; premature wrinkles; gum disease; yellow fingernails. No one starts smoking to acquire any of these, but they come with the habit—along with far more serious

TABLE 8.4 Alternatives to Alcohol and Drugs

People drink and use drugs for many reasons, including to alter normal, waking consciousness and get high. Yet drugs aren't the only—and certainly not the best—way to achieve exhilarating and enduring highs. Here are other non-compulsive, non-chemical ways of achieving each of the following:

Physical relaxation	Meditation, exercise, yoga, and so on.
Sensory stimulation	Hiking a forest trail, swimming, star-gazing, and so on.
Feeling happier	Talk with a friend, join a service organization, see a counselor, exercise, and so on.
Escape from boredom	Campus clubs and activities, discussion groups, travel, and so on.
Greater creativity	Visit art galleries, attend concerts, take a non-credit photography class, and so on.
Kicks	Sign up for a wilderness survival course, take up rock or wall climbing, learn to tango, and so on.

health consequences. About half of all those who continue to smoke will end up dying from a smoking-related illness. Even today, with smoking rates lower than they have been in decades, tobacco kills more people than AIDS, alcohol, drug abuse, car crashes, murders, suicides, and fires combined. You don't have to be in this unfortunate number.

About one in ten college students reports smoking in the last 30 days—often as a way of managing stress.[27] Students who've had traumatic experiences are more likely to smoke to alleviate symptoms such as difficulty concentrating and irritability, and typically find it more difficult to quit.[28] White students have the highest smoking rates, followed by Hispanic, Asian, and African American students. About equal percentages of college men and women smoke, although women are somewhat more likely than men to report smoking daily.[29] Other forms of tobacco use, such as electronic cigarettes, have become more popular on college campuses. Although they can help smokers quit, "vaping" poses health risks of its own.

Maybe you don't think of yourself as a smoker because you only smoke at parties, during finals, or with particular friends; maybe you've cut back or are thinking about quitting; maybe you've quit several times already. If you smoke at all—a cigarette a week or a pack a day, in social settings or anywhere you can—there is nothing more important that you can do for yourself, your health, and your future than to quit. Do it now.

 Stress Reliever: If You Want to Quit

Start the morning by saying, "I am not a smoker." Repeat this phrase to yourself 20 times. Write it down 20 times. Repeat it as you go through your day—while taking a shower, making coffee, walking up the stairs, waiting for the light to change, downloading music, looking up the weather report. Be sure to repeat this mantra morning and night and as often as possible during the day.

Make this statement even if you are tapering down your tobacco use and continuing to smoke. Your mind will register the discrepancy between the message you are sending yourself and your behavior. In time you will find it easier not to smoke because you see yourself as a nonsmoker.

Strengthening Your Coping Muscles

Just like physical health, psychological well-being involves more than an absence of problems. By developing your inner strengths and resources, you become the author of your life, capable of confronting challenges and learning from them. You have greater control over how happy, optimistic, upbeat, and lovable you are than anyone or anything else. But only by consciously taking charge of your life can you find happiness and fulfillment.

Think of yourself as an athlete in training. If you decide to run a charity 5-kilometer race, you don't head for the gym or track and go the full distance. You build up your muscles and your aerobic capacity by starting with a lap or two and gradually increasing your distance and pace. The same is true for stress management. You need to acquire and enhance fundamental skills that lay the foundation for developing all kinds of new, more complex habits and skills. Here are some suggestions for your training sessions:

- Be on task. By all means, set goals, following the steps in Chapter 7. But don't stop there. Use your goals to guide you. Talk to yourself about them. Note how you are progressing toward them; if you drift, come back with a vengeance. Lock in on them like a heat-seeking missile.

- Think back to times in the last week or so when you managed stress well. Write down the practical skills you used. Go further into the past and think about other times you handled stress successfully. Keep adding to your list of strengths.

- Review the times in the past when you did not handle stress well. Write down why you think you handled stress badly in certain situations. Identify specific steps or skills that would have enabled you to handle the situations better.

- In assessing your strengths and weaknesses in handling stress, separate what you did, especially any mistakes you made, from who you are. Instead of saying, "I'm so stupid," tell yourself, "That wasn't the smartest move I ever made, but I learned from it."

- Use affirmations, positive statements that help reinforce the most positive aspects of your personality and experience. Every day, you might say, "I am a loving, caring person," or "I am honest and open in expressing my feelings." Write down a few affirmations, and read them at least once a day, every day.

- Psychologically healthy men and women can cope with the stressors of everyday living, value themselves, strive toward happiness and fulfillment, accept life's limitations as well as its possibilities; and feel a sense of meaning and purpose that makes the gestures of living worth the effort required. Emotional health includes feelings and moods.

- Emotional intelligence consists of recognition and expression of emotions while feeling them, the ability to create and maintain healthy interpersonal relationships and to control and marshal emotions in order to remain focused and reach goals; understanding of what others are feeling; and the ability to manage emotions, regulate moods, handle stress, and rebound from emotional setbacks.

- Among the aspects of emotional intelligence that most benefit students, particularly when under stress, are focusing on clear, manageable goals and identifying and understanding emotions rather than relying on gut feelings.

- Positive psychology (the scientific study of ordinary human strengths and virtues) and positive psychiatry (which promotes positive psychosocial development in those with or at high risk of mental or physical illness) focus on the aspects of human experience that lead to happiness and fulfillment—in other words, on what makes life worthwhile.

- Positive emotions can expand our ways of thinking and acting and lead to new adaptive behavior. Various approaches, such as recalling positive memories, using your unique or signature strengths in new ways, and cultivating gratitude and acceptance, bolster positivity.

- Positive emotions help shorten the after-effects of the stress response by relieving tension and cleansing your body of stress hormones. Unlike panic and fear, which narrow focus and attention, positive emotions enable us to be more flexible and open in our thinking.

- A sense of self-esteem, of belief or pride in ourselves, gives us confidence to dare to attempt to achieve at school or work and to reach out to others to form friendships and close relationships.

- College students who rate high in conscientiousness (striving for competence and achievement, self-discipline, orderliness, reliability, deliberativeness) and low in extraversion (being active, talkative, assertive, social, stimulation- seeking)—are more likely to manage stress well.

- Self-compassion is a healthy form of self-acceptance that encompasses favorable and unfavorable attitudes about ourselves and others.

- The humanist theorist Abraham Maslow believed that human needs are the motivating factors in personality development. First, we must satisfy basic physiological needs, such as those for food, shelter, and sleep. Only then can we pursue fulfillment of our higher needs—for safety and security, love and affection, and self-esteem.

- Happiness is not the absence of stress, but an abundance of eustress that induces stress-reducing changes in the brain. Researchers distinguish between two types of happiness: hedonic, which involves accumulating material things and enjoying pleasurable activities, and eudaemonic, which is based on a sense of higher purpose and service to others.

- Mental health professionals define optimism as the "extent to which individuals expect favorable outcomes to occur." Optimism breeds hope, another life-affirming positive emotion.

- Grateful people feel more frequent and intense positive emotions, have more positive views of their social environment, use more productive coping strategies, sleep better, and appreciate their lives and possessions more.

- Negative emotions outnumber positive feelings four to one. The most effective way to banish a sad or bad feeling is by changing what caused it in the first place.

- If you peel away all the layers of emotions involved in stress, at its innermost core you'll find the same thing: fear. If you work with fear correctly, fear will become your ally in managing stress.

- Whatever its trigger, anger inevitably unleashes the stress response, which revs the body into a state of combat readiness, increasing the risk for bodily harm, stroke and heart attack—even in healthy individuals.

- Addictive behaviors and substances may seem like quick escapes from stress, but they can intensify the stress in your daily life and create unforeseen and unpredictable new stresses.

- About half of students who gamble at least once a month experience significant problems related to their gambling, including poor academic performance, heavy alcohol consumption, illicit drug use, unprotected sex, and other risky behaviors.

- About two thirds of students drink alcohol, most often to relax. Because it depresses the central nervous system, alcohol can make people feel less stressed—even though it does nothing to relieve the cause of the stress and may make some stressors worse.

- A binge is a pattern of drinking alcohol that brings blood-alcohol concentration (BAC) (discussed later in this chapter) to 0.08 gram-percent or above. For a typical adult man, this pattern corresponds to consuming five or more drinks in about two hours; for a woman, four or more drinks.

- Substance abuse is a serious health risk for the minority of undergraduates who do use drugs. Every aspect of substance abuse generates stress, ranging from short-term consequences to long-term physical and psychological problems.

- About one in every four to five students currently smokes—often as a way of managing stress. About equal percentages of male and female students smoke, although women are somewhat more likely than men to report smoking daily.

🔧 STRESS RELIEVERS

The XYZ Technique
How do you put difficult emotions into words? Think "X-Y-Z":

- I felt X (frustrated, hurt, disappointed)

- when you did Y (didn't follow through, made fun of me, didn't call)

- in situation Z (at the meeting, when you promised, in front of my parents).

Accentuate the Positive
Do's:

- Smile. A happy face makes for a happy spirit.

- Focus. By being fully present in the moment, you'll experience it more intensely.

- Share your joy. Talking about and celebrating good experiences extends positive feelings.

- Travel through time. Vividly remembering or anticipating positive events—a technique called "positive mental time travel"—boosts levels of happiness and life satisfaction.

Don'ts:

- Don't hide your feelings. Suppressing positive feelings— because of shyness or a sense of modesty, for instance— diminishes them.

- Don't get distracted. Unrelated worries and thoughts detract from the here-and-now of a positive experience.

- Don't find fault. Paying attention to negative aspects of otherwise positive experiences sabotages levels of happiness, optimism, self-esteem, and life satisfaction.

- Don't go there. "Negative mental time travel"—reflecting on what went wrong or what may go wrong—can lower self-esteem and foster depressive symptoms.

Reframe
Think of something that is stressing you out. Can you look at it in a more positive way? Try incorporating some of the following attitude-adjusting strategies:

- Accept that some things are out of your control.

- Challenge your negative thoughts.

- Be compassionate and forgiving, both to yourself and to those around you.

- Keep it real. Don't let your expectations become unreasonable or catastrophic.

- Avoid extremes. Thinking in absolute terms such as "always" or "never" is bound to bring you down.

Make Deposits in Your Happiness Bank
At the end of each day, think of one thing that made you happy and describe it in words (written or recorded). When you're feeling down, tap into this happiness fund to lift your spirits.

Step Outside
Being puts the irritations of daily living into perspective. Let your gaze linger on silvery ice glazing a branch or an azalea bush in wild bloom. Follow the flight of a bird; watch clouds float overhead. Gaze into the night sky and think of the stars as holes in the darkness letting the light of heaven shine through. Breathe deeply and fully inhabit the moment. Let your anger blow away in the breeze. If you can't go outdoors, visualize a natural scene.

Reappraise
Ask:

_____ What lessons did this teach me?
_____ What would I have done differently?
_____ Could there be a silver lining or hidden benefit?

Set a Drinking Quota and Write it Down
"My limit is ___ drink(s) whenever I drink."
Sign and date the entry.

When "No" Isn't Enough
Being with people who are drinking doesn't mean you have to drink as much as they are. Here are some effective ways to get your message across. Visualize situations in which you might use them. Rehearse before you go out:

_____ "Just have one beer."

"I have a bet with someone (no need to say it's you) to see I can go without drinking."

"I can't stop at one, and I'm not going there tonight."

_____ "How about a round of tequila shooters for everyone?"

"No, the last time I tried tequila I swore I'd never do it again."

_____ "Why aren't you drinking?"

"I don't drink."

"I've got practice/work/a job interview/whatever/first thing tomorrow."

_____ "Can I buy you a drink?"

"Not tonight, thanks. Maybe next time."

⊜ YOUR PERSONAL STRESS MANAGEMENT TOOLKIT

REFLECTION: How Grateful Are You?

Look at each item in the following list, and put a check beside each one for which you were grateful today in some conscious way.

_____ Health
_____ Finances
_____ Father
_____ Mother
_____ Other family members
_____ Friends
_____ Your intelligence
_____ Your talents
_____ Your bed
_____ Your room
_____ Your roommates if you have them. (Remember, even if are not fond of a roommate, you learn a great deal from having one.)
_____ Your professors
_____ Your classes
_____ Your books
_____ What you ate today
_____ Your senses
_____ Your personal freedom
_____ Your choices
_____ Air conditioning and its inventor(s)
_____ Heating
_____ Farmers who raise the food you eat
_____ Factories that make your furniture and clothing
_____ If you took transportation today, the type and those who developed and built it
_____ Exams
_____ Assigned papers
_____ Seat belts
_____ Books
_____ Any road you took
_____ Any bridge you passed over
_____ Love
_____ Loyalty
_____ Integrity

_____ Commitment
_____ Art
_____ Beauty
_____ Feelings
_____ Animals
_____ Life
_____ Guides
_____ Intuition
_____ Your toothbrush
_____ Shoelaces
_____ Ice cream
_____ Fruit
_____ Chocolate
_____ Your smartphone and every person whose efforts led to its development
_____ The drivers of the cars that stopped for you and did not hit you while you were in the last crosswalk you passed through
_____ Traffic lights and the cooperation involved in ensuring our safety.
_____ Jet planes
_____ Automobiles
_____ The constitution of the United States
_____ Your citizenship
_____ Your feet
_____ Your hands
_____ Your thumbs
_____ Your fingers
_____ Your toes
_____ Your fingernails
_____ Your arms and legs
_____ Your digestive system
_____ The sea
_____ The sky
_____ A full moon
_____ Shooting stars
_____ Fireflies
_____ Spring
_____ Other…

Continue adding to this list every day for at least a week.

TECHNIQUE: Taming a Toxic Temper

In order to control your anger, you must recognize subtle cues that you are becoming angry as soon as possible.

How Does Your Anger Feel?

What is the earliest sign of anger you experience in your body? When do you first notice it? Describe what you feel when you get angry, for instance:

_____ Do you clench your fists?

_____ Do you hold your breath?

_____ Do you tighten your jaw?

_____ Do you feel heat?

_____ Does your chest burn?

_____ Does your voice change?

_____ Does your heart pound?

_____ Do you talk louder?

_____ Do you become quiet?

Usually people experience several cues, but one is often the very first sign that they're getting angry. Your job is to identify and tune into this cue. Whenever you feel the first sensation, look for something subtle that comes before it—a thought, perhaps, or a perception of something about another person that does not set right with you. The earlier you sense that something is beginning to make you angry, the greater the opportunity to engage your rational mind. Even a couple of milliseconds can be enough to hold your temper in check.

What Are Your Anger Triggers?

When you know you are about to confront a situation that sets you off, you have the opportunity to get ready internally to maintain your calm. Make a list of all the things that can set you off, for instance:

_____ Bad or discourteous drivers

_____ Someone cutting in front of you in line

_____ Poor service

_____ Disrespect

_____ Any delays

_____ Talking during a movie

_____ Someone not picking up after a dog

_____ Roommates who trash the bathroom and don't clean it up

_____ Anyone who keeps you waiting

_____ _____

_____ _____

_____ _____

Talk Yourself Down

When you experience a trigger and feel an anger cue, remind yourself what is at stake and why you don't want to let anger control you. Develop a list of your own reminders—ones that will make a difference to you when you say them to yourself—and write them down. Here are some examples of the kinds of things you might say to yourself:

_____ "I could get in trouble." "I could get kicked off the team." "This time my partner may walk out for good."

_____ Repeat to yourself a phrase like one of the following:

_____ He's not worth it.

_____ She's not worth it.

_____ "It's not worth it."

_____ Remind yourself, "I've got so much else going on in my life. I can let this go."

_____ Ask, "Is it worth going there?"

Rely on Anger-Reducers

Build up a repertoire of anger-control techniques. Try each of the suggestions below in real life, and describe the experience of doing so in words. Here are some examples:

- Count backwards.

- Breathe in through your nose slowly and deeply, pushing your abdomen out so your diaphragm contracts maximally. Hold your breath for a few seconds. Exhale slowly through your mouth, thinking, "Relax." Repeat the sequence five to 10 times, concentrating on breathing slowly and deeply.

- Visualize a place where you usually enjoy yourself, like a favorite vacation spot. See yourself in a hammock or on a sunny beach, feeling serene and tranquil.

- Fast-forward yourself twenty years into the future, and ask if you'll even remember what made you angry. Better yet, laugh about it.

- Repeat a simple affirmation: "I am going to stay in control." Remind yourself that by getting angry, you give control to the person pushing your buttons.

- Backing off and taking the high road may seem harder, but it is healthier and more satisfying in the long run and eliminates anger's negative consequences.

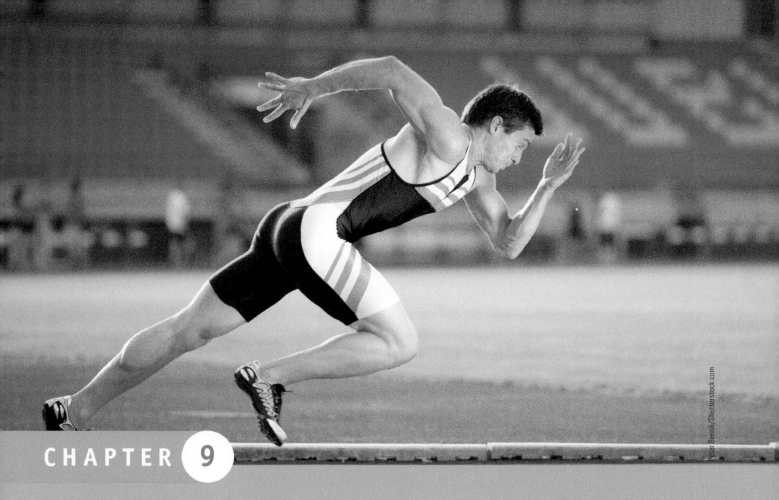

Petar Bennik /Shutterstock.com

CHAPTER (9)

Stress-Resistant Health Habits

After reading this chapter, you should be able to:

9.1 Describe ways in which physical activity lowers stress and enhances wellbeing.

9.2 Summarize the significance of a good night's sleep.

9.3 Identify the components of good nutrition and the roles played by macronutrients and micronutrients.

9.4 Discuss gender, racial, and ethnic differences in relation to body image.

9.5 Identify factors related to weight gain for students on campus.

9.6 Describe the forms of disordered eating and of eating disorders.

9.7 Employ strategies related to physical activity, sleep, and eating to develop a stress-resistant lifestyle.

	Yes	No
Do you exercise regularly?		
Do you usually get enough sleep to feel refreshed in the morning and alert during the day?		
Do you eat a balanced diet that includes vegetables, fruit, whole grains, and protein, and limits sugar and salt?		
If you drink alcohol, do you limit the amount you consume?		
Do you refrain from any tobacco use?		

Individuals whose lifestyles include these fundamental behaviors are less likely to be overwhelmed by stress or to suffer poor mental health. If you didn't check all five, this chapter will help improve your score—and your stress resistance.

Along with the rest of the soccer team, Matt worked out every day and fueled up with nutritious meals. Then a sprained Achilles tendon sidelined him. The season ended before he was cleared for exercise. Even after he recovered, Matt rarely managed to get to the gym or go out for a run.

The time pressure intensified when Matt, struggling through organic chemistry, signed up for free tutoring sessions and make-up lab work. He wolfed down burritos and burgers and guzzled energy drinks to stay alert. Even when he collapsed into bed, he'd toss and turn His jeans felt so snug that he mainly wore sweatpants. As finals approached, his skin broke out, and his stomach felt tied in knots.

"You sound stressed," his mother said when they talked on the phone. "Are you taking care of yourself?"

"Not really," Matt replied. For the first time in his life, he realized, he was neglecting his body's basic needs—and paying the price.

Like Matt, many college students find themselves sitting more, exercising less, sleeping poorly, eating junk food, and putting on unwanted pounds. It's easy to blame stress, but the fact is that you always have choices. You decide when to take a quick walk or jog, when to go to bed and get up in the morning, when to say no to junk food, how often to weigh yourself. Healthy choices can help you withstand the inevitable challenges of daily life; unhealthy ones can increase the stressors you encounter and intensify their consequences. By the time they graduate, one in four college students has at least one major risk factor for diabetes or heart disease, such as high blood glucose or high blood pressure—all affected by exercise, diet, weight, and stress.

The best defense against stress-related health problems begins with a good offense—or, more precisely, a proactive plan that includes regular physical activity, consistent sleep patterns, good nutrition, and weight management. As you take better care of your body, you will gain a sense of internal commitment and achievement. The sheer pleasure of living in a physically fit, rested, well-nourished body will become a powerful stress reducer in itself.

Physical Activity and Exercise

✔ Check-in: How physically active are you?

You are designed to move. Your body is a biomechanical marvel with every cell primed for action. You have toes that wiggle, a heart that pumps, muscles that stretch, hands that reach, lungs that expand. But without the activity it craves, your body grows weaker, your energy runs out, and you're more susceptible to stress.

Physical activity lowers stress and enhances well-being via several mechanisms, including the following:

- Blunting the hormonal stress response systems, such as the hypothalamus-pituitary-adrenal axis and the sympathetic nervous system (described in Chapter 2). This reduces emotional, physiological, and metabolic reactivity (responsiveness) and also increases positive mood and well-being.[1]

- Minimizing excessive inflammation. As discussed in Chapter 2, chronic psychological stress has been associated with persistent, systemic (body-wide), low-grade inflammation, which can contribute to many chronic diseases.

- Increasing levels of KAT, an enzyme that helps rid the body of a stress-induced amino acid (kynurenine) associated with depression

and other mental disorders.[2] This may be one reason why exercise has proven as effective as psychotherapy or antidepressant medication in relieving depression.

According to the American College Health Association (ACHA's) national surveys, fewer than half of undergraduates (45.4 percent) meet the current recommendations for moderate or vigorous exercise.[3] Students are more likely to exercise if they don't have full- or part-time jobs, live on campus, are single rather than married, separated, or divorced, do not have children or, if they do, are not single mothers and fathers.

The Stress of Sedentary Living

Doing nothing may seem the opposite of being stressed, but it can end up causing significant, even life-threatening harm. A sedentary lifestyle, particularly combined with a diet high in fat and calories, can add unhealthy pounds to your frame and inches to your waist. Inactivity doubles the risk of cardiorespiratory diseases, diabetes, and obesity and increases the risk of colon cancer, high blood pressure, osteoporosis, depression, and anxiety. As a risk factor for heart disease, a sedentary lifestyle is as perilous as elevated cholesterol or high blood pressure. The more time spent in "recreational sitting" in front of a television or computer screen, the greater the risk of obesity, chronic diseases, and early death.

 Stress Reliever: Take an Exercise Break

Getting up and walking for a few minutes every hour can reverse the negative effects of prolonged sitting. In one study, a short burst of activity such as walking or going up and down stairs boosted the longevity of people who were sedentary more than half of their day.[4]

Exercise, Stress, and the Brain

Exercise itself is a form of stress. In fact, intense exercise is the greatest physiological stress that our bodies experience. During maximum exertion, an elite athlete's heart can pump eight times more blood than when at rest. Its effects on the brain are equally dramatic.

Just as exercise makes muscles stronger and more resilient, it stimulates production of neurochemicals that protect the brain from damage and raises our brain's stress reaction threshold. It also enhances neuroplasticity, the brain's ability

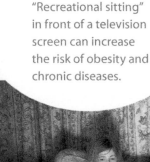

"Recreational sitting" in front of a television screen can increase the risk of obesity and chronic diseases.

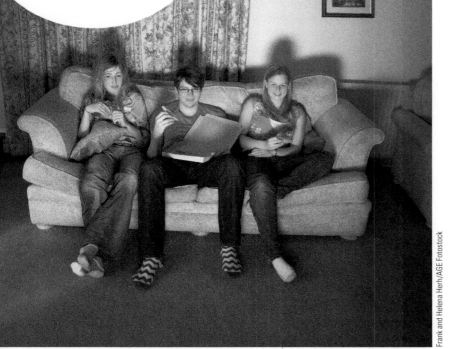

Frank and Helena Herh/AGE Fotostock

to change and produce new cells and connections, thereby improving mood and thinking.[5] In animal studies, distance running proved particularly beneficial in generating new neurons in the hippocampus, a key area of the brain for learning and memory.[6] (See Chapter 3 for more on stress and the brain.)

As always, the key is balance between overexertion and underexertion. Some researchers compare exercise's effects on neurons to the training of military forces in peacetime. Soldiers work out and drill regularly to remain in optimum condition and constant readiness. However, they avoid overexertion so they don't deplete their energy and reserves.[7]

In addition to its long-term benefits, exercise has an immediate payoff: It makes you feel good. When you go for a brisk walk or jog, you activate so many neurons and circuits that, as neuroimaging reveals, your brain literally lights up as it produces neurochemicals called endorphins that induce the state of eustress called "runner's high."[8]

....

✔ **Check-in:** Make time to move

....

When was the last time you stretched? Went for a walk? Worked out at the gym?

....

Stop waiting until you have the time. Make an appointment to exercise, and mark it on your schedule.

....

Fitness Fundamentals

The terms *physical activity* and *exercise*, although often used interchangeably, are not the same. **Physical activity** refers to any movement produced by the muscles that results in expenditure of energy (measured in calories). **Exercise** is a type of physical activity that requires planned, structured, and repetitive bodily movement with the intent of improving one or more components of physical fitness. You can be physically active without exercising—and reap health rewards. An "active lifestyle" that incorporates short stretches of activity, such as walking several blocks during the day, has proven as effective as structured exercise in lowering cortisol and stress levels.[9]

The simplest definition of **physical fitness** is the ability to respond to routine physical demands with enough reserve energy to cope with a sudden challenge. Fitness affects your ability, not only to lift a backpack onto a luggage rack, but also to handle stress and other challenges. Its components include:

- Cardiorespiratory fitness, the ability of the heart to pump blood through the body efficiently, which is achieved by aerobic activities, such as brisk walking or swimming.

- Metabolic fitness, which refers to reduced risk for diabetes and cardiovascular disease and can be achieved through moderate-intensity exercise.

- Muscular strength, the force within muscles measured by the absolute maximum weight you can lift, push, or press in one effort, and endurance, measured by counting how many times you can lift, push, or press a given weight.

- Flexibility, the range of motion around certain joints—for example, the stretching you do to touch your toes or twist your torso.

- Body composition, the relative amounts of fat and lean tissue (bone, muscle, organs, water) in the body.

> 🔧 **Stress Reliever:** Build Physical Activity Into Your Daily Routine. How?
>
> ....
>
> Walk to class instead of taking the shuttle.
>
> Opt for the stairs rather than the elevator.
>
> Get up from your cubicle in the library every 30 minutes and walk around the stacks.
>
> Dance during a study break.
>
> By all means, schedule regular workouts. Just don't think that the only place to get physical is the gym.

As Figure 9.1 illustrates, physical activity and exercise affect every aspect of your life, including its duration.[10] Physical activity reduces unhelpful stress hormones that can dampen resistance to disease and enhances the circulation of natural killer cells that fight off viruses and bacteria. Regular exercise—such as walking, running, or lifting weights—relieves anxiety and depression, brightens mood, boosts positive feelings, improves memory, concentration, and alertness, and protects the brain from dementia. It also increases flexibility in the joints, improves digestion, speeds up metabolism, and builds lean body mass, so the body burns more calories and body fat decreases. Exercise heightens sensitivity to insulin (a great benefit for diabetics) and may lower the risk of developing diabetes. In addition, it boosts clot-dissolving substances in the blood, helping to prevent strokes, heart attacks,

physical activity Any movement produced by the muscles that results in expenditure of energy.

exercise A type of physical activity that requires planned, structured, and repetitive bodily movement with the intent of improving one or more components of physical fitness.

physical fitness The ability to respond to routine physical demands with enough reserve energy to cope with a sudden challenge.

FIGURE 9.1

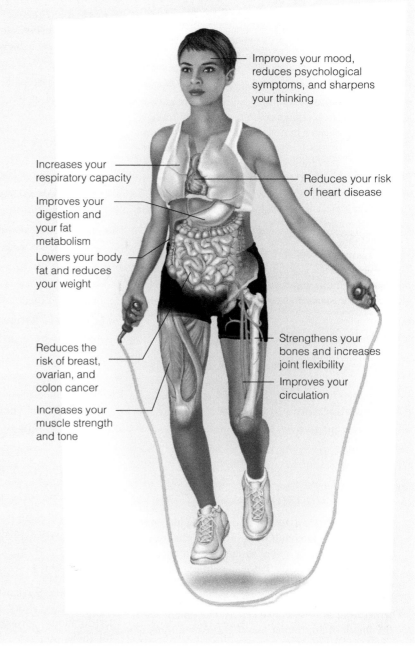

Health Benefits of Physical Activity—A Review of the Strength of the Scientific Evidence

Strong Evidence

- Lower risk of early death
- Lower risk of coronary heart disease
- Lower risk of stroke
- Lower risk of high blood pressure
- Lower risk of adverse blood lipid profile
- Lower risk of type 2 diabetes
- Lower risk of metabolic syndrome
- Lower risk of colon cancer
- Lower risk of breast cancer
- Prevention of weight gain
- Weight loss, particularly when combined with reduced calorie intake
- Prevention of falls
- Reduced depression
- Better cognitive function (for older adults)

Moderate to Strong Evidence

- Better functional health (for older adults)
- Reduced abdominal obesity

Moderate Evidence

- Lower risk of hip fracture
- Lower risk of lung cancer
- Lower risk of endometrial cancer
- Weight maintenance after weight loss
- Increased bone density
- Improved sleep quality

Source: U.S. Department of Health and Human Services, www.hhs.gov

Improves your mood, reduces psychological symptoms, and sharpens your thinking

Increases your respiratory capacity

Reduces your risk of heart disease

Improves your digestion and your fat metabolism

Lowers your body fat and reduces your weight

Strengthens your bones and increases joint flexibility

Improves your circulation

Reduces the risk of breast, ovarian, and colon cancer

Increases your muscle strength and tone

and pulmonary embolisms (clots in the lungs), and lowers the risk of certain cancers.[11]

Guidelines for Physical Activity and Exercise

A single bout of intense aerobic exercise can sharpen your memory. This may be because exercise, an acute stressor, focuses attention and intensifies brain activity.[12] Low-intensity workouts also can help: Just 20 minutes of any physical activity can alleviate stress by reducing muscle tension and cortisol secretion. Regular and consistent exercise produces more and more lasting benefits, including psychological ones. When exercise is part of your daily routine, you take control of one aspect of your life, which boosts your confidence in what else you can do and strengthens your stress resilience.

The most recent U.S. Department of Health and Human Services *Physical Activity Guidelines for Americans,* based on the latest research findings on the health benefits of physical activity, recognize that some activity is better than none. However, the *Guidelines* emphasize that more activity—consisting of both aerobic (endurance) and muscle-strengthening (resistance) workouts—is more beneficial.[13]

Here are the government's key recommendations:

- Avoid inactivity. Any amount of physical activity yields some health benefits.

- For substantial health benefits, do at least 150 minutes (2 hours and 30 minutes) a week of moderate-intensity, or 75 minutes (1 hour and 15 minutes) a week of vigorous-intensity, aerobic physical activity, or an equivalent combination of moderate- and vigorous-intensity aerobic activity.

- For additional health benefits, increase aerobic physical activity to 300 minutes (5 hours) a week of moderate-intensity, or 150 minutes (2 1/2 hours) a week of vigorous-intensity aerobic physical activity, or an equivalent combination of moderate- and vigorous- intensity activity.

- Do muscle-strengthening activities of moderate or high intensity that involve all major muscle groups on two or more days a week.

Get F.I.T.T.

To get the maximum benefits from exercise, sports medicine specialists recommend following the F.I.T.T. Formula (for frequency, intensity, time, and type):

Frequency: How Often Should You Exercise?

Face it: A Saturday morning hike or an hour at the gym every week won't whip you into shape. You need to exercise more often to reap the greatest benefit: a minimum of three to five days of aerobic or cardiovascular training and two days of resistance and flexibility training.

Intensity: How Hard Should You Work Out?

Whether you're doing an aerobic exercise or working on muscle strength, you need to meet a greater-than-normal challenge. If you're walking or running, move fast enough to speed up your heart rate. Start with a 15-minute walk or jog, and increase time and distance gradually as you go farther and faster. For strength training, you can increase the amount of weight you lift, the resistance you work against, or the number of repetitions.

Time: How Long Should You Work Out?

The answer depends on how hard you're working. If you're exercising at high intensity (such as biking uphill or jogging at a ten-minute-a-mile pace), you don't need to continue as long as when you're biking on flat terrain or walking at a slower pace. For strength and flexibility training, pay attention to the number of repetitions of doing chest presses or biceps curls rather than total time.

Type: What Kind of Exercise Should You Do?

Both aerobic and resistance exercise have proven useful in lessening stress, boosting mood, and relieving depression. Ideally, your weekly workout should include a mix of aerobic activities, strength training, and flexibility exercises. (See Table 9.1 on Exercise Options.) Consider all the options you have and choose those you enjoy most. If you hate running, try cycling or swimming. See if there are climbing walls, yoga, kickboxing, tennis, or other activities offered nearby.

Many college campuses have club or social sports teams (such as club soccer or social kickball leagues) that are a great way to get in physical activity, as well as meet new people. If you feel uncomfortable at a gym or health club, download a workout video and exercise at home or ask a friend to start going for regular walks or hikes.

Sleep and Stress

You stay up late cramming for a final; you drive through the night to visit a friend at another campus; you get up for an early class during the week but stay in bed until noon on weekends. And you wonder: "Why am I so tired?" The answer: You're not getting enough sleep. According to the American College Health Association's national survey, only about one in ten undergraduates reported getting enough sleep in the previous week to feel rested every morning. About six in ten report feeling tired, dragged out, or sleepy three or more days a week[14] (see Table 9.2).

....

✔ **Check-in:** Are you getting enough sleep?

....

The National Sleep Foundation recommends seven to nine hours for men and women ages 18 to 25. How do you compare?

....

The Toll of Stress

If, as Shakespeare put it, sleep "knits up the raveled sleeve of care," stress unravels it, making it

TABLE 9.1 Exercise Options

AEROBIC (Cardiovascular)	STRENGTH TRAINING	FLEXIBILITY (See Part III/Glossary for descriptions of some of these mind-body disciplines)
Jogging/running	Free weights	Stretching
Swimming	Resistance machines	Pilates
Biking	Body-sculpting classes	Yoga
Spinning	Rock or wall climbing	Fitball
Kayaking/canoeing	Circuit training	Tai chi
Dance	Weighted pulleys	
Tennis		
Handball		
Cross-country skiing		
Basketball		
Soccer		
Skipping rope		
Stair climbing		
Cardio-kickboxing		
Zumba		

HconQ/Shutterstock.com

✔ **Check-in:** What's your favorite form of activity: walking, jogging, swimming, dancing, hiking, biking, yoga, Pilates, tai chi, Zumba, rollerblading, snowboarding, or something else entirely? Why do you like this way of being in motion? How does it make you feel?

hard to fall and often even harder to stay asleep. By disrupting a night's rest, stress deprives you of crucial hormones secreted during sleep and keeps you yawning through the day.

Here are some of the ways in which poor sleep affects your health and your ability to cope with stress:

- **Learning and memory.** When you sleep, your brain consolidates new information so you are more likely to retain it in your memory. It's harder to master and remember material when you're sleepy, stressed, or both.

- **Poor academic performance.** Poor or irregular sleep lowers grades, reduces ability to focus in class, and undermines assimilation of new material.[15]

- **Metabolism and weight.** The less you sleep, the more weight you may put on.[16] Chronic sleep deprivation may alter metabolism (for example, changing the way you process and store calories) and stimulate excess stress hormones, such as cortisol, that contribute to weight gain. Loss of sleep also

reduces levels of the hormones that regulate appetite, which may encourage stress-eating.[17]

- **Mood/quality of life.** Too little sleep—whether just for a night or two or for longer periods—can cause psychological symptoms, such as irritability, impatience, inability to concentrate, moodiness, and lower long-term life satisfaction.

- **Cardiovascular health.** Serious sleep disorders such as insomnia and sleep apnea (impaired breathing during sleep) increase stress hormones and inflammation, which may play a role in heart disease.

- **Immunity.** Stress itself dampens immunity; too little sleep may have a similar effect. If you get less than seven hours of sleep a night, you may be three times more likely to catch a cold.

- **Susceptibility to physical and mental disorders.** Without adequate sleep, your risk of diabetes, obesity, depression, anxiety, obesity, hypertension, high cholesterol, and traumatic stress disorders increases.

TABLE 9.2 Sleepless on Campus

Percentage of Students Getting Enough Sleep to Feel Rested in the Morning (Past Seven Days)

Time	Male (Percent)	Female (Percent)	Average (Percent)
0 days	10.4	14.1	13.0
1–2 days	27.7	33.3	31.5
3–5 days	48.9	43.2	45.0
6+ days	13.0	9.4	10.5

Percentage of Students Often Feeling Tired, Dragged Out, or Sleepy During the Day (Past Seven Days)

Time	Male (Percent)	Female (Percent)	Average (Percent)
0 days	13.2	6.3	8.6
1–2 days	34.2	27.4	29.5
3–5 days	39.6	45.7	43.7
6+ days	13.1	20.5	18.1

Impact of Sleepiness on Daytime Activities Reported by Students

Severity of Problem	Male (Percent)	Female (Percent)	Average (Percent)
No problem	13.0	6.9	9.0
A little problem	48.4	45.5	46.3
More than a little problem	24.8	27.2	26.4
A big problem	9.7	14.2	12.8
A very big problem	4.0	6.2	5.6

Source: American College Health Association. American College Health Association–National College Health Assessment II: Reference Group Executive Summary, Fall 2015, Hanover, MD: American College Health Association, 2016.

Student Night Life

College students are notorious for their erratic sleep schedules and late bedtimes. About one in five college students say that sleep difficulties have affected their academic performance, ranking only behind stress and anxiety.[18] The sleep-related difficulties that students report include greater daytime sleepiness, overall fatigue, depression, anxiety, slower reaction times, and more traffic accidents.

On average, today's college students go to bed 1–2 hours later and sleep 1–1.6 hours less than students of a generation ago. In comparisons of exhaustion levels reported by workers in various occupations, college students consistently score high. Women experience more sleep disturbances than men and are at greater risk for poor academic performance and more physical, social, and emotional problems. Students reporting poor sleep feel more stressed, irritable, anxious, depressed, angry, and confused than others.

Alcohol compounds many students' sleep problems. Poor-quality sleepers report drinking more alcohol than good sleepers and are twice as likely to use alcohol to induce sleep as are better sleepers. Students who drink more alcohol go to bed later, sleep less, and show greater differences between weekday and weekend sleep timing and duration. In general, students who do not adhere to a regular bedtime and rising schedule are more likely to be poor sleepers.

✔ **Check-in:** Are you a poor sleeper?

About six in ten college students report poor sleep—often the result of irregular sleep-wake schedules, late bedtimes, or a noisy/bright/disruptive sleep environment.

How Much Sleep Do You Need?

College students report an average sleep time of slightly less than seven hours, with little difference between men and women. To figure out your sleep needs, keep your wake-up time the same every morning and vary your bedtime. Are you groggy after six hours of shut-eye? Does an extra hour give you more stamina? What about an extra two hours? Since too much sleep can make you feel sluggish, don't assume that more is always better; listen to your body's signals, and adjust your sleep schedule to suit them.

Are you better off pulling an all-nighter before a big test or closing the books and getting a good night's sleep? According to researchers, that depends on the nature of the exam. If it's a test of facts—Civil War battles, for instance—cramming all night works. If you will have to write analytical essays in which you compare, contrast, and make connections, however, you need to sleep to make the most of your reasoning abilities.

Stress-induced Insomnia

Stress-induced **insomnia** (a lack of sleep so severe that it interferes with functioning during the day) can take different forms:

- problems falling asleep.
- waking frequently in the night.
- waking too early.
- not getting enough sleep to feel alert and energetic the next day.

Most often insomnia is transient, typically occurring before or after a stressful life event (such as a big game or internship interview) and lasting for three or four nights. During periods of prolonged stress (after a breakup, for instance, or during recovery from an injury), short-term insomnia may continue for several weeks.

Chronic insomnia, often triggered by a life crisis or stress, can begin at any age and persist long after the stressor has faded. About 15 percent of those seeking help for chronic insomnia suffer from "learned" or "behavioral" insomnia. While a life crisis may trigger their initial sleep problems, each night they try harder and harder to get to sleep, but they cannot—although they often doze off while reading or watching a movie.

Sleeping pills may be used for a specific, time-limited problem—always with a physician's supervision. In the long term, behavioral approaches, including the following, have proved more effective:

insomnia A lack of sleep so severe that it interferes with functioning during the day.

- **Relaxation therapy,** which may involve progressive muscle relaxation and diaphragmatic breathing (see Chapter 12).
- **Cognitive therapy,** which challenges misconceptions about sleep and helps shift a poor sleeper's mind away from anxiety-inducing thoughts (see Chapter 3).
- **Stimulus control therapy,** in which individuals who do not fall asleep quickly must get up and leave their beds until they are very sleepy.
- **Sleep restriction therapy,** in which sleep times are sharply curtailed in order to improve the quality of sleep.

How to Get a Good Night's Sleep

✔ **Check-in:** Are you sleep smart?

Read the following questions, and check whichever description applies to you:

_____ I get up at the same time most weekdays.

_____ I go to bed at the same time most weeknights.

_____ I exercise regularly, but never within two hours of my bedtime.

_____ I never drink caffeinated beverages after 6:00 P.M.

_____ I don't smoke.

_____ I keep my bedroom dark, quiet, and cool.

_____ I never drink alcohol before getting into bed.

_____ I allow a transition time from work or chores before going to bed.

_____ I don't read troubling or scary books or articles right before bed.

_____ I don't take long naps, especially in the evening.

A perfect 10 is an A+; a 0 or 1 is an F.

It's not rocket science. Often simple changes in your surroundings and your behaviors can take the stress out of getting the sleep you need. Remember that quality matters more than quantity. Try to get as much sleep as you need, not more. The longer people stay in bed, the shallower and more fragmented their sleep becomes.

Your Sleep Environment

Answer the following questions:

- Where do you sleep? In a dorm room with one or more roommates? In your room at your parents' house? In an apartment?

- What do you do in your bed? Sleep, study, eat, listen to music, answer e-mails, do homework?
  - Find an alternative location for everything except sleeping and sex. Getting into bed should be a cue for getting a good night's sleep.

- What is the state of your bed? The mattress may be old, but do you have a comfortable pillow? Are the sheets clean? How often do you change them?
  - Your bed should be a beckoning, comfortable cocoon for your nights.

- How dark and quiet is your bedroom?

If you live in a noisy dorm or apartment or if your roommate snores, buy inexpensive earplugs. If your roommate stays up all hours with his desk light on, use an eyeshade.

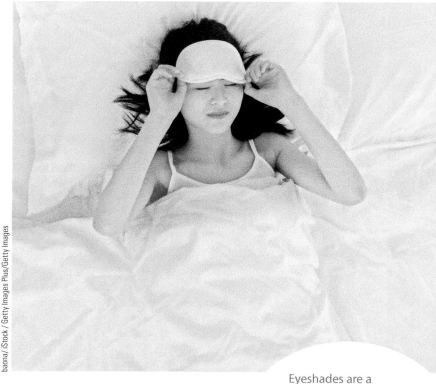

baona / iStock / Getty Images Plus/Getty Images

Eyeshades are a simple way to block any light that could disrupt your sleep.

 Stress Reliever: Try Aromatherapy

Essential oils and scents can calm and soothe mind and body by sending a message of comfort and relaxation to the limbic system, the area of the brain associated with emotion and mood. Those recommended for improving sleep are lavender, rose, chamomile, sage, jasmine, and vanilla. You can mix scents together or choose your favorite one. Try placing a few drops on your pillow, on your pulse points, or in a diffuser by your bed. You can also try scented sachets or pillow sprays. (See Chapter 15 for more on aromatherapy.)

Your Curfews

The time to start planning a good night's sleep is long before you get into bed. Keep in mind that caffeine, a common sleep saboteur, has a half-life of five to seven hours in the body. If you have an energy drink at 5:00 P.M., half of the caffeine from that beverage is still in your system at 10:00 P.M. Technological devices—televisions, computers,

or cell phones—can also interfere with sleep because artificial light disrupts the body's natural circadian rhythm and blocks production of the sleep hormone melatonin.

Because of individual variability, you have to experiment with your body's sensitivity to various types of stimuli. However, start with the following guidelines:

4:00 P.M.	No more caffeine, including coffee, tea, soda, energy drinks, and so on.
6:00 P.M.	No more decaffeinated beverages or chocolate
Two hours before bedtime	No more vigorous exercise
One hour before bedtime	No more alcohol
30 minutes before bedtime	No more work or chores
30–60 minutes before bedtime	No phones, no computer, no tablet except for reading

Your Worries

Meditation, deep-breathing, and mindfulness exercises can relax the body, calm mind and spirit, and enable you to rest more easily at night (See Chapters 12 and 13). If you find that your mind can't let go of certain anxieties once you get into bed, set a daily worry time. Use this designated period to problem-solve, write in your journal, make notes, or talk through the issue. If something new pops into your mind when you get into bed, tell yourself you'll deal with it at tomorrow's regular session.

Your Sleep Ritual

Before you can slide into sleep, you've got to shift gears. Your transition from day to night can be as simple or as elaborate as you choose. You might start with some gentle stretches to release knots of tension in your muscles or with a warm bath. Maybe you like to listen to some quiet music, do a little tidying up, or curl up with a not-too-thrilling book. Whatever you choose, do the same things every evening until they become cues for your body to settle down for the night. Once you've established a routine for yourself, your brain will rewire itself to associate these actions and sounds with shutting down for the night.

If you've had problems sleeping for a while, the ritual meant to calm you down may be having the opposite effect. As you go through the familiar motions of getting ready for bed, you may also start to worry about how or whether you'll sleep. If that's the case, change your sleep ritual. Switch off the nightly news you usually watch, and lay out your clothes for the next day. Rather than reading in bed, listen to music. These subtle changes carry an important message: You're breaking out of your old cycle of sleeplessness and can and will rest easier.

> **Stress Reliever:** Put Yourself to Sleep
>
> Get into bed for the night and close your eyes, imagining a peaceful place, such as a quiet beach. Focus on the serenity around you as you practice mindful breathing. If thoughts from the day or tomorrow's to-do list pop into your consciousness, acknowledge them and then refocus on your place of peace. Fall asleep in this beautiful scene.

Napping

✔ **Check-in:** Do you nap at least once a week?

Four in ten college students say they do.

Is napping good or bad for you? That depends. In a recent study, a late-afternoon nap proved to reverse the negative impact on hormones and immunity of a lost night of sleep.[19] However, in a study of college students, quantity and quality of sleep as well as GPA and class attendance suffered in those who napped more than three days a week, for longer than two hours at a time, or between 6:00 and 9:00 P.M.[20]

As researchers have demonstrated, you can train yourself to take efficient daytime naps. Here are some basic guidelines:

Power Napping

A "power nap" of about 15 to 20 minutes can boost mood, motivation, and performance, lower stress, and improve memory and learning. Some people use power naps when they don't get enough sleep at night. Others nap even when they get a full night's sleep for the extra boost in energy.

- Try a nap in the late morning or just after lunch. Because of daily biological rhythms, if you nap in the late afternoon, you're likely to wake up groggy.

- In the hour or two before your nap, avoid caffeine or foods that are heavy in fat and sugar. Instead, choose foods high in calcium and protein, which promote sleep.

- Find a clean, quiet place. Your dorm room or apartment might be ideal if you can return between classes.

- Darken your sleep space, or wear an eyeshade. Darkness stimulates production of melatonin, the sleep-inducing hormone.

- Since body temperature drops when you fall asleep, raise the room temperature or use a blanket.

- Set your alarm or cell phone to ring 20 minutes from the time you lie down.

Fast Naps

If you don't have time or can't find a place for a power nap, try the following:

- **A mini-nap.** Just 5 to 15-minutes of sleep can increase alertness and stamina.

- **A micro-nap.** If you're tired but can't take a real nap, give yourself two to five-minutes of rest, which is enough to reduce sleepiness.

- **A nano-nap.** Just 10 to 20 seconds of closing your eyes, breathing deeply, and releasing all thoughts and tension from your body provides a breather for your brain.

Healthy Eating

✔ **Check-in:** Do any of the following sound familiar?

Always rushed, you look for food that's fast and filling. Yes, you want it to taste good and not cost a lot, but you don't pay much attention to what it contains or how it's made.

Struggling to keep up with assignments while working an evening shift, you chug energy drinks and snack on chocolate bars. Your hands tremble; you feel wound up and can't focus.

Feeling low, you comfort yourself with foods you loved as a child: hot chocolate, mac and cheese, Cheetos. Long after your hunger subsides, you keep eating and eating.

Keep your answers in mind as you continue reading.

Both body and mind require good nutrition to run efficiently. Poor eating habits—skipping meals, wolfing down snacks, munching on junk foods—contribute to stress by making us physically uncomfortable and psychologically uneasy and unable to concentrate on the tasks at hand, relax, or enjoy being with others. A healthful, balanced diet is essential to a feeling of well-being as well as to good health and a healthy weight.

Essential Nutrients

Every day your body requires certain essential nutrients that it cannot manufacture for itself. They provide energy, build and repair body tissues, and regulate body functions. The six classes of essential nutrients are:

- **Water** carries nutrients; maintains temperature; lubricates joints; helps with digestion; and rids the body of waste through urine and perspiration.

- **Protein** serves as the basic framework for our muscles, bones, blood, hair, and fingernails, and is essential for growth and repair (especially during illness).

- **Carbohydrates** are the organic compounds that provide our brains and bodies with glucose, their basic fuel.

- **Fats** carry the fat-soluble vitamins A, D, F, and K; aid in their absorption in the intestine; protect organs from injury; regulate body

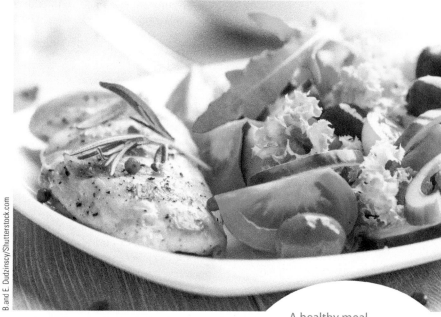

B. and E. Dudzinscy/Shutterstock.com

A healthy meal includes a variety of foods, including vegetables and proteins.

temperature; and play an important role in growth and development.

- **Vitamins** help put proteins, fats, and carbohydrates to use; they are essential for regulating growth, maintaining tissue, and releasing energy from foods.

- **Minerals** play a key role in building bones and teeth; aid in muscle function; maintain normal heartbeats; make hormones; and help our nervous systems transmit messages.

Healthy Eating Guidelines

There is no one "right" way to eat. In its most recent *Dietary Guidelines*, the United States Department of Agriculture (USDA) recommended that Americans customize a "healthy eating pattern" that can accommodate cultural, ethnic, traditional, and personal preferences as well as food costs and availability.[21] It should include the following:

- A variety of vegetables—dark green, red, and orange, legumes (beans and peas), starches

- Fruits, especially whole fruits

- Grains, at least half of which are whole grains

- Fat-free or low-fat dairy, including milk, yogurt, cheese, and/or fortified soy beverages

- A variety of protein foods, including seafood, lean meats and poultry, eggs, legumes (beans and peas), and nuts, seeds, and soy products

- Oils

- Limited amounts of saturated fats and *trans* fats, added sugars, and sodium

- No more than one drink per day for women and no more than two drinks per day for men—and only if they are of legal drinking age.

The guidelines also recommend that Americans:

- Consume less than 10 percent of calories per day from added sugars

- Consume less than 10 percent of calories per day from saturated fats

- Consume less than 2,300 milligrams (mg) per day of sodium

> **Stress Reliever:** Make Stress-Smart Choices
>
> Do:
>
> Choose healthy snacks: an apple, peanut butter on whole-wheat crackers, a small handful of nuts, sunflower seeds, or dried fruit instead of a bag of chips.
>
> Add a salad with low-fat dressing to your lunch or dinner.
>
> Drink water, tea, or skim milk with your meals rather than soda or a sweetened beverage.
>
> Don't:
>
> Supersize fries or burgers.
>
> Eat when feeling lonely or sad, regardless of whether you're hungry.
>
> Choose a candy bar at the vending machine; opt for nuts or trail mix instead.

Mindful Eating

Too often we rush through our meals and scarf whatever food is in front of us, hardly aware of what we're consuming. Not only is speed-eating stressful on your stomach, but it commonly leads to overeating, gastrointestinal discomfort, and heartburn. Remind yourself that we eat with more than just our mouths. We eat with our eyes, our noses, our ears—with our entire body. And our entire body is affected by what we eat.

If you want to transform your three daily meals from mundane chores to life-enhancing experiences, learn to eat with your mind too. When you bring your mind to the table, you are making conscious choices, nourishing itself, lowering stress, and adding another dimension of pleasure to your life.

Whatever your eating circumstances, you always have choices. Maybe you eat in the dining hall every day; maybe you commute home for dinner with your family. Even when you feel you can't completely control *what* you eat, you can control *how* you eat.

While enjoying a snack or meal, eat each bite slowly and pay attention to its smell, texture, and taste. Ask yourself, "Do I really need to finish all of this or am I satisfied with just a bit?" Pausing in between bites to be mindful can aid your digestion and prevent overeating. (See the Get a Grip on Stress Eating technique in the Personal Stress Management Toolkit on page 191).

> **Stress Reliever:** How to Eat Mindfully
>
> Choose foods that are both pleasing to you and nourishing for your body.
>
> Use all your senses to explore, savor, and taste the foods you eat.
>
> Acknowledge your responses to food (likes, dislikes, neutral) without judgment.
>
> Tune into physical cues of hunger and satiety. Let them guide your decisions on when to begin and when to stop eating.

Nutrition and Mood

Many people associate terms such as "well-balanced diet" and "vitamins and minerals" with tasteless food, weird diet trends, or chalky pills sold at the drugstore. Certain nutrients, however, not only help the body manage and reduce stress, but also improve your sleep, balance your mood, and improve memory, concentration, and attention. You can get nutrients such as folic acid, GABA, magnesium, the B vitamins, and vitamin C, in a wide variety of delicious foods (see Table 9.3).

Liquid Stress

What you drink, like what you eat, has an effect on how much stress you experience. Inadequate hydration stresses the body—and you. You lose about 64 to 80 ounces of water a day—the equivalent of eight to ten 8-ounce glasses—through perspiration,

TABLE 9.3 Good Sources of Nutrients for a Healthier Mind and Body

Nutrient	What It Can Help	Where to Find It
Folic Acid	anxiety depression memory	spinach, lettuce, asparagus, beets, cabbage, bok choy, broccoli, peas, Brussels sprouts, avocados, cauliflower, cod, tuna, salmon, halibut, shellfish, turkey, peanuts, sesame seeds, hazelnuts, cashews, walnuts, yeast, lentils, chickpeas, beans, oranges, and strawberries
GABA	anxiety depression stress	cherry tomatoes, kimchi, whole grains, (e.g., oats, brown rice, wheat germ, bran, barley, rye), yogurt, kefir, most fermented foods, and green, oolong, and black teas
Magnesium	anxiety depression insomnia irritability stress	spinach, watercress, avocados, peppers, broccoli, Brussels sprouts, cabbage, nuts, seeds, yogurt, beans, bananas, kiwi, strawberries, blackberries, oranges, raisins, dark chocolate.
Omega 3 Fatty Acids	depression memory	spinach, broccoli, kidney beans, soy beans, shellfish, salmon, sardines, mackerel, scallops, tuna, halibut, cod, trout, flaxseed, pumpkin seeds, walnuts, and pecans
Selenium	depression irritability	mushrooms, onions, whole grains, yeast, tuna, halibut, sardines, flounder, salmon, shellfish, beef, lamb, pork, chicken, turkey, eggs, brazil nuts, and sunflower seeds
Tyrosine	memory depression	avocados, chicken, turkey, tuna, almonds, pumpkin seeds, yogurt, cheese, bananas
Vitamin B (B1,B3, B5, B6 ,B12)	attention/concentration depression irritability memory stress	peppers, cabbage, broccoli, asparagus, lettuce, bok choy, squash, eggplant, peas, mushrooms, sweet potatoes, beans, lentils, whole grains, tuna, salmon, trout, halibut, cod, shellfish, pork, chicken, turkey, strawberries, oranges, tangerines, kiwi, cantaloupe, papaya, cranberries, pineapple, raspberries, lemon, watermelon, bananas, mango, nuts and seeds
Vitamin C	depression irritability stress	kale, Brussels sprouts, peppers, broccoli, cabbage, spinach, mustard greens, squash, watercress, papaya, strawberries, pineapple, kiwi, oranges, cantaloupe, cranberries, tangerines
Zinc	depression memory	spinach, peas, mushrooms, squash, asparagus, broccoli, lentils, miso, chickpeas, beans, oats, beef, lamb, turkey, pork, sesame seeds, pumpkin seeds, blackberries, and kiwi

During a stressful time, combine foods rich in these nutrients in your meals—perhaps salmon with brown rice and asparagus, or chicken with avocado and beans, followed by a piece of dark chocolate and berries. Both your mind and body will benefit.

urination, bowel movements, and normal exhalation. You lose water more rapidly if you exercise, live in a dry climate or at a high altitude, drink a lot of caffeine or alcohol (which increases urination), skip a meal, or become ill. To ensure adequate water intake, nutritionists advise drinking enough so that your urine is not dark in color.

Don't assume that bottles of water labeled "fortified" or "enriched" actually contain anything better. There is no evidence that most of these supposedly added benefits confer any health benefits. Often these drinks contain sugar and sodium, making dehydration more likely than hydration. If the prospect of eight glasses of water a day sounds dull and unappealing, try infusing water with fresh fruit, vegetables, and herbs.

You'll stay hydrated and get the benefit of stress-relieving nutrients.

Some beverages, particularly if consumed in excess, may undermine health and stress resilience in different ways.

Soft Drinks

Sugar-sweetened beverages add an estimated 300 calories a day to Americans' daily intake—and do nothing to lighten your stress load. Researchers have linked soft drink consumption with higher body weight, lower consumption of essential vitamins and minerals, and greater risk of serious medical problems, such as diabetes. Soft drinks, whether diet or regular, also have been linked to greater risk of metabolic syndrome and heart disease, damaged tooth enamel, and thinning of the bones in women.[22] The bottom line: Drink them sparingly. Find healthy alternatives you can choose to enjoy instead.

Caffeine

✔ **Check-in:** How much caffeine do you consume every day?

More than ninety percent of college students consume caffeine. Their reasons include wanting to feel awake, taste, social aspects, improved concentration, physical energy, improved mood, and alleviating stress.[23] The main source of caffeine on campus is coffee, which contains 100 to 150 milligrams of caffeine per cup.

For most people, caffeine poses few serious health risks. As a stimulant, caffeine improves performance and concentration, reduces fatigue, and sharpens awareness—when used judiciously. Moderate amounts of caffeinated or decaffeinated coffee may also lower the risk of type 2 diabetes and cardiovascular disease.[24]

Doctors recommend that adults limit their caffeine intake to no more than five cups a day, with lesser amounts for those who have heart problems, high blood pressure, or trouble sleeping, or who are taking medications. Higher doses of daily caffeine can produce caffeine intoxication, which can lead to potentially life-threatening conditions, such as acute kidney injury, hepatitis, seizures, strokes, coronary spasms, and heart attack (see Table 9.4). Over-consumption of

caffeine can also lead to dependence. Symptoms of caffeine withdrawal include headache, fatigue, drowsiness, irritability, anxiety, depression, nausea, vomiting, and compromised ability to concentrate.

Energy Drinks

Energy drinks, the fastest-growing part of the beverage market in the United States, have become extremely popular on college campuses. In a study of full- and part-time students at two- and four-year colleges and technical schools, 80 percent reported using energy drinks in the preceding year. Although many students drink caffeine-fueled concoctions for a physical or mental edge, there is little scientific evidence to back up such claims. In fact, medical experts have come to view these beverages as a serious public health danger.

Some energy drinks contain caffeine levels 15 times those in a 12-ounce serving of cola. Red Bull, for instance, contains nearly 80 mg of caffeine per can, about the same amount as a cup of brewed coffee and twice the caffeine of a cup of tea. Other energy drinks contain several times this amount (see Table 9.5).

The high levels of caffeine in these drinks can predispose users to a higher rate of anxiety and panic attacks, depression, aggression, and substance abuse. Unlike soft drinks, which typically contain only 35 mg of caffeine per serving,

TABLE 9.4 Signs and Symptoms of Caffeine Intoxication

Ringing in the ears
Flashes of light
Restlessness
Nervousness
Excitement
Insomnia
Flushed face
Increased urination
Digestive disturbances
Muscle twitching
Rambling thoughts or speech
Rapid or irregular heart rate
Periods of inexhaustibility

Source: From An Invitation to Health Table 12.1, p. 355

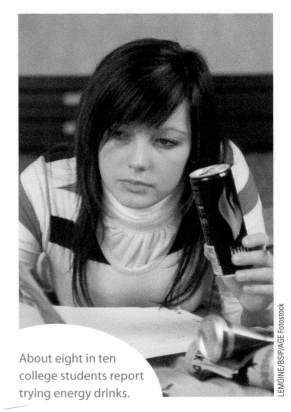

About eight in ten college students report trying energy drinks.

LEMOINE/BSIP/AGE Fotostock

TABLE 9.5 Caffeine Counts

Drink	Company	Milligrams of Caffeine in 12 oz.
Soft Drinks		
JOLT	Wet Planet	72
Mountain Dew Code Red	PepsiCo	55
Mountain Dew	PepsiCo	55
Mello Yello	Coca-Cola	51
Diet Coke	Coca-Cola	45
Dr Pepper	Cadbury	41
Pepsi-Cola	PepsiCo	38
Energy Drinks		
Redline Power Rush	Vital Pharmaceuticals	1,680
JOLT Endurance Shot	Wet Planet	900
Cocaine Energy Drink	Redux Beverages	400
Blow (Energy Drink Mix)	Kingpin Concepts	360
Monster	Monster Beverage	120
Red Bull	Red Bull	116

Jeffrey Blackler/Alamy Stock Photo

AmED Alcohol mixed with energy drinks: Any combination of alcohol with caffeine and other stimulants.

A distorted body image can cause stress and lead to disordered eating.

energy drinks can contain 500 mg or more. Many contain herbs and additives that enhance the effects of caffeine and can interact with medications, causing harmful effects.

Alcohol mixed with energy drinks—**AmEd** in the medical literature—presents even greater dangers. Students mixing alcohol and caffeine engage in more high-risk drinking behaviors and are twice as likely to report being hurt or injured as those who don't. Many students adding alcohol to energy drinks assume that the caffeine counteracts the adverse effects of alcohol. Caffeine may reduce sleepiness, but it leads to a state of "wide-awake drunkenness," in which drinkers cannot fully assess their level of impairment and are more likely to endanger themselves with behaviors such as driving while intoxicated.

Body Image and Stress

✔ **Check-in:** What do you see when you look in the mirror?

A clean, strong, healthy body? Or do you compare yourself with the idealized bodies—sleek, slim, sculpted—that appear in advertisements, commercials, and movies?

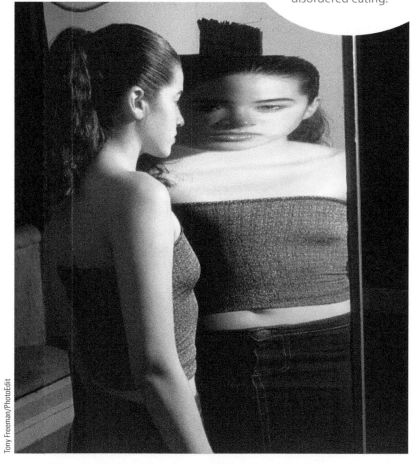

Tony Freeman/PhotoEdit

The airbrushed, touched-up, computer-enhanced images in the media bear little resemblance to the human beings you see every day. The gap between ideal and real can foster a common and insidious form of stress based on body image.

Women have long been bombarded by idealized images in the media of female bodies that bear little resemblance to the way most women look. Increasingly, more advertisements and men's magazines are featuring idealized male bodies that bear little resemblance to the bodies most men inhabit. As the gap between reality and ideal grows, both genders struggle with issues related to body image, although men and women report different concerns:

- Women express greater worry about thinness and more dissatisfaction with their lower rather than their upper bodies.

- College women are more likely to overestimate their weight, while men tend to underestimate their actual weight.

- The greater the discrepancy between a woman's current view of her body shape and the ideal she considers most attractive to men, the more likely she is to worry about how others will view her and to doubt her ability to make a desirable impression.

College students of different ethnic and racial backgrounds express as much concern about their body shape and weight as whites—and sometimes more. African American and Caucasian men are similar in their ideals for body size and in their perceptions of their own shapes. Both African American and white women perceive themselves as smaller than they actually are and desire an even smaller body size. However, African American women are more accepting of larger size.

Female college students who spend a lot of time on Facebook tend to be more likely to be concerned about their body image and could be at increased risk for eating disorders, a recent study suggests. More so than other students, they placed greater importance on receiving comments and "likes," frequently untagged photos of themselves, and compared their photos to pictures of friends.[25] Athletes in sports involving pressure either to maintain ideal body weight or to achieve a weight that might enhance their performance—such as gymnastics, distance running, diving, figure skating, wrestling, and cycling—are more likely to develop eating disorders. Male and female performers, dancers, and models are also at risk.

"Fat Talk"

✔ **Check-in:** Have you heard—or made—statements like these?

_____ "I'm so fat."

_____ "I can't fit into my jeans anymore."

_____ "My butt looks enormous."

_____ "I don't want anyone to know what size I wear."

_____ "I haven't been to the gym in weeks."

All of these statements are examples of what researchers call "fat talk," or informal conversations about body image, weight, and shape. Such discussions are especially common on college campuses. Regardless of their weight, undergraduates perceive body talk, including negative comments about size and fitness, as normal. Typically, one woman complains about her size or weight, while her peers insist that she is not too fat or too big and argue that they are heavier or have flabbier arms or an extra chin. Women rarely express satisfaction with their appearance or body parts, perhaps because they fear such comments will sound arrogant or unsympathetic to women who are dissatisfied with their bodies.

Regardless of whether women are expressing unhappiness with their own bodies, comparing themselves to others, or denying that another woman is or looks fat, the conversation itself increases stress. When students with low to moderate levels of stress engaged in fat talk, they reported greater body dissatisfaction and desire for thinness—not strength and healthiness, but skinniness.

College men talk about their bodies but in different ways, focusing most often on their abdomens, chests, and overall muscularity. These discussions are most likely to occur at the gym or while working out with friends, talking about women, or engaging in an activity such as swimming that involves removal of clothing. Often male friends disguise their body image talk with jabs and jokes, like "I bet you can't bench press 120 pounds," or "Don't ask me for help moving—I can barely lift my laptop."

Men's comments about their own bodies—unlike women's—are as likely to be positive as negative. This may be because it seems more acceptable in our culture for men to praise their appearance without sounding arrogant. Men also are more likely than women to validate a friend's bodily concerns—for instance, to agree that another man needs to lose weight or has gotten out of shape. Yet hearing their peers engage in muscle or fat talk results in lower body satisfaction and self-esteem for men as well as women.

Social Physique Anxiety

A specific type of stress called "**social physique anxiety**" occurs most often in women who feel

social physique anxiety A type of distress that occurs most often in women who feel they do not measure up to what they or others consider most desirable in terms of weight or appearance.

they do not measure up to what they or others consider most desirable in terms of weight or appearance. Women may be more susceptible because they compare their appearance to that of celebrities, models, and peers more frequently than men, and they worry more that others will think negatively about their looks. The greater the discrepancy between a woman's current view of her body shape and the ideal she considers most attractive to men, the more likely she is to worry about how others will view her and to doubt her ability to make a desirable impression. Those reporting the greatest distress because of body image are at highest risk of eating disorders.

Men are as likely as women to engage in efforts to improve their bodies. But while women are most dissatisfied with their weight and their lower bodies, men want to be bigger and have more muscular upper bodies. According to recent studies, male college students overwhelmingly associate greater muscularity with feeling sexier, more confident, and more attractive to women. However, the quest for extremely low body fat and extremely high levels of lean muscle mass can lead to a dangerous obsession called **muscle dysmorphia**, or reverse anorexia, that puts men at risk for depression, anxiety, and abuse of substances such as anabolic steroids.

Weight and Stress

As many students discover, it's easy to gain weight on campuses, which are typically crammed with vending machines, fast-food counters, and cafeterias serving up hearty meals. Only about 5 percent of students gain the legendary "freshman 15." The average weight gain may be closer to ten or eleven pounds, although some students actually lose weight their first year. Among male freshmen, increased alcohol consumption accounts for extra pounds. In women, the strongest correlation of weight gain is often an increased workload, which may lead to more stress-related eating, greater snacking, or less exercise. On some campuses, about half of students—usually more men than women—are overweight or obese.[26]

Stress Fat

Regardless of whether you consume fat, protein, or carbohydrates, if you take in more calories than required to maintain your size and don't work them off in some sort of physical activity, your body will convert the excess to fat. Some people, perhaps those who are genetically hypersensitive to cortisol, put on "belly" or visceral fat (deposited deep in the central abdominal area of the body) when stressed regardless of whether they consume more calories. This type of fat poses a greater health threat than subcutaneous (under-the-skin) fat because it enters the bloodstream more readily, raises levels of harmful cholesterol, and heightens the risk of diseases such as diabetes, high blood pressure, and stroke.

Even if your scale shows that you haven't gained a pound, your waist may widen if you've been under stress. Because of the physiological impact of stress hormones, fat may accumulate around your midsection in times of tension and turmoil.

A widening waist, or "apple" shape, is a warning signal (See Figure 9.2.). Unlike fat in the thighs or hips, abdominal fat increases the risk of high blood pressure, type 2 diabetes, high cholesterol, and metabolic syndrome (a perilous combination of excess weight, high blood pressure, and high levels of cholesterol and blood sugar).

muscle dysmorphia
A dangerous obsession, primarily among men, characterized by the belief that one's own body is too small, too skinny, and not muscular or lean enough. Also known as refers anorexia, this obsession puts men at risk for depression, anxiety, and abuse of substances such as anabolic steroids.

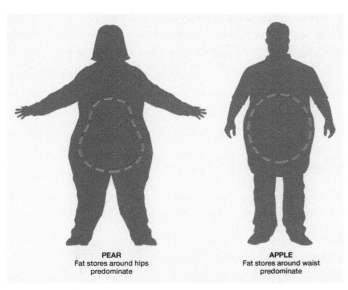

PEAR
Fat stores around hips
predominate

APPLE
Fat stores around waist
predominate

FIGURE 9.2 Pear-shaped versus apple-shaped bodies.

✔ **Check-in:** Is your waist too wide?

To measure your waist circumference, place a tape measure around your bare abdomen just above your hipbone. Be sure that the tape is snug but does not compress your skin. Relax, exhale, and measure. A waist measuring more than 35 inches in a woman or more than 40 inches in a man may signal greater health risks.

Excess Weight

Extra pounds usually mean extra stress—physically and psychologically. Here are some reasons why:

- Overweight young adults have a 70 percent chance of becoming overweight or obese as they get older.

- They are two to three times more likely to have high total cholesterol levels and more than 43 times more likely to have cardiovascular disease risk factors such as elevated blood pressure.

- They have a higher prevalence of type 2 diabetes and a significantly increased the risk of dying before age 55.

- Being overweight or obese at age 25 increases your likelihood of difficulties in walking, balance, and rising from a chair.

The effects of obesity on health are the equivalent of 20 years of aging. They include increased risk of cardiovascular disease, diabetes, and cancer, as well as rheumatoid arthritis, sleep apnea, gout, and liver disease. Obesity robs people of about 2.5 healthy, pain-free years. Total medical costs, both direct and indirect, amount to more than $117 billion a year.

In our calorie-conscious and thinness-obsessed society, obesity also affects quality of life, including stress. Many see excess weight as a psychological burden, a sign of failure, laziness, or inadequate willpower. Overweight men and women often blame themselves for becoming heavy, feel guilty, become depressed, and consider suicide.[27] In fact, the psychological problems once considered the cause of obesity may be its consequence.

> **Stress Reliever:** Become Your Own Cheerleader
>
> Dieters who use positive affirmations lose more pounds and more inches than those who don't. To affirm your way to a lower weight, construct a simple statement that is positive and clear and uses the present tense, such as, "I am choosing to become thinner."
>
> Repeat your affirmation at least 15 to 20 times morning and evening every day. In addition, say your affirmation to yourself while taking a shower, sitting in traffic, standing in line, riding an elevator. As you keep repeating it, you'll feel less of an urge to reach for a macaroon with your coffee.

Who's in Control of Your Weight?

If you eat less and exercise more, you will lose weight—at least for a while. Unfortunately, most people regain the pounds they lose. The reason is that diets aim for the wrong target: the belly. To lose weight and keep it off, you have to target the brain, especially your sense of control and self-efficacy.

✔ **Check-in:** How do you rate on locus of control and self-efficacy in terms of your weight? Read the following questions, and answer true or false.

	True	False
1. I am overweight because I eat too much.	___	___
2. Weight problems run in my family.	___	___
3. Diet pills are my best hope for losing weight.	___	___
4. I would keep weight off if I exercised regularly.	___	___
5. I wouldn't overeat if I didn't have to cook for the people I live with.	___	___
6. Some people are born thin and never have to diet.	___	___
7. I lose weight when I eat only diet shakes or prepared foods.	___	___
8. I could make time for exercise if I really wanted to.	___	___
9. My doctor will make sure I'm at a healthy weight.	___	___
10. I'm determined to lose weight, and I know I will.	___	___

"True" answers to numbers 1, 4, 8, and 10 indicate that you take responsibility for and see yourself in control of your weight. "True" answers to numbers 2, 3, 5, 6, 7, and 9 suggest that you credit or blame others for your weight. The more that you see external forces as being in charge, the more difficult you will find it to make changes and lose weight permanently.

Beyond Diets

Every year, sometimes every season, seems to bring a breakthrough diet that promises to take off pounds, reshape your body, and recharge your life. Some popular diets are high in protein; others, in complex carbohydrates. Some allow no fat; others ban all sugar. Which ones work?

As long as you are burning more calories than you consume, they all do. But not every diet is practical, inexpensive, easy to stick with, or good for your overall nutrition and health. There is no one perfect diet that will work for everyone who needs to lose weight. Rather than trying one diet after another, focus on finding ways to eat that you can stick with for the rest of your life.

Stress Reliever: Lessen Weight Loss Stress

Be realistic. Trying to shrink to an impossibly low weight dooms you to defeat.

Focus on the parts of your body you like. Take pride in your powerful shoulders or large eyes.

Treat yourself with the respect you'd like to receive from others. Don't put yourself down or joke about your weight.

Don't put off special plans, such as learning to kayak or signing up for an exchange program, until you reach a certain magical weight. Do what you want to do now.

Intuitive Eating

Intuitive eating emphasizes recognizing and responding to hunger signals and eating without guilt or ethical dilemmas. Its basic principles include:

- Rejecting the diet mentality. Give up the false hopes of the current dietary craze.

- Honor your hunger. Eat when your body signals that it needs nourishment.

- Make peace with food. Give yourself unconditional permission to eat the foods you prefer without telling yourself that you should or shouldn't have them.

- Challenge your internal food police. Reject guilt-provoking self-criticism, hopeless phrases, and snarky remarks.

- Feel your fullness. Pause in the middle of a meal or snack and ask yourself if you are still hungry. If you aren't, stop eating.

- Savor satisfaction. When you eat without guilt and stop when you're full, you'll find that it takes less food than you might guess to decide that you've had enough.[28]

Stress and Disordered Eating

Stress directly affects what researchers call our "drive to eat." [29] We eat more, binge more, and choose sweets like candy and cookies or salty treats like chips and pretzels rather than healthier options.[28] However, sweet treats can propel you from a brief sugar rush to a miserable sugar crash. Salty snacks also pose health risks, especially if you are not getting enough water and other key nutrients. While acute stress may trigger a brief bout of overeating, episodic or chronic stress can contribute to a pattern of unhealthy eating.

Stress Eating

Occasionally all of us seek solace from food. However, many people habitually use food as a way of coping with stress, anger, frustration, boredom, or fatigue. Whatever its trigger, stress eating always involves eating for reasons other than physiological hunger, such as sensory gratification, comfort, or distraction.

In a study of college students who said they ate for emotional reasons, men and women varied in their reasons for stress eating and their reactions to it. Female students ate more when stressed about school, while male students ate less. Although both sexes hoped that eating—usually chocolate or another treat—would make them feel better, it often had the opposite effect. Women in particular felt "overwhelming feelings of guilt" afterward. Men felt aware of having eaten too much but experienced less acute guilt.[33]

Stress eating cycles often begin when an individual eats to deal with stress and negative emotions (see Table 9.6). Then the person typically feels worse, reaching for another sugary treat to cope with the uncomfortable feelings. In the short term stress eating has negative effects on mood and stress levels. In the long term subsequent weight gain increases stress and sadness.[28] (See the Personal Stress Management Toolkit on page 190.)

Compulsive Overeating

People who eat compulsively cannot stop putting food in their mouths. They eat fast, and they eat a lot. They eat even when they're full. They may eat around the clock rather than at set mealtimes, often in private because they are embarrassed about how much they consume. Some mental health professionals describe compulsive eating as a food addiction. According to Overeaters Anonymous (OA), an international 12-Step program, many women who eat compulsively view food as a source of comfort against feelings of stress, inner emptiness, low self-esteem, and fear of abandonment.

The following behaviors may signal a potential problem with compulsive overeating:

- **Turning to food** when depressed or lonely, when feeling rejected, or as a reward.
- **A history of failed diets** and anxiety when dieting.
- **Thinking about food** throughout the day.
- **Eating quickly** and without pleasure.
- **Continuing to eat** even when no longer hungry.
- **Frequently talking or refusing to talk about food.**
- **Fear of not being able to stop** eating after starting.

Binge Eating

Binge eating—the rapid consumption of an abnormally large amount of food in a relatively short time—often occurs in compulsive eaters. The 25 million Americans with a binge-eating disorder typically eat a larger-than-ordinary amount of food during a relatively brief period, eat rapidly and feel a lack of control over eating, eat alone because they are embarrassed by how and how much they eat, and binge at least once a week for at least a three-month period.[30]

If you occasionally go on eating binges, use the behavioral technique called *habit reversal*

binge eating The rapid consumption of an abnormally large amount of food in a relatively short time.

TABLE 9.6 Is it hunger or stress?

Physical Hunger	"Pseudo-hunger"
Builds gradually	Develops suddenly
Strikes below the neck (e.g., growling stomach)	Strikes above the neck (e.g. a "taste" for ice cream)
Occurs several hours after a meal	Unrelated to time
Goes away when full	Persists despite fullness
Eating leads to satisfaction	Eating leads to guilt and shame

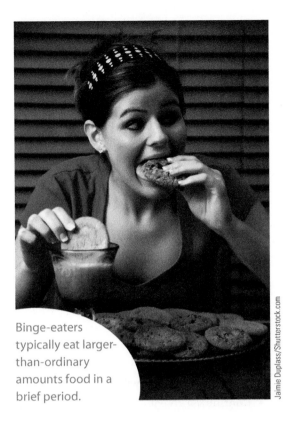

Binge-eaters typically eat larger-than-ordinary amounts food in a brief period.

Jaimie Duplass/Shutterstock.com

and replace your bingeing with a competing behavior. For example, every time you're tempted to binge, immediately do something—text-message a friend, play solitaire, check your e-mail—that keeps food out of your mouth. If you binge once a week or more for at least a three-month period, you may have **binge-eating disorder**, a recently recognized psychiatric disorder that can require professional help.[34] Short-term talk treatment, such as cognitive behavioral therapy, either individually or in a group setting, has proven most effective for binge eating.

Eating Disorders

Researchers estimate that only about one third of college women maintain healthy eating patterns. Some college women have full-blown eating disorders; others develop "partial syndromes" and experience symptoms that are not severe or numerous enough for a diagnosis of **anorexia nervosa** (a psychological disorder in which refusal to eat and/or an extreme loss of appetite leads to malnutrition, severe weight loss, and possibly death) or **bulimia nervosa** (episodic binge eating, often followed by forced vomiting or laxative abuse, and accompanied by a persistent preoccupation with body shape and weight).

Among the factors that increase the risk are:

- Genetic predisposition.
- Preoccupation with a thin body.

- Social pressure.
- Perfectionism and excessive cautiousness, which can reflect an obsessive-compulsive personality.
- Life transitions, such as puberty and the transition from adolescence to adulthood.
- Distress about body image increases the risk of all forms of disordered eating.

Creating a Stress-Resistant Lifestyle

If anyone could capture the benefits of regular exercise, sound sleep, good nutrition, and a healthy weight in a pill, it would be a miracle medicine. But you have the ability to put their miraculous powers to work for you every day. You don't have to transform your life or make over your entire schedule. All you must do is begin:

Physical Activity

- Add an extra ten minutes of activity to your day.
- Add one more workout to your weekly exercise regimen.
- Don't allow yourself to sit for more than thirty to sixty minutes before getting up to walk, stretch, or bend.
- Make exercise part of your daily routine. If you can, block out a half hour for working out at the beginning of the day, between classes, or in the evening. Write it into your schedule as if it were a class or doctor's appointment. A written plan encourages you to stay on track.
- If you can't find 30 minutes, look for two 15-minute or three 10-minute slots that you can use for "mini-workouts."

Better Sleep

- Rise and shine. Resist the temptation to sleep in on mornings when you don't have an early class or appointment.
- Make your bed. Yes, the room will look neater. But you also are sending your brain a message that this is a place reserved for sleep.
- Visualize yourself going through the day's routine filled with energy and vitality.
- Keep regular hours for going to bed and getting up in the morning. Stay as close as

binge-eating disorder
A psychiatric disorder characterized by bingeing once a week or more for at least a three-month period.

anorexia nervosa
A psychological disorder in which refusal to eat and/or an extreme loss of appetite leads to malnutrition, severe weight loss, and possibly death.

bulimia nervosa
A psychological disorder characterized by episodic binge eating, often followed by forced vomiting or laxative abuse, and a persistent preoccupation with body shape and weight.

possible to this schedule on weekends as well as weekdays.

- Eat breakfast. Easy-to-prepare breakfasts include smoothies, cold cereal with fruit and low-fat milk, whole-wheat toast with peanut butter, yogurt with fruit, or whole-grain waffles.

Healthier Eating

- Don't eat too much of one thing. Your body needs protein, carbohydrates, fat, and many different vitamins and minerals from a variety of foods.

- Don't ban any food. Fit in a higher-fat food, like pepperoni pizza at dinner, by choosing lower-fat foods at other meals. And don't forget about moderation. If two pieces of pizza fill you up, don't eat a third.

- Make every calorie count. Load up on nutrients, not on big portions. Choosing foods that are nutrient dense will help protect against disease and keep you healthy.

- Adopt the 90 percent rule. If you practice good eating habits 90 percent of the time, a few lapses won't make a difference.

- Look for joy and meaning beyond your food life. Make your personal goals and your relationships your priorities, and treat food as the fuel that allows you to bring your best to both.

After a few months, take stock. Do you have more energy you have at the end of the day? Ask yourself if you're feeling any less stressed, despite the push and pull of daily pressures. Enjoy the pure pleasure of living in the body you deserve.

Chapter Summary

- A sedentary lifestyle, particularly combined with foods high in fat and calories, is as perilous to health as elevated cholesterol or high blood pressure.

- The more time spent in "recreational sitting" in front of a television or computer screen, the greater the risk of obesity, chronic diseases, and early death.

- Physical activity refers to any movement produced by the muscles that results in expenditure of energy (measured in calories).

- Exercise is a type of physical activity that requires planned, structured, and repetitive bodily movement with the intent of improving one or more components of physical fitness.

- Physical fitness is the ability to respond to routine physical demands with enough reserve energy to cope with a sudden challenge. Its components include cardiorespiratory fitness; metabolic fitness; muscular strength and stamina; flexibility; and body composition.

- Regular exercise relieves anxiety and depression, brightens mood, boosts positive feelings, improves memory, concentration, and alertness, and protects the brain from dementia.

- The *Physical Activity Guidelines for Americans* recommendations, for substantial health benefits, are at least 150 minutes (2 hours and 30 minutes) a week of moderate- intensity, or 75 minutes (1 hour and

15 minutes) a week of vigorous-intensity, aerobic physical activity; and muscle-strengthening activities of moderate or high intensity that involve all major muscle groups two or more days a week.

- To get the maximum benefits from exercise, sports medicine specialists recommend the F.I.T.T. (frequency, intensity, time, and type) Formula.

- Only about one in ten undergraduates gets enough sleep every night to feel rested in the morning. Six in ten report feeling tired, dragged out, or sleepy three or more days a week.

- Poor or irregular sleep can lower student grades, reduce ability to focus in class, and interfere with learning new material.

- Serious sleep disorders such as insomnia and sleep apnea (impaired breathing during sleep) increase stress hormones and inflammation, which may play a role in heart disease. Without adequate sleep, the risk of diabetes, obesity, depression, anxiety, obesity, hypertension, high cholesterol, and traumatic stress disorders increases.

- Daytime sleepiness may affect academic performance as well as daily tasks such as driving.

- To figure out your sleep needs, keep your wake-up time the same every morning and vary your bedtime. Listen to your body's signals, and adjust your sleep schedule to suit them.

- Stress-induced insomnia can take different forms, including problems falling asleep, waking frequently in the night, waking too early, and not getting enough sleep to feel alert and energetic the next day.

- During periods of prolonged stress , short-term insomnia may continue for several weeks. Chronic insomnia, often triggered by a life crisis or ongoing stress, can begin at any age and persist long after the stressor has faded.

- Sleeping pills may be used for a specific, time-limited problem—always with a physician's supervision. In the long term, behavioral approaches have proved more effective.

- To get a good night's sleep, set curfews for caffeine, exercise, alcohol, work, and technology use and establish a sleep ritual.

- A short nap of about 15 to 20 minutes can boost mood, motivation, and performance, lower stress as well as improve memory and learning.

- Poor eating habits—skipping meals, wolfing down snacks, munching on junk foods—contribute to stress by making us physically uncomfortable and unable to concentrate on the tasks at hand, relax, or enjoy being with others.

- Mindful eating means savoring each bite and paying attention to its smell, texture, and taste.

- Certain nutrients not only help the body manage and reduce stress, but also improve your sleep, balance your mood, and improve memory, concentration, and attention.

- Inadequate hydration stresses the body—and you. To ensure adequate water intake, nutritionists advise drinking enough so that your urine is not dark in color.

- Sugar-sweetened beverages add an estimated 300 calories a day to Americans' daily intake—and do nothing to lighten your stress load.

- For most people, caffeine improves performance and concentration, reduces fatigue, and sharpens awareness—when used judiciously.

- The high levels of caffeine in energy drinks can predispose users to a higher rate of anxiety and panic attacks, depression, aggression, and substance abuse.

- Alcohol mixed with energy drinks—AmEd in the medical literature—can lead to more high-risk drinking behaviors and increases the risk of injury.

- "Fat talk" consists of informal conversations about body image, weight, and shape. Regardless of their weight, undergraduates perceive body talk, including negative comments about size and fitness, as normal.

- Social physique anxiety occurs most often in women who feel they do not measure up to what they or others consider most desirable in terms of weight or appearance.

- Some people put on "belly" or visceral fat (deposited deep in the central abdominal area of the body) when stressed regardless of whether they consume more calories.

- The effects of obesity on health are the equivalent of 20 years of aging. Obesity also affects quality of life and increases stress.

- Stress directly affects what researchers call our "drive to eat." Under any type of stress, we eat more, binge more, and choose sweets or salty treats rather than healthier options.

- Intuitive eating emphasizes recognizing and responding to hunger signals and eating without guilt or ethical dilemma.

- Stress eating always involves eating for reasons other than physiological hunger.

- Binge eating—the rapid consumption of an abnormally large amount of food in a relatively short time—often occurs in compulsive eaters.

- Two common eating disorders on campus are anorexia nervosa, characterized by a refusal to eat and/or an extreme loss of appetite, and bulimia nervosa, episodic binge eating, often followed by forced vomiting or laxative abuse.

STRESS RELIEVERS

Take an Exercise Break

Getting up and walking for a few minutes every hour can reverse the negative effects of prolonged sitting. In one study, a short burst of activity such as walking or going up and down stairs boosted the longevity of people who were sedentary more than half of their day.[29]

Build Physical Activity into Your Daily Routine. How?

- Walk to class instead of taking the shuttle.

- Opt for the stairs rather than the elevator.

- Get up from your cubicle in the library every 30 minutes and walk around the stacks.

- Dance during a study break.

- By all means, schedule regular workouts. Just don't think that the only place to get physical is the gym.

Try Aromatherapy

Essential oils and scents can calm and soothe mind and body by sending a message of comfort and relaxation to the limbic system, the area of the brain associated with emotion and mood. Those recommended for improving sleep are lavender, rose, chamomile, sage, jasmine, and vanilla. You can mix scents together or choose your favorite one. Try placing a few drops on your pillow, on your pulse points, or in a diffuser by your bed. You can also try scented sachets or pillow sprays. (See Chapter 15 for more on aromatherapy.)

Put Yourself to Sleep

Get into bed for the night and close your eyes, imagining a peaceful place. such as a quiet beach. Focus on the serenity around you as you practice mindful breathing. If thoughts from the day or tomorrow's to-do list pop into your consciousness, acknowledge them and then refocus on your place of peace. Fall asleep in this beautiful scene.

How to Eat Mindfully

- Choose foods that are both pleasing to you and nourishing for your body.

- Use all your senses to explore, savor, and taste the foods you eat.

- Acknowledge your responses to food (likes, dislikes, neutral) without judgment.

- Tune into physical cues of hunger and satiety. Let them guide your decisions on when to begin and when to stop eating.

Love the Body You're In

You may not be able to avoid comparisons and conversations that make you feel bad about your body. You may think that the only way to feel better is to lose weight or build up muscle. But you don't have to wait to improve your body esteem. Answer the following questions to remind you of why your body deserves love and appreciation.

- Do your feet take you where you want to go?

- Does your tongue allow you to talk with your friends?

- Do your eyes allow you to see the people you love?

- Do your ears allow you to hear laughter and music?

- Do all your senses fill your life with beauty and wonder?

Take a deep breath. Remind yourself that you are not your freckles, or wrinkles, or hips, or belly, or butt. You are more than the sum of your body parts. Celebrate your glorious being.

Become Your Own Cheerleader

Dieters who use positive affirmations lose more pounds and more inches than those who don't. To affirm your way to a lower weight, construct a simple statement that is positive and clear and uses the present tense, such as "I am choosing to become thinner."

Repeat your affirmation at least 15 to 20 times morning and evening every day. In addition, say your affirmation to yourself while taking a shower, sitting in traffic, standing in line, riding an elevator. As you keep repeating it, you'll feel less of an urge to reach for a macaroon with your coffee.

Lessen Weight Loss Stress

- Be realistic. Trying to shrink to an impossibly low weight dooms you to defeat.

- Focus on the parts of your body you like. Take pride in your powerful shoulders or large eyes.

- Treat yourself with the respect you'd like to receive from others. Don't put yourself down or joke about your weight.

- Don't put off special plans, such as learning to kayak or signing up for an exchange program, until you reach a certain magical weight. Do what you want to do now.

⊜ YOUR PERSONAL STRESS MANAGEMENT TOOLKIT

REFLECTION: Stress Eating

Ask yourself the following questions:

- Do you eat when you're not hungry?

- Do you eat or continue eating even if the food doesn't taste good?

- Do you eat when you're emotionally vulnerable—tired, frustrated, or worried?

- Do you eat after an argument or stressful situation to calm down?

- Do you eat as one of your favorite ways of enjoying yourself?

- Do you eat to reward yourself?

- Do you keep eating even after you're full?

Each "yes" answer indicates that you're eating in response to what you feel, not what you need. Since neither stress nor food ever go away, you have to learn to deal with both for as long as you live.

TECHNIQUE: Get a Grip on Stress Eating

Try this three-step plan:

Step 1. Know your triggers.
Whatever its specific motivation, stress eating always involves eating for reasons other than physiological hunger. The first step to getting it under control is awareness:

Ask yourself: What are the feelings that set off an eating binge?

- Anger? Many people swallow their anger by eating because they're afraid of what might happen if they express it.

- Guilt? Some people eat because they feel they're always falling short or failing in some way.

- Rebellion? Eating may be the only way some individuals give themselves permission to take a break from duties and responsibilities.

- Deprivation? At the end of a long day, some justify turning to food as a well-deserved reward, maybe the first nice thing they've done for themselves all day.

If any of these possibilities hit home, train yourself to take a step back and ask yourself a series of questions before you take a bite:

- Are you hungry?

- If not, what are you feeling: stressed, tired, anxious, sad, happy?

- Once you identify your true feelings, push deeper and ask why you feel this way.

- Write down your answers in your online journal. This is an even more effective way to help make sure that every bite you take is a conscious one.

Step 2: Put your body, not your emotions, in charge of what you eat.
To keep mind and body on an even keel, avoid getting so hungry and feeling so deprived that you become desperate. If you're facing an intensely stressful period—your first visit home, perhaps—plan your meals and snacks in advance, and try, as much as you can, to stick to your program. Rather than swearing off any much-loved food forever, work indulgences into your weekly routine. You can enjoy a brownie on Sundays if you skip sugary desserts during the week.

Step 3: Focus on your feelings.
Feel whatever you're feeling without eating. Be present with your body and the food in front of you. Breathe deeply for a minute or two. Focus on the places in your body that feel tense. Rate the intensity of the emotion on a scale from ten (life or death) to one (truly trivial). Ask yourself: What's the worst-case scenario of feeling this way? Is food going to make it better in any way? Will it make it worse?

When you're tempted to eat but aren't hungry, write down the circumstances and try to discern the underlying reasons. If you eat a bag of chips, ask, "What does it get me?" The answer might be that it relaxes you. Once you realize that the chips are a means to an end, you can figure out something else you can do, such as a breathing or visualization exercise, to get the same emotional benefits.

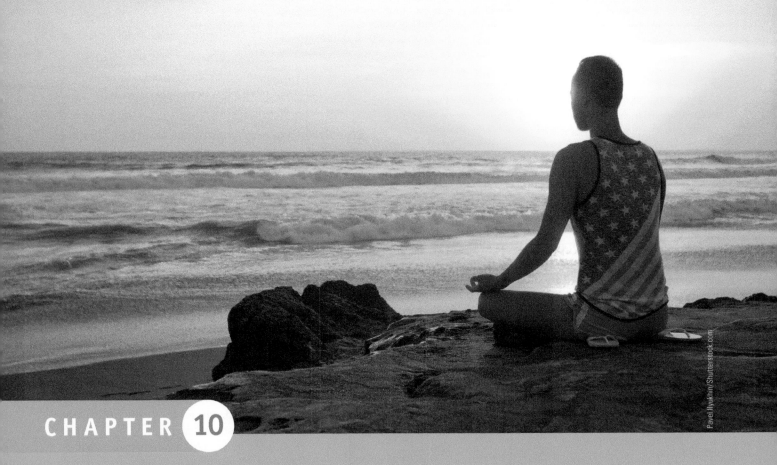
Pavel Ilyukhin/Shutterstock.com

CHAPTER 10

Spirituality, Life Balance, and Resilience

After reading this chapter, you should be able to:

10.1 Discuss the impact of spirituality on individuals.

10.2 Outline the relationship between values and spiritual growth.

10.3 Identify some components of a fulfilling, happy, balanced life.

10.4 Evaluate strategies that strengthen resilience.

10.5 Describe the benefits of techniques for effective stress management.

10.6 Explain strategies for supporting resilience to stress throughout life.

This scale consists of five statements that you may agree or disagree with. Using the following 1–7 scale, indicate your agreement with each item by placing the appropriate number on the line preceding that item. Be open and honest in responding.

7–Strongly agree; 6–Agree; 5–Slightly agree; 4–Neither agree nor disagree; 3–Slightly disagree; 2–Disagree; 1–Strongly disagree

____ In most ways my life is close to my ideal.

____ The conditions of my life are excellent.

____ I am satisfied with my life.

____ So far I have gotten the important things I want in life.

____ If I could live my life over, I would change almost nothing.

Scoring: 35–31: Extremely satisfied
26–30: Satisfied
21–25: Slightly satisfied
20: Neutral
15–19: Slightly dissatisfied
10–14: Dissatisfied
5–9: Extremely dissatisfied

If you got a high score, you're already on the right track. If you scored at only "slightly satisfied" or "neutral," you need to focus on doing more of the things that you value most and that bring you the greatest satisfaction. If you are dissatisfied, it's time to consider a course correction.

Source: Diener, E. D. et al. (1985) "The Satisfaction with Life Scale." *Journal of Personality Assessment* 49(1): 71–75.

As a high school student, Caitlin enjoyed singing in her church choir. She also volunteered at a local shelter for homeless women and children. Reading stories or helping with homework lifted her spirits as well as brightening their day.

In college, academics and a part-time job take up so much of Caitlin's time that she doesn't get to church as regularly as she once did. She'd like to do volunteer work, but every week of the term seems more stressful than the one before. During the long holiday break, she returns to her family's church and to the homeless women's shelter where she had worked. And she realizes that something is missing in her life—the experiences that had nurtured her spirit.

Whether or not you pray, worship, or believe in God or a hereafter, you are more than a body of a certain height and weight occupying space on the planet. Just as you have a mind that equips you to learn and a body that carries you through the world, you have a spirit that animates everything you say and do. Sometimes overshadowed by the speed and loud talk all around, this sensitive, quieter part of you is invisible but no less real. In fact, it constitutes what is always and most essentially you. It can be ignored or overlooked, but not for long without cost to your totality.

When nurtured, your spirit can help you to resist and recover from stress. Both Eastern and Western philosophies agree that a spiritual path transforms consciousness and counters the forces that create suffering and stress in ourselves and the world.

The key to connecting mind, body, and spirit and juggling all the demands on your energy and time is balance. In order to survive and thrive, every person needs to find his or her own personal combination of exertion, achievement, stimulation, variety, novelty, activity, and social contact *along with* their opposites: repose, detachment, serenity, sameness, familiarity, solitude, inactivity. No one formula fits all—or fits you throughout your life.

If you feel you are stressed out, running too hard, or are in some way seeking to make better contact with your deeper self, this chapter will help you provide the food your soul needs and the balance a well-rounded life requires. Remember that this life is your gift to yourself. Open it; use it; delight in it.

Spirituality

✔ **Check-in:** How would you describe your spiritual life?

Spirituality is a belief in what some call a higher power, in someone or something that transcends the boundaries of self. It gives rise to a strong sense of purpose, values, morals, and ethics. More than six billion people around the world identify with a particular religion: Christianity, Judaism, Hinduism, Buddhism, Islam, or one of dozens of other faiths.

You may have been raised in a religious tradition in which you find strength and renewal. Or your past religious experiences may have been more limited, less positive, even negative. You may be a seeker for spiritual enlightenment and curious about all religions. Or you may have no particular interest in formalized religion or spiritual practices. Yet throughout life you make choices and decide to behave in one way rather than another because your spirit serves as both a compass and a guide.

The terms *religiosity* and *religiousness* refer to various spiritual practices. That definition may seem vague, but one thing is clear. According to thousands of studies on the relationship between religiosity and health, religious individuals are less depressed, less anxious, and better able to cope with stress and crises such as illness or divorce than are nonreligious ones.

Spirituality and Health

Spiritual health refers to our ability to identify our basic purpose in life and experience the fulfillment of achieving our full potential. Spiritual practices—such as prayer, meditation, or attending services—can produce a range of health benefits, including:[1]

- increased calmness and inner strength.

- improve self-awareness.

- enhanced sense of well-being.

- lower risk of depression, alcohol abuse,[2] and eating disorders.[3]

- greater life satisfaction beyond the benefits of social support from friends and family.[4]

- lower risk for heart disease, stroke, brain deterioration, and premature death.[5]

Prayer and other spiritual experiences, including meditation (see Chapter 13), may actually change the brain—for the better. Using neuroimaging techniques, scientists have documented alterations in various parts of the brain that are associated with stress and anxiety. This effect may slow down the aging process, reduce psychological symptoms, and increase feelings of security, compassion, and love.[6]

Whatever role religion plays in your life, you have the capacity for deep, spiritual experiences that can add great meaning to everyday existence. You don't need to enroll in theology classes or commit to a certain religious preference to gain such personal richness. Try the following exercise:

🔄 Stress Reliever: An Infinity Experience

Have you ever been in a place—atop a high building or mountain, in a sunlit forest glade, on a windswept beach or cliff—where you sensed something timeless and eternal?

Visit this place in your imagination several times each week. Linger there for ten or more minutes. Bathe in the feelings you associate with it, and reflect on life as you are currently living it. Expand your horizons. From the perspective of this place, allow something to become clearer about the big picture of your life and what you might want to add or subtract.

Spiritual Intelligence

Spiritual intelligence is defined as the capacity to sense, understand, and tap into the highest parts of ourselves, others, and the world around us. Unlike spirituality, it does not center on the worship of a God above, but on the discovery of a wisdom within. All of us are born with the potential to develop spiritual intelligence, but many aren't aware of it—and do little or nothing to nurture it. Part of the reason is that we confuse spiritual intelligence with religion, dogma, or old-fashioned morality.

You don't have to go to church or even believe in God to be spiritually intelligent. Spiritual intelligence allows you to use the wisdom you have when you're in a state of inner peace. You access it by listening less to what's in your head and more to what's in your soul.

Enriching Your Spiritual Life

Spirituality exists in every cell of the body, not just in the brain, whether or not you are religious.

spirituality A belief in someone or something that transcends the boundaries of self.

spiritual health The ability to identify one's basic purpose in life, to engage in meaningful pursuits, and to achieve one's full potential.

spiritual intelligence The capacity to sense, understand, and tap into ourselves, others, and the world around us.

Here's how you can deepen this dimension of your health and being:

If You Are Not Religious:

- **Sit quietly.** The process of cultivating spiritual intelligence begins in solitude and silence. "There is an inner wisdom," says Dr. Dean Ornish, the pioneering cardiologist who incorporates spiritual health into his mind–body therapies, "but it speaks very, very softly." To tune into its whisper, turn down the volume in your busy, noisy, complicated life and force yourself to do nothing at all. This may sound easy; it's anything but.

- **Start small.** Create islands of silence in your day. Don't turn on the radio as soon as you get in the car. Leave your earbuds on as you walk across campus, but turn off the music. Shut the door to your room, take a few huge deep breaths, and let them out very, very slowly. Don't worry if you're too busy to carve out half an hour for quiet contemplation. Even 10 minutes every day can make a difference.

- **Ask questions of yourself.** Some people use their contemplative time to focus on a line of scripture or poetry. Others ask open-ended questions, such as: What am I feeling? What are my choices? Where am I heading?

- **Connect with nature.** Being outdoors or simply looking at the horizon puts the little hassles of daily living into perspective. As you wait for the bus or for a traffic light to change, let your gaze linger on silvery ice glazing a branch or an azalea bush in wild bloom. Follow the flight of a bird; watch clouds float overhead; gaze into the night sky.

- **Tap into your spirit in creative ways.** As a student, you devote much of your day to mental labor. For your spirit's sake, try a less cerebral activity, such as singing, dancing, gardening, walking, arranging flowers, or immersing yourself in a simple process like preparing a meal. You can find many more stress-reducing techniques in Part IV of this book.

- **Keep an open mind** about the value of religion or spirituality. Consider visiting a church or synagogue. Read the writings of inspired people of deep faith, such as Rabbi Harold Kushner and Rev. Martin Luther King, Jr.

If You Are Religious:

- Set aside a time for prayer or meditation as part of your daily routine—perhaps first thing in the morning, last thing at night, or both.

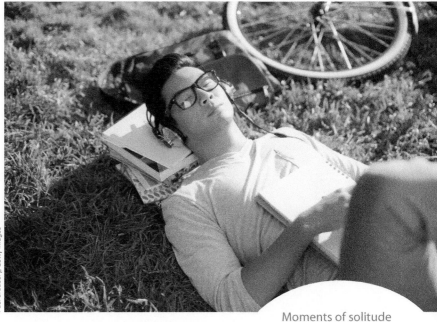

Moments of solitude can refresh your spirit throughout the day.

- Make a regular habit of reading scriptures, sacred texts, or writings related to your chosen faith or practice. Or read the works of philosophers or spiritual leaders, such as the Dalai Lama, Confucius, or Aristotle.

- Designate a physical location for your daily spiritual practice—a particular space in your room, a quiet bench on campus, even your car.

- Try a physically active form of spirituality, such as walking meditation or yoga.

- Practice a creative form of spirituality, such as singing or playing sacred music, painting or drawing to express sacred ideals, or writing spiritually inspired poetry.

- Become part of a group, either physical or virtual, that worships or practices together—such as a congregation, meditation circle, or scriptural study group.

The Power of Prayer

Petitionary prayer—praying directly to a higher power—boosts morale; lowers agitation, loneliness, and life dissatisfaction; and enhances ability to cope. Much like exercise and diet, prayer is one of the best and most cost-effective ways of protecting and enhancing health.

The benefits of regular praying include:

- significantly lower blood pressure.
- stronger immune systems.
- fewer hospitalizations.
- less likelihood of drinking or smoking heavily.[7]

Inspire Yourself

A man who views the world the same at fifty as he did at twenty has wasted thirty years of his life.
Muhammad Ali

The real voyage of discovery consists not in seeking new landscapes but in having new eyes.
Marcel Proust

Just think how happy you'd be if you lost everything you have right now - and then got it back again.
Anonymous

Knowing others is intelligence; knowing yourself is true wisdom. Mastering others is strength; mastering yourself is true power.
Lao Tzu

Don't judge each day by the harvest you reap but by the seeds that you plant.
Robert Louis Stevenson

The forces of fate that bear down on man and threaten to break him also have the capacity to ennoble him.
Viktor Frankl

Permanence, perseverance, and persistence in spite of all obstacles, discouragements, and impossibilities: It is this in all things that distinguishes the strong soul from the weak.
Sir Frances Drake

No bird soars too high if he soars with his own wings.
William Blake

If we had no winter, the spring would not be so pleasant: if we did not sometimes taste adversity, prosperity would not be so welcome.
Anne Bradstreet

Character is what you have when nobody is looking.
Marie Dressler

Nothing is all wrong. Even a clock that has stopped running is right twice a day.
Anonymous

The most wasted of all days is one without laughter.
e. e. cummings

Korpithas/Shutterstock.com

The quotations above can provide inspiration and solace in challenging times. Are there other quotes you find meaningful and uplifting?

Forgiveness

 Stress Reliever: Forgiving

Is there someone who you feel wronged you in some way and you've never forgiven?

Imagine saying, "I forgive you."

Try saying it out loud. Write it down. Reflect on how you feel.

"I forgive you"—three of the most difficult words to say—are among the most powerful for the body as well as the soul. Being angry, harboring resentments, or reliving hurts over and over again creates chronic stress that is bad for your health in general and your heart in particular.

The word "forgive" comes from the Greek for "letting go," and that's what happens when you forgive. You let go of all the anger and pain that have been demanding your time and wasting your energy. To some people, forgiveness seems a sign of weakness or submission. People may feel more in control and powerful when they're filled with anger, but forgiving instills a much greater sense of power. Forgiving a friend or family member may be more difficult than forgiving a stranger because the hurt occurs in a context in which people deliberately make themselves vulnerable. Forgiving yourself may be even harder.

When you forgive, you reclaim your power to choose. It doesn't matter whether someone deserves to be forgiven; you deserve to be free. Forgiveness is not a one-time thing, but rather a process that takes a lot of time and work involving both the conscious and unconscious mind.

Forgiveness-based interventions for individuals, couples, and groups, and for specific conditions such as bereavement and alcohol abuse, have resulted in greater self-esteem and hopefulness, positive emotions toward others, less depression and anxiety, and improved resistance to drug use. In college students, such interventions have helped relieve stress and related symptoms.

Here are some suggestions for finding a way to forgive another person:

- **Compose an apology letter.** Address it to yourself and write it from someone who's hurt you. This simple task enables you to get a new perspective on a painful experience.

- **Leap forward in time.** In a visualization exercise, imagine that you are very old, meet a person who hurt you long ago, and sit down together on a park bench on a beautiful spring day. You both talk until everything that needs to be said finally is said. This allows you to benefit from the perspective time brings without having to wait years to achieve it.

- **Talk with "safe" people.** Vent your anger or disappointment with a trusted friend or counselor, without the danger of saying or doing anything you'll regret later. If you can laugh about what happened with a friend, the laughter helps dissolve the rage.

- **Forgive the person, not the deed.** In themselves, abuse, rape, murder, and betrayal are beyond forgiveness. But you can forgive people who couldn't manage to handle their own misery, confusion, and desperation.

Naikan

Naikan is a Japanese method of self-reflection that encourages one to "look inside." According to its principles, three simple questions can free you from focusing on your problems and shift your attention to feelings of appreciation for others. As this internal shift occurs, your troubles and stress become less important.

To try Naikan, think of a person close to you (partner, spouse, colleague, parent, sibling, teacher, friend) and answer the following three questions:

- What have I received from this person?
- What have I given to this person?
- What difficulties or troubles have I brought to this person?

Write down your reflections. Repeat this exercise each day over the next several months, choosing a new person each time. This activity provides a better understanding of your connection to others and an increased sense of behaving responsibly with others and within yourself. As this desire to act responsibly increases, you will find a spillover to all parts of your life. In a unique and gentle way, Naikan can lighten your stress and keep you moving toward greater spiritual fulfillment.

Karma

In the Buddhist and Hindu traditions, karma means that nothing happens by itself. Everything is a result of what has gone before. If bad choices and unhealthy behavior came before, what follows is almost sure to be stressful. If what came before is good and worthy, what follows will be satisfying. Being true to yourself and making good choices determines your lot in the future.

When you reflect on the idea of karma in connection with stress, think of what has gone before. Have you taken good care of your body? Have you kept it fit and fed it well? Have you invested in meaningful relationships? Have you treated others with respect and kindness? Have you committed yourself to your studies and work? Have you faced challenges head on? Have you nourished your spirit? Have the choices and habits of your past created bad or good karma?

In addition to the karma of your past, there is the karma that will shape your future. Consider:

- Are you creating more stress for yourself by continuing to neglect or abuse your body?

- Are you sabotaging fulfilling relationships by not treating others as well as you could?

- Are you undermining your spiritual development by trying to numb or avoid painful issues?

- Is the karma that your current lifestyle is creating the one that you want?

You can have a different, more satisfying, and less stressful life. As you begin or continue to make better conscious choices, you will be creating good karma both for the present and the future.

Your Values

✔ **Check-in:** The tombstone test

Imagine an old-fashioned tombstone with your name on it. What would you like written on it to summarize who you were and what you did in life?

Your **values** are the criteria by which you evaluate things, people, events, and yourself; they represent what's most important to you. In a world of almost dizzying complexity, values can provide guidelines for making decisions that are right for you. If understood and applied, they help give life meaning and structure.

Identifying or clarifying your values is crucial to your spiritual growth—and to how you think about and cope with stressful experiences. Individuals who are connected with their values are more likely to take positive action and less likely to try to avoid stress by denying a problem or delaying its resolution.

values The criteria by which one makes choices about one's thoughts, actions, goals, and ideals.

compassion Desire to help another on the basis of feelings of empathy.

empathy Ability to take the perspective of and feel the emotions of another person.

altruism Helping or giving to others promote someone else's welfare, even at a risk or cost to ourselves.

Clarifying Your Values

Values clarification is not a once-in-a-lifetime task, but an ongoing process of sorting out what matters most to you. If you believe in protecting the environment, do you shut off lights or walk rather than drive in order to conserve energy? Do you vote for political candidates who support environmental protection? Do you recycle newspapers, bottles, and cans? Values are more than ideals you would like to attain; they should be reflected in the way you live day by day.

Tapping into your values changes the story you tell yourself about stress. If you see yourself as strong and able to grow from adversity, you are more likely to confront challenges rather than avoid them and to see meaning in difficult circumstances.

Compassion

Compassion literally means "to suffer together." Among emotion researchers, it is defined as the feeling that arises when you are confronted with another's suffering and feel motivated to relieve that suffering. Compassion is not the same as **empathy** or **altruism**, although the concepts are related. Empathy refers more generally to our ability to take the perspective of and feel the emotions of another person; compassion emerges when those feelings and thoughts include the desire to help. Altruism, in turn, is the kind, selfless behavior often prompted by feelings of compassion.

Compassion may serve a deep evolutionary purpose. When we feel compassion, our heart rate slows down, we secrete the "bonding hormone" oxytocin, and regions of the brain linked to caring, empathy, and feelings of pleasure light up, which often results in our wanting to care for others. Here is a simple exercise that may have a similar effect:

 Stress Reliever: Five-Finger Exercise

Touch your thumb to your index finger. As you do, go back to a time when your body felt healthy and strong after a swim, a run, or another exhilarating activity.

Touch your thumb to your middle finger. As you do, go back to a time when you felt loved and loving. Remember the details of a romantic moment or a warm embrace by a friend or family member.

Touch your thumb to your ring finger. As you do, recall the nicest compliment you were ever given. Accept it now. Bask in this praise as you also recall the person who said it.

Touch your thumb to your little finger. As you do that, go back to the most beautiful place you have ever been. Dwell in it for a while.

Stretch all your fingers, and feel warmth and relaxation spread from them throughout your body.

Altruism

Like gratitude (discussed in Chapter 8), altruism (helping or giving to others promote someone else's welfare, even at a risk or cost to ourselves) enhances self-esteem, relieves physical and mental stress, and protects psychological well-being.[8] Giving to or doing for others helps those who give as well as those who receive. People involved in community organizations, for instance, consistently report a surge of well-being called *helper's high*, which they describe as a unique sense of calmness, warmth, and enhanced self-worth.

College students who provided community service as part of a semester-long course reported changes in attitude (including a decreased tendency to blame people for their misfortunes), self-esteem (primarily a belief that they can make a difference), and behavior (such as a greater commitment to do more volunteer work). Volunteering also may lower risk factors for cardiovascular disease.

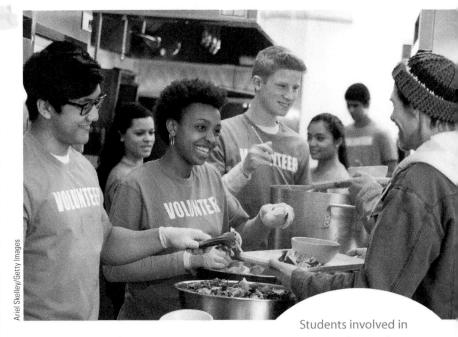

Ariel Skelley/Getty Images

Other benefits of altruism include:

- fewer aches and pains.
- better overall physical health.
- less depression.
- improvements in chronic illness.
- less risk of relapse in addictions.

Like other social behaviors, altruism is contagious: An altruistic act spurs a ripple effect of generosity, spreading from person to person to person so that a single kindness can influence dozens or even hundreds of people.[9]

Students involved in community service report greater compassion as well as a "helper's high" of positive feelings.

Volunteering provides an opportunity to make a difference in other people's lives.

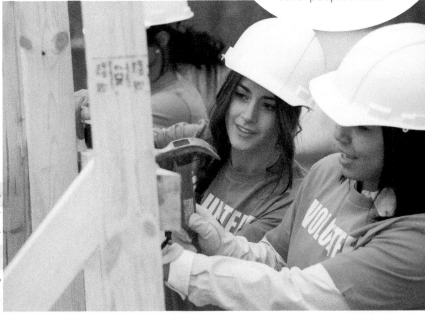

Blend Images/Ariel Skelley/Getty Images

In addition to our families, friendships, and social networks, we are part of communities—our campus, our neighborhood, our town or city. (Chapter 11 discusses the global community in which we all hold citizenship: planet Earth.) Contributing to your community can take many forms, from serving meals at a homeless shelter to joining a park cleanup. By giving to others, you get a great deal in return. Helping or giving to others enhances self-esteem, relieves physical and mental stress, and protects psychological well-being.

 Stress Reliever: Day By Day

Record the nicest thing that happens to you every day. It might be as small as a bus driver's hearty hello or as big as making a team.

Also track something you did to make someone else's day. Again, it can be as small as wishing a janitor a good day or as big as planning a surprise birthday party for a friend.

Do at least some of your carefully thought-out and well-targeted acts of kindness anonymously so that you do not know whether your kindness was appreciated or noticed. In other words, do the kindness for its own sake, not for the "feel good" you will receive.

A balanced life involves a mixture of activity and rest, work and play, socializing and solitude.

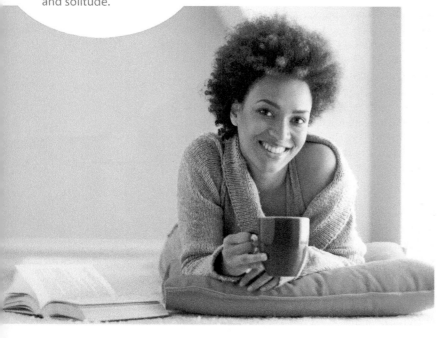

luminaimages/Shutterstock.com

A Life in Balance

As you've learned, the key to stress management is homeostasis or balance. In order to survive and thrive, you need to find your own mixture of exertion, achievement, stimulation, variety, novelty, activity, and social contact along with their opposites: repose, withdrawal of effort, serenity, sameness, familiarity, solitude, inactivity. No one formula fits all—or fits you throughout your life.

Balance is not necessarily a matter of perfectly symmetrical similar days all lined up in a row. Your interests and preferences wax and wane. You don't want to make every single day the same, but to include in your life enough exertion along with restorative practices to keep your life balanced and anchored. The majority of new college graduates say that a balanced life is their top priority. Learning how to create balance now can prepare you to maintain balance and increase satisfaction and fulfillment in the future.

Positive psychology has identified the key components of a fulfilling, happy, balanced life. Does your life include all of the following?

Close, Supportive Relationships

People who have a committed intimate relationship or a network of supportive friendships consistently rank themselves as happier than others. The quality of their close relationships marks the difference between people who are merely happy and those who are positively joyous.

Spirituality or a Higher Purpose in Life

As noted earlier in this chapter, by deepening the spiritual dimension of their lives, individuals can identify their own basic purpose in life; develop a strong sense of purpose, values, morals, and ethics; experience greater peace and fulfillment; and help themselves and others achieve their full potential.

Positive Traits

As the burgeoning field of positive psychology has resoundingly proved, people who are happy, appreciative, and altruistic are more creative and productive, earn more money, attract more friends, enjoy better marriages, suffer fewer illnesses, and even live longer. None of these positive qualities are bestowed at birth by fairy godmothers. All grow with practice, persistence, and genuine commitment.

Hope

Individuals who rate high in hope aren't immune to negative experiences, but they are less likely to be depressed by them. In studies of college students, the "high-hopers" tended to solve problems more effectively than those with low hope, in part because they avoid ineffective coping strategies, such as social withdrawal and self-criticism. People who are high in hope may deal with stress more effectively because they tend to anticipate greater well-being in the future, are more confident, and are flexible enough to find alternative pathways to their goals.

Engagement

A passionate pursuit—for family, work, sport, or other experiences—also adds great satisfaction to a life. Psychologist Mihaly Czikszentmihalyi coined the word *flow* to describe a zone in which people become so absorbed in an activity that they lose consciousness of space and time. Do you become so engrossed in an activity that hours fly by? Do you experience creative highs or profound satisfaction when you're concentrating on a task, walking on a beach, singing in a choir?

Resilience

✔ **Check-in:** How resilient are you?

	YES	NO
During and after life's most stressful events, I tend to find opportunity for growth.		
I have at least one close and secure relationship that helps me when I am stressed.		
When there are no clear solutions to my problems, sometimes fate or God can help.		
During and after life's most stressful events, I know how to calm and comfort myself.		

If you checked four "yes's," you've already mastered the fundamentals of resilience. If you checked one or more "no's," focus on building these specific elements of stress resilience.

Physicists describe materials and objects that resume their original shape upon being bent or stretched as resilient. The American Psychological Association defines human **resilience** as "the process of adapting well in the face of adversity,

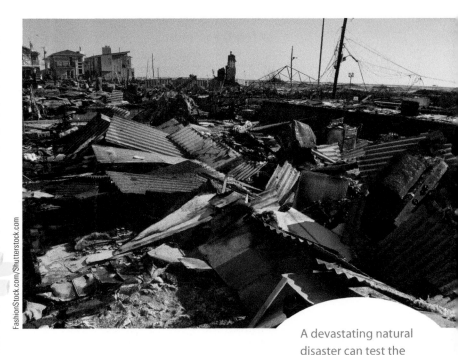

A devastating natural disaster can test the resilience of an entire community.

trauma, tragedy, threats, and even significant sources of stress—such as family and relationship problems, serious health problems, or work place and financial stresses."

However careful you are, you can't dodge every danger. You will inevitably face serious stressors. As many as 50 to 90 percent of Americans, by various estimates, experience one or more major traumas, such as violent crime, rape, child abuse, a serious automobile accident, a natural disaster, or combat. Yet even when confronted by the same threat or crisis, no two people respond in the same manner.

A hurricane may submerge an entire town, sweeping away houses and disrupting lives. One sorrowful family may leave the home they once loved. Another may move in with relatives and take their time deciding their next step. Others never consider any option but rebuilding and getting on with their lives. Although they may be temporarily distressed, many eventually bounce back—some as if the ordeal never happened, others managing to cope in healthy ways despite lingering issues. The most vulnerable are those who had experienced or witnessed a previous traumatic event. [10]

Resilient people who've weathered past stresses keep their eye on the ball and maintain determination, no matter what goes on around them. While everyone else is stuck on the problems, they look for solutions and focus on one overriding goal: moving forward. They don't waste time worrying about what they can't change, but rather build on what they can. "I've survived other rough spots," they tell themselves. "I can handle this."

resilience The process of adapting well to adversity and significant sources of stress.

You can be like them. You have abundant internal resources you can develop and turn to in tough times. Just as you take sensible precautions to safeguard your health and work out regularly to increase your fitness, you can take a similar approach to stress management: Prevent as many potential problems as possible and strengthen your coping mechanisms so you can deal more effectively with those you cannot avoid. Go inward, connect with your strength, and be your own lifeline.

Lessons from Resilient People

In dozens of studies of survivors of natural catastrophes, train wrecks, plane crashes, terrorist attacks, bombings, kidnappings, and imprisonment as POWs, researchers have discovered that resilient individuals are ordinary in many ways. They come from every race, ethnic and economic group, educational and social background. But in the face of a crisis, resilient people turn right back into adversity and feed off it as a source of energy. [11]

Instead of allowing external events or circumstances to crush them, resilient individuals choose to draw inspiration and renewed force from the very extreme challenge that they confront. They do not allow themselves to be defeated; they do not even entertain such thoughts. Instead, they not only learn from stress, but also thrive on responding to it. And if—more likely when—another crisis looms before them, they respond better, faster, and more effectively. In a process psychologists refer to as "stress inoculation," each experience with stress toughens them in various ways, such as teaching them skills that enhance their ability to cope and boosting their confidence in their ability to weather a rough patch. (See Table 10.1.)

Resilient individuals also may be more tuned into their body's signals. In research studies, elite athletes, soldiers, and individuals who scored high in resilience underwent brain scanning while wearing face masks that temporarily made it difficult to breathe. Those who paid more attention to changes in their breathing during this

TABLE 10.1 Characteristics of Resilient People

From extensive studies of survivors of all sorts of traumas, psychologists have identified common characteristics of those who bounce back from serious setbacks. Resilient people typically:

Confront their fears directly

Maintain an optimistic but realistic attitude

Are resourceful and flexible

Believe that they have a right to survive and thrive

Seek, accept, and make the most of social support

Imitate inspiring role models

Rely upon their own inner moral compass

Have goals

Make positive statements

Turn to religious or spiritual practices

Find a way to accept the things that they cannot change

Attend to their health and well-being

Train intensively to stay physically fit, mentally sharp, and emotionally strong

Are active problem-solvers

Look for meaning and opportunity in the midst of adversity

Sometimes find humor even in the darkest hours

Accept personal responsibility for their own emotional well-being

✔ **Check-in:** How do you compare with the resilient individuals we've described?

At first glance resilient people may seem larger-than-life, more heroic and courageous than you can imagine being. But rest assured that they were not born this way. Like other behaviors, resiliency can be acquired and developed.

highly stressful experience didn't over-react and were better able to return to homeostasis—a sign of physical and mental resilience.[12] (The breathing techniques in Chapter 12 can help increase breath awareness and control.)

Some describe resilient individuals as embodying **hardiness**, a personality trait characterized by three C's:

- *Commitment*—being committed to something that is meaningful, for example, work, community, or family, and staying engaged and involved in ongoing events, even in the most trying of circumstances, rather than feeling isolated.

- *Control*—believing in their ability, through their own efforts, to turn events to their advantage rather than adopting a passive and powerless victim mode.

- *Challenge*—viewing change, whether positive or negative, as an opportunity to learn rather than as a threat.

The first step is a purposeful decision to interpret obstacles as challenges and as a source of lessons. Simply make the conscious choice to see setbacks and hardships in this way. Then decide that nothing will crush you.

Develop the stress-resistant attitude that tough experiences are a source of valuable lessons. Purposely cultivate an internal approach to difficulties that is oriented to learning and coping rather than feeling victimized and blaming circumstances or others. If you are momentarily thrown off by setbacks, obstacles, or adversity, talk and coach yourself back to this perspective. Resolve to learn from your setback, make the necessary adjustments, and continue, knowing you are the stronger for it.

 Stress Reliever: Ask Yourself

If the present moment is difficult but . . .

- if you know the pain you are feeling now won't kill you, are you willing to withstand it?

- if you know that what you're feeling now won't last, are you willing to experience it?

- if you know this episode is not the last chapter of the book, can you find the strength to carry on?

- if you know that your future is going to be better than your past or present, are you willing to keep going?

Dealing with Setbacks

We don't always get what we want. Even when we do, nothing lasts forever. The best-laid plans unravel. You come down with bronchitis; you find out that your cat was hit by a car. You're closed out of the prerequisite classes for your major; you get laid off; someone steals your phone. Mom may have warned you that there would be days like this. Be happy and enjoy it when things are going well—but the honeymoon won't last forever.

By its very nature, life presents you with surprises, roadblocks, detours, and delays. If they blindside you or come at you in quick succession, they may hit you harder. It's okay to say "Ouch!"—just don't decide to interpret a bump in the road as evidence that you can't handle stress or that you're back at square one.

A setback is nothing more than something that sets you back a bit. In your life to date, temporary setbacks have undoubtedly accompanied all the progress you have made. "Temporary" is the key. You are the one who decides whether you will allow any setback to become a reason to stop moving forward. Your perspective can make all the difference. For the rest of your life, you can turn to the techniques learned in this class to keep you on track and help you refocus where you're going by redirecting you to the goals you value most. They will help you swerve around some common roadblocks and steer toward your deepest values.

 Stress Reliever: Remind Yourself . . .

Roses have thorns. If you like roses, you learn to work around the thorns.

Simply resolve to learn from your setbacks, make necessary adjustments, and continue on, knowing that overcoming each setback makes you stronger.

Whatever you do, do not even consider a stumble as a failure. The only failure will be failing to mine the situation to discover as much information as you can. Mistakes and setbacks teach exactly what you need to move forward—especially if you think you have hit the wall or crashed and burned.

Do a post-mortem on a recent misstep. Then regroup, reload, and launch Plan B. Avoid drama. Don't get caught in a thinking trap. Consider all of this as nothing more than a mid-course correction. When you drive, you make hundreds of tiny

hardiness
A personality trait characterized by being committed to something that is meaningful, believing it is possible to take control, and viewing change, whether positive or negative, as an opportunity to learn.

course corrections in order to travel in a straight line. It is the same with managing stress.

Block Your Escape Routes

✔ **Check-in:** What are some of the escape routes you've tried in the past? Where did they lead?

Nearly all rough patches, obstacles, and setbacks provide one dangerously addictive possibility: the chance to look for a way out. Think back. Have you abandoned your goals or retreated from an ambitious project because you ran into a rough patch? If so, when the going gets difficult, you may again be tempted to take some well-trod escape routes. You may already know what they are because you have used them so frequently. Do you veg out, overeat, drink, take drugs, procrastinate, hook up, or go to bed and pull the blankets over your head?

Escape "works" only in the sense that it provides immediate though short-lived relief from anxiety. This relief is its seduction—what makes escape tempting. As an actual solution, escape is a complete failure. It can even create more problems. The only way to get over or around any difficult situation is to go *through* it so you can learn from it.

Resist any temptation to make small obstacles big in order to justify quitting and not changing. Would you abandon your car if you lost the keys? Drop out of school because you blew a test? Of course not. If you indulge in self-pity when you confront obstacles now, you could be running for the exits before you know it.

No Failure to Fear

As we've said before and will say again, the biggest source of stress is fear, often a fear of failure that prompts you to step away from risks and look for a way out. But escape involves more downside risks than the failure you fear.

A life well lived is marked by one failure after another. This is nothing to mourn or evade. "Nothing is a failure," an old Italian proverb says. "Everything is a lesson." You must embrace this reality to begin the journey toward a real life. Real life is filled with day and night, light and dark, summer and winter. Only by taking risks and experiencing failure as well as success can you gain sufficient knowledge to live fully.

Learning and growing require failure. If you have always accomplished whatever you set out to do with ease and without failure, either your ambitions are modest or you have confined yourself to familiar territory. If your primary objective is to avoid failure, you put an immediate lid on how far you can go. If you do not take risks into account, you will not survive. If you make evading risks your only concern, you will miss opportunities. Failures, in fact, are exactly the opportunities you need. And you need as many as it takes to grow accustomed to thinking this way.

The inventor Thomas Edison systematically tried over 16,000 different materials in search of a filament for what he hoped would be an electrical source of light. Only after over 16,000 failures did he find one—tungsten—that worked. Learn to consider failure the ore from which you extract success, for failure is a richer source of information and enlightenment than quick success.

When your idea of what constitutes success and failure changes, your fear of failure dissipates. Failure is nothing more than evidence that you are learning something new—unless you make it more. You decide when to consider a failure a learning experience or a wipe-out.

Our opinion is that the only two things to run from are: characterizing a setback or mistake as a failure or calling *yourself* a failure for experiencing one. And our ideas of failure? Hanging back and avoiding stress or quitting.

Everything else is just part of the learning process. Remember your first time on a snowboard or trying your hand at cooking? You probably weren't a natural at either. The absence of failure is often evidence of sticking to the tried and true, and quite possibly boring, safety of no risks.

 Stress Reliever: Your Best Mistake

Describe a recent stressful situation and what you learned from handling this setback, what strengths and strategies helped you through it, what you adjusted, and how much stronger you are for overcoming it.

The Power of Plan B—and C

In order to manage whatever stress comes your way, you need backup support at every turn. Developing Plan B in case Plan A fails isn't enough; you need Plan C too. Your best backups grow from your own experience. Let's say that when you got stressed over a calculus assignment, you would stop working on it because you became increasingly anxious. But you can decide that as soon as that kind of frustration starts to build, you will focus your attention on your breathing and count your breaths until you calm down.

What if you soon start feeling stressed again? This is a critical moment. Without another backup plan, you are at risk. You need other strategies in place in case the first one fails. Don't imagine you will stay cool and come up with a plan on the spot. Improvising opens the gates for old, automatic behavior patterns, such as fleeing the situation. Know your next steps in advance.

In this case, you might take a break and visualize a favorite tranquil place—a beach, say, or a garden—that you associate with relaxation and well-being. Once you compose yourself, you could resolve to take up where you left off with renewed energy.

If you do not know in advance what to do when you hit an obstacle, you are more likely to waffle and, as a consequence, head in the direction of giving up. If, instead of taking the easy way out, you calmly survey the situation, make midcourse corrections, and rejoin the battle more fully, you hugely increase your chances of success.

Relapse Rehearsals

Since setbacks, lapses, and even dreaded relapses come with the territory of stress management, you need to recognize them for what they are: brief sidetracks into old, deeply carved behaviors that, if not caught quickly, automatically lead to other dead ends. Therapists who help individuals, families, and groups deal with unhealthy behavior such as addictions have developed specific techniques to lower the likelihood of relapses. One of the most powerful is rehearsal.

How does a recovering alcoholic get ready for a Super Bowl party? Or a problem gambler survive a night in Las Vegas without blowing a wad of money? Or a dieter stick to a weight loss plan over the holidays? All can prepare for these stress-inducing situations and prevent relapses by rehearsing their new behavior.

The ex-drinker can begin with new operating instructions, such as "Whenever I am at any party where alcohol is available, I will always drink fruit juice, sparkling water, or another non-alcoholic beverage." The ex-drinker plays out in his mind a step-by-step approach for dealing with his friends on Super Bowl Sunday and may actually practice standing around chatting with a non-alcoholic drink in hand. The ex-gambler in Vegas for a car show imagines himself walking past the bright lights and dark poker rooms of the casinos. The dieter visualizes politely declining whipped cream for Grandma's pecan pie and eating just three bites. All of them imagine themselves in control and confidently making good decisions.

The following exercise can help you rehearse your way around a potential relapse.

 Stress Reliever: Virtual Rehearsal

Think of a situation that is likely to lead to a stressful setback or relapse. Visualize yourself in the scene. See yourself, for instance, being invited to join some friends as they head out for the evening when you should be studying for a midterm. Then in vivid detail, see yourself hitting the books because the wiser part of your mind prevails.

Tools for Finding Meaning and Joy

Mental health professionals have developed an array of sophisticated therapeutic approaches that can help in managing stress. Two of the most effective behaviors—expressive writing and journaling—seem simple but can have a profound impact.

Expressive Writing and Journaling

Without reflection and contemplation, we are highly likely to repeat what we have always done—and to continue to feel stressed. We are far more susceptible to following instead of leading and to acting on impulse or habit instead of reason. **Expressive writing** (disclosing one's deepest thoughts and feelings about a stressful life event) and **journaling** (translating thoughts and feelings into words, photos, or video) create an opportunity to reflect. And reflection is a crucial part of stress management.

Have you ever tried but failed to communicate the excitement of a truly extraordinary experience? Maybe the best you could manage was "You had to be there." Journaling is another "had to be there" phenomenon; you have to do it to understand it. You don't need to put pen to paper; you can create a new computer file, or you can talk into a tape recorder. However, seeing words in print carries a more powerful subconscious impact. Whatever the method, as long as you put your thoughts and feelings into words on a regular basis, you will benefit. Simply keeping track of your experiences and observations can lead to a profound inner exploration. Expressive writing after a traumatic experience has proven effective in treating stress-related disorder.[6]

expressive writing Disclosing one's deepest thoughts and feelings about a stressful life event.

journaling Translating thoughts and feelings into words, photos or video.

Certain individuals—men more than women—resist expressive writing until a stressful experience, such as a breakup, serious illness, or the death of a friend or loved one, forces them to seek deeper understanding. But don't wait for a crisis; even everyday frustrations and victories can provide topics for your writing. Journaling works every time you use it—not just in emergencies. Journaling provides the opportunity to step back. It's another way of getting to know yourself and of acquiring a bird's-eye view on where you are now and where you want to go from here.

Your journal is personal, not for public display. Make sure that the people you live with—family members or roommates—know that your journal is your private property. You will find that others will be respectful of your writing, especially when you ask them to treat it that way.

The Benefits of Expressive Writing and Journaling

We are drowning in information. Facts of every conceivable type are at our fingertips. Want to know the temperature in Prague? You know how to get it—just Google. Want to settle a bet on which league won the most World Series titles in the last 20 years? All it takes is a couple of keystrokes. Yet we are profoundly short of self-knowledge. Communicating your innermost thoughts, if you stay with it, taps into deeper understanding and wisdom and takes you beyond just emotional intelligence to weave a tapestry of personal reflections that inform all your decisions and judgments.[10]

Expressive writing is an antidote to media saturation, gimmickry, and blind materialism.

Regular journaling can provide insight into your feelings and behaviors.

Massonstock/iStock /Getty Images

Commercials screech at you; news teasers bait you; the Internet beckons you. But none leads to depth or understanding. There is more to life than news, weather, sports, celebrity gossip, games, and reality shows. You already know this, but journaling is a power tool for getting to what else exists. Deeper satisfactions arise from self-knowledge than from any TV show or video game.

When practiced regularly, expressive writing taps your unconscious and your creativity in ways that are surprising and not immediately clear. Do you have to understand electricity to flip a switch and turn on lights? No. Nor do you have to understand why journaling can improve your grades, your relationships, or your coping skills. But it may do all of this and more.

Types of Journaling

You can journal about any topic: relationships, dreams, emotions (negative and positive), goals. If you write about the same subject day after day, you will penetrate that topic to an unprecedented degree. As you write about a topic long enough, you will write about the way it relates to your life, your career, and your goals. Eventually you can move to different topics and aspects of your life.

For example, if you do not understand your emotional reactions, keep a running record of intense feelings you have in the course of the day. Do not immediately look for patterns. As you write over time, they will clearly emerge and you will begin to see what you have been allowing to set you. Experiment with different ways of capturing your innermost thoughts and feelings in words, including the following:

Stream-of-Consciousness Journaling

In stream-of-consciousness journaling, you simply record whatever thoughts come into your mind. Sit quietly and breathe deeply. Once relaxed and settled, begin to write. Don't be surprised at the number and intensity of thoughts and feelings that emerge. As they become part of your awareness, they may lead to insights that have eluded you in the past because you are not taking the time to "hear" what you are thinking.

Journaling for Specific Solutions

You also can use your journal to tackle specific stressors. Here's how:

- Write when you need to sort out complicated feelings about an issue in your life.
- Write when you're caught up in a major life change and struggling to persist.
- Write before an event or activity that you believe will be stressful.

- Write afterward or the next day to chronicle the good choices you made or to note what you'll do differently the next time.

Reflective Journaling

Write about yourself and your life in the third person. You might begin with the phrase, "It was a time when…" Describe an event or experience in detail, using as many of your senses as possible. Write down the sounds, sights, smells, and feelings as if you were writing a novel. Use "he" or "she," rather than "I," as if you were an outside observer. Often this provides a new perspective on what you're going through.

Cathartic Writing

Let it all out. Put your pain, fear, anger, frustrations, and grief down on paper. Say what you want or need to say on the page. The journal is a safe place where no one will judge or criticize you. Begin with the phrase "Right now I feel . . .", and then let yourself write whatever comes out. If you run out of feelings, reread what you've just written and then write the next thing that comes to mind.

After you release deep emotions, you may choose to throw away your writing or burn it as a rite of letting go of an event or feeling that disrupted your life. Follow your intuition's lead as to what to do with the words once you've written them.

You don't have to wait until you're feeling bad to write; Use your journal to celebrate feelings of joy and gratitude as well.

Third-Person Writing

Although traditional therapeutic writing has used the first person, writing about yourself in the third person—"the child was all alone," rather than "I was all alone"— may be more beneficial when describing traumatic events. Shifting pronouns also shifts perspective so it is possible to write about painful experiences with greater detachment and fewer intrusive emotions. Experiment with both as you create narratives about your life.[11]

Letters You Never Send

Write a letter to a person, place, event, even an attitude. By allowing you to express emotions that you may not feel comfortable venting more directly, this technique can help you resolve issues with someone who is far away or dead or to process difficult emotions, such as anger or frustration, that come up in a relationship.

Begin with a salutation, just as you would if you were writing a letter: "Dear . . . .". Then let your fingers lead you. You may be surprised at the power and clarity you experience from your writing. While you are writing or afterward, you may feel deep emotions. Accept them as normal and healthy. In fact, the emotional release contributes to the healthy impact of journaling. If you want to do more with what you've written, share it with a trusted friend or counselor.

Dialogue Journaling

In dialogue journaling, you split yourself into two or more identities. In essence, you compose a script with at least two characters. One character might talk only of the difficulties you're facing. Another might mention the support and resources available to you. A third might comment on the exchange between the other two. Write a back-and-forth conversation, giving each character equal opportunity to make points and counterpoints.

> **⚙ Stress Reliever:** Make the Most of Journaling
>
> Write first thing in the morning or last thing at night—or better yet, both. If you write first thing in the morning, you tap directly into your mind when it is fresh, rested, and free of the distractions and mechanical habits of the day. If you write at night, you have a chance to survey the day and process what happened. While you sleep, the mind can assimilate and work without interference on the material you just provided.
>
> Write regularly. More is better than less. You don't have to write every day, although we do suggest a minimum of four or five times a week. On the other hand, would you brush your teeth only four or five days a week? Think of journaling as brushing your mind.

Humor or Laughter Therapy

Laughter is a powerful antidote to stress, pain, and conflict. Nothing works faster or more dependably to bring your mind and body back into balance than a good laugh. Laughter makes you feel good, and this good feeling remains with you even after the laughter subsides. More than just a respite from sadness and pain, laughter gives you the courage and strength to find new sources of meaning and hope. In the most difficult of times,

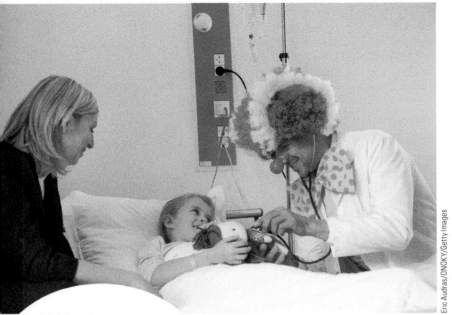

Visiting clowns ease anxiety and boost the spirits of hospital patients.

score highest in ratings of self-esteem and well-being.[12]

✔ **Check-in:** What types of humor do you use most? Do you see yourself as a humor endorser, denier, or enhancer?

a laugh—or even a smile—can go a long way toward making you feel better. And laughter really is contagious. Just hearing laughter primes your brain, readies you to smile and join in the fun, and allows you to see situations in a more realistic, less threatening light.

Types of Humor

Researchers have identified different humor styles:

- Affiliative humor, which uses humor to enhance relationships with others, for instance, by telling jokes and funny stories.

- Self-enhancing humor, in which a humorous outlook is used to cheer oneself up.

- Aggressive humor, a hostile form of humor that enhances feelings of self-worth at the expense of others, often by sarcasm or mockery.

- Self-defeating humor, which enhances relationships with others by disparaging or making fun of oneself or laughing along with others when being made fun of.[7]

Individuals also use humor in different ways:

- Humor endorsers score high on all types of humor and tend to be cheerful, look on the sunny side of life, and not take things too seriously.

- Humor deniers rarely engage in any form of humor, especially self-enhancing humor—and score lowest in self-esteem.

- Humor enhancers use humor to cheer themselves up even when not in the company of others and engage in more self-enhancing humor and less self-defeating humor. They

humor or laughter therapy The use of humor and laughter to promote overall health and relieve stress.

therapeutic humor Any intervention that uses the power of smiles, laughter, and playfulness to help heal physical or mental illness.

Humor or laughter therapy uses the power of smiles, laughter, and playfulness to help heal people with physical or mental illness. Laughter stimulates the heart, alters brain wave patterns and breathing patterns, reduces perceptions of pain, lowers levels of stress hormones, and strengthens the immune system.[13] Even in the face of dire stress, such as chemotherapy for cancer patients, **therapeutic humor** (any intervention that enhances health or facilitates healing or coping through humor) can defuse tension and physiological arousal and overcome dread and doubt.[14] Clowns who visit hospital patients, for instance, leave them with lighter, brighter spirits as well as smiling faces.[15]

Since we laugh as often, if not more, with others than by ourselves, humor also helps in forging supportive relationships. Humor helps you keep a positive, optimistic outlook through difficult situations, lightens your burdens, inspires hope, connects you to others, and keeps you grounded, focused, and alert. A humorous perspective creates psychological distance, which can help a person feel in control of a situation and make it seem more manageable.

Anyone can use humor therapy, either preventively or as part of treatment for a disease. In the treatment of long-term (chronic) diseases, especially those made worse by stress, humor therapy lessens anxiety and helplessness. Incorporating more humor and play into your daily interactions can improve the quality of your connections with co-workers, family members, and friends. See Table 10.2.

 Stress Reliever: Lighten Up!

Click on a link of favorite funny clips.

Watch a funny movie or TV show.

Go to a comedy club.

Share a good joke or a funny story.

Play with a pet.

Goof around with children.

Do something silly.

Make time for fun activities (e.g. bowling, miniature golf, karaoke).

Eric Audras/ONOKY/Getty Images

TABLE 10.2 The Benefits of Humor Therapy

Laughter can truly be the best medicine. Here are some of the reasons:

Physical Benefits

Boosts immunity

Lowers levels of stress hormones

Decreases pain

Relaxes muscles

Prevents heart disease

Reduces cholesterol

Psychological Benefits

Adds joy and zest to life

Triggers the release of feel-good endorphins

Dissolves anxiety and fear

Relieves stress

Improves mood

Enhances resilience

Social Benefits

Strengthens relationships

Attracts others to us

Enhances teamwork

Helps defuse conflict

Promotes group bonding

Coping with Life's Ups and Downs

Despite very real difficulties, most people adjust to life's ups and downs. They at least try to treat others with respect, to love their circle of family and friends, to find ways to contribute to society and the welfare of others, and to live with honesty and integrity. But some people do more. Rather than holding on for dear life and surviving, they flourish and thrive, even in the face of stress. Below are some steps you can take to prepare for life challenges and strengthen your stress resilience muscles.

When Something Good Happens:

- Acknowledge the part you played in making it happen. Allow yourself a "Way to go!" or a pat on the back.

- Feel grateful to whomever or whatever was responsible for the part you didn't play in your good fortune—even if it was just simple good luck.

- Enhance the experience. Think of ways to expand the scope or lengthen the duration of the positive event or situation.

- Record what happened. Write down exactly what happened in as much detail as possible, including what you did or said and, if others were involved, what they did or said. Include your feelings at the time, later, and now as you remember it. Explain what you think caused this event to occur.

When Something Bad Happens:

- Take one day or, if necessary, just one hour at a time. Even if you feel nothing but pain at the moment, remind yourself that over time good things will return.

- Compartmentalize. Rather than letting the traumatic event or difficult situation pervade all areas of your life, keep it within limits.

- Identify strengths and resources you can use to deal with the problem.

- Pay deliberate attention to what is good around you—for instance, to the kindness of others or to the beauty of a sunset.

- When criticisms or self-blame intrude, challenge your internal critic. If you are catastrophizing or over-generalizing, ask "What good does it do to beat myself up?"

Chapter Summary

- Spirituality is a belief in what some call a higher power, in someone or something that transcends the boundaries of self. It gives rise to a strong sense of purpose, values, morals, and ethics.

- Spiritual health refers to our ability to identify our basic purpose in life and experience the fulfillment of achieving our full potential. Spirituality is a belief in what some call a higher power, in someone or something that transcends the boundaries of self.

- Spiritual intelligence is "the capacity to sense, understand, and tap into the highest parts of ourselves, others, and the world around us." Spiritual intelligence, unlike spirituality, does not center on the worship of a God above, but on the discovery of a wisdom within.

- Prayer, a spiritual practice of millions, is the most commonly used form of complementary and alternative medicine. As brain imaging shows, prayer and meditation cause changes in blood flow in particular regions of the brain that may lower blood pressure, decrease anxiety, and enhance well-being.

- Forgiveness means letting go of anger and pain that waste energy. Forgiveness is not a one-time thing, but rather a process involving both the conscious and unconscious mind.

- Naikan is a Japanese method of self-reflection that encourages one to "look inside" to shift your attention to feelings of appreciation for others.

- Karma means that everything is a result of what has gone before. Being true to yourself and making good choices determine your lot in the future.

- Values are the criteria by which you evaluate things, people, events, and yourself; they represent what's most important to you. If understood and applied, values help give life meaning and structure.

- Compassion is the feeling that arises when you are confronted with another's suffering and feel motivated to relieve that suffering.

- Altruism (helping or giving to others), which promotes someone else's welfare even at a risk or cost to

ourselves, enhances self-esteem, relieves physical and mental stress, and protects psychological well-being.

- The key components of a fulfilling, happy, balanced life are close, supportive relationships, spirituality or a higher purpose in life, positive traits, hope, and engagement.

- Resilience is the process of adapting well in the face of adversity, trauma, tragedy, threats, and even significant stressors—such as family and relationship problems, serious health problems, or workplace and financial stressors.

- A setback sets you back temporarily. You are the one who decides whether you will allow any setback to become a reason to permanently stop moving forward.

- Resilient people typically are resourceful, believe that they have a right to survive and thrive, are able to attract and use support, extract the maximum benefit from the support they receive, keep in mind images of figures who have provided support in the past, are flexible, have goals, embody a fighting spirit, and tend to make positive statements.

- Journaling is a way of getting to know yourself and of acquiring a bird's-eye view on where you are now and where you want to go from here.

- Humor or laughter therapy uses the power of smiles, laughter, and playfulness to help heal people with physical or mental illness. Therapeutic humor is any intervention that promotes health and wellness by stimulating expression or appreciation of the absurdity or incongruity of life's situations.

⬛ STRESS RELIEVERS

An Infinity Experience

Have you ever been in a place—atop a high building or mountain, in a sunlit forest glade, on a windswept beach or cliff—where you sensed something timeless and eternal?

Visit this place in your imagination several times each week. Linger there for ten or more minutes. Bathe in the feelings you associate with it, and reflect on life as you are currently living it. Expand your horizons. From the perspective of this place, allow something to become clearer about the big picture of your life and what you might want to add or subtract.

Forgiving

Is there someone who you feel wronged you in some way and you've never forgiven?

Imagine saying, "I forgive you."

Try saying it out loud. Write it down. Reflect on how you feel.

Your Adjective Audit

Make a list, in no particular order, of the adjectives that might describe a person. Here are some ideas, but keep going until you fill an entire page or can't think of any more:

_____ generous
_____ thoughtful
_____ deceitful
_____ cheerful
_____ mean-spirited
_____ frugal
_____ cowardly
_____ crabby
_____ courageous
_____ loving
_____ miserly
_____ hard-working

_____ hostile

_____ indifferent

_____ committed

_____ cynical

_____ optimistic

_____ passionate

_____ whiny

_____ lonely

_____ friendly

_____ quiet

_____ kind

_____ vindictive

_____ joyful

Circle the adjectives you would like others to use to describe you. Cross out any that you hope are not used. Reflect on how you could live your life to earn the positive descriptors and avoid the negative ones. Pick one adjective daily that you want to describe you. Weave that quality into your actions that day.

Your Signature Behaviors

When someone dies, acquaintances often summarize the individual in terms of a characteristic behavior: "She had a smile for everyone." "He treated everyone with respect."

What one-liners might people use to describe you?

List five behaviors you'd like attributed to you. Consciously choose to insert each those five behaviors into your activities at least once each day.

Five-Finger Exercise

- Touch your thumb to your index finger. As you do, go back to a time when your body felt healthy and strong after a swim, a run, or another exhilarating activity.

- Touch your thumb to your middle finger. As you do, go back to a time when you felt loved and loving. Remember the details of a romantic moment or a warm embrace by a friend or family member.

- Touch your thumb to your ring finger. As you do, recall the nicest compliment you were ever given. Accept it now. Bask in this praise as you also recall the person who said it.

- Touch your thumb to your little finger. As you do that, go back to the most beautiful place you have ever been. Dwell in it for a while.

- Stretch all your fingers, and feel warmth and relaxation spread from them throughout your body.

Day By Day

Record the nicest thing that happens to you every day. It might be as small as a bus driver's hearty hello, or as big as making a team.

Also track something you did to make someone else's day. Again, it can be as small as wishing a janitor a good day, or as big as planning a surprise birthday party for a friend.

Do at least some of your carefully thought-out and well-targeted acts of kindness anonymously so that you do not know whether your kindness was appreciated or noticed. In other words, do the kindness for its own sake, not for the "feel good" you will receive.

Ask Yourself

If the present moment is difficult, but . . .

- you know the pain you are feeling now won't kill you, are you willing to withstand it?

- you know that what you're feeling now won't last, are you willing to experience it?

- you know this episode is not the last chapter of the book, can you find the strength to carry on?

- you know that your future is going to be better than your past or present, are you willing to keep going?

Remind Yourself . . .

Roses have thorns. If you like roses, you learn to work around the thorns.

Simply resolve to learn from your setbacks, make necessary adjustments, and continue on, knowing that overcoming each setback makes you stronger.

Your Best Mistake

Describe a recent stressful situation and what you learned from handling this setback, what strengths and strategies helped you through it, what you adjusted, and how much stronger you are for overcoming it.

Virtual Rehearsal

Think of a situation that is likely to lead to a stressful setback or relapse. Visualize yourself in the scene. See yourself, for instance, being invited to join some friends as they head out for the evening when you should be studying for a midterm. Then in vivid detail, see yourself hitting the books because the wiser part of your mind prevails.

Make the Most of Journaling

Write first thing in the morning or last thing at night—or better yet, both. If you write first thing in the morning, you tap directly into your mind when it is fresh, rested, and free of the distractions and mechanical habits of the day. If you write at night, you have a chance to survey the day and process what happened. While you sleep, the mind can assimilate and work without interference on the material you just provided.

Write regularly. More is better than less. You don't have to write every day, although we do suggest a minimum of four or five times a week. On the other hand, would you brush your teeth only four or five days a week? Think of journaling as brushing your mind.

Lighten Up!

_____ Click on a link of favorite funny clips.

_____ Watch a funny movie or TV show.

_____ Go to a comedy club.

_____ Share a good joke or a funny story.

_____ Play with a pet.

_____ Goof around with children.

_____ Do something silly.

_____ Make time for fun activities (e.g. bowling, miniature golf, karaoke).

⊜ YOUR PERSONAL STRESS MANAGEMENT TOOLKIT

REFLECTION: A Day in Your Life

Answer yes or no to the following questions, based on the last 24 hours:

- Did you look at the sky?

- Did you notice any smells of the season?

- Did you listen to music that delighted you?

- Did your eyes linger on something—a ray of sunshine, a reflection in a puddle, a splash of color—that intrigued or pleased them?

- Did you consciously feel the swish of your hair against your neck or your sleeves along your arms?

- Did you taste something absolutely yummy?

- Did you sing to yourself?

- Did you talk to someone you care for?

- Did you learn something new?

- Did you make someone smile?

- Did you laugh?

- Did you say "I love you"?

- Did you say "Thank you"?

- Did you stop to clear your mind, pray, or meditate?

- Did you exercise your body?

- Did you text, call, or email a friend?

- Were you kind to someone?

- Did you pick up after yourself?

- Were you patient?

- Did you open your mind to a new idea?

- Did you smile at a child?

- Were you kind to yourself in at least one conscious way?

- Did you experience something—a stunning sunset, a poetic image, a chord of music—that lifted your spirit to a higher plane, if only for a few minutes?

The more often you answered "yes," the more fully you lived the last 24 hours. Use this assessment to make even more of the next 24.

TECHNIQUE: Pie Chart

Draw a pie chart of how big the different parts of your life are (school, family, friends, work, sports, exercise, hobbies, and so on). Are you happy with how big or small each piece of the pie is?

Draw another pie chart that depicts what an ideal "life pie" would look like.

What are the differences between the two?

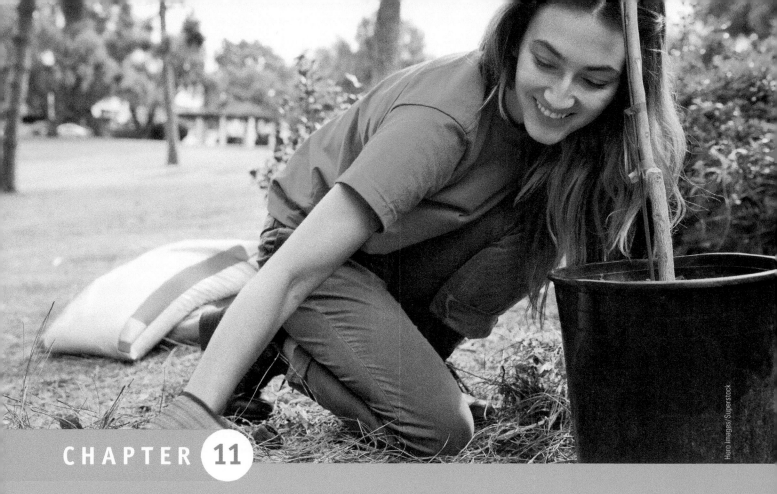

CHAPTER **11**

Occupational and Environmental Stress

After reading this chapter, you should be able to:

11.1 Develop tools to set the stage for a successful future.

11.2 Explain the importance of a resume in finding a job.

11.3 Evaluate the impact of job-related stressors.

11.4 Discuss the effects of high job strain on physical and mental health.

11.5 Describe the ways in which human health depends on the health of the environment.

PRE-CHAPTER CHECK-IN: RATE YOUR JOB STRESS

If you have or have had a job, take the following self-survey:

Enter a number from the sliding scale:

STRONGLY DISAGREE				AGREE SOMEWHAT			STRONGLY AGREE		
1	2	3	4	5	6	7	8	9	10

I can say what I really think or feel at work. _____

I have authority to make decisions. _____

I make the most of the time I have to complete a task. _____

I regularly receive acknowledgement for good work. _____

I am satisfied with my job. _____

I don't feel that I am picked on or discriminated against at work. _____

My workplace is pleasant and safe. _____

My job does not interfere unduly with my family and social life. _____

I get along well with superiors, coworkers, or customers. _____

Most of the time I feel I have control over my life at work. _____

TOTAL JOB STRESS SCORE: _____

70-100: handling job stress well
40-60: handling job stress moderately well
Less than 40: high-stress problems that need to be resolved

Lauren got her first paying job when she was ten and started walking the neighbor's dog. At 13, she took a babysitting course and soon was working for several families in her neighborhood. At 16, she became a lifeguard at the community center. As a college freshman, she worked at the library on a work-study grant.

Something changed when Lauren got a summer job at a "green" store selling products made with recycled materials. Inspired by the global vision of the shop's owners, she joined an environmental action group whose activities included planting trees, setting up recycling centers, and launching energy-conservation makeovers on campus. As she looks beyond graduation, Lauren is applying for jobs where she can make, not just a living, but also a difference.

Like Lauren, you may have worked off and on for years—in offices, restaurants, schools, summer camps, community pools, construction crews. You may have or may find yourself with a terrific job or one that exhausts, stresses, frustrates, or bores you. Your workplace may be stimulating and serene or noisy, disorganized, and plagued with inequality, discrimination, even harassment. Regardless of what you do and where you end up working, stress—positive and negative—will come with the job. The coping strategies you master in college will help you maintain a healthy balance.

Many college students are also like Lauren in their commitment to create a healthier environment. Although issues such as climate change and pollution may seem so enormous that nothing any individual can do will have an effect, this is not the case. All of us, as citizens of the world, can help find solutions to the challenges confronting our planet. The first step is realizing that you have a personal responsibility for safeguarding the health of your environment and, thereby, your own well-being.

As you read this chapter, think ahead to your future. Where do you see yourself working? What might you be doing? Which types of stressors might you encounter? What about your lifestyle? Do you see yourself walking or biking to work? Living in a house powered by solar panels? Driving an electric car? In a world of possibilities, all these could happen, but the chances of their becoming reality depend on the decisions you make and the behaviors you choose—starting now.

✔ **Check-in:** What do you want to be when you grow up?

People may have started asking you that question when you were five. What did you say then? What do you say now?

Preparing for Your Future

The time to start developing tools to navigate the work world is sooner rather than later. As a first step, create a professional-quality resume. You also need to master skills such as writing introductory e-mails, preparing for interviews, and making a positive impression on potential employers.

Balancing Work and School

An estimated 60 to 70 percent of college students have jobs. If you're among them, your financial aid package may require several hours of work study per week, or you may be working off-campus to cover your expenses. Despite the extra demands on time and energy, earning money while in school pays off in more than dollars and cents.

Jobs of any sort can teach the responsibilities that come with being an adult. If you can find one related to your major, you also gain valuable experience. If not, look for a position that plays to your strengths and interests. If you're extroverted and have a decent car, try driving for a car-sharing company. If you enjoy sports, apply for a job in a store selling running shoes or athletic gear. If you like kids, find babysitting gigs through local ads or childcare agencies. Jobs in retail or restaurants teach important skills, such as how to be part of a team, interact with customers, and think on your feet.

Your immediate goal may simply be to bring in money, but while supporting yourself, you are also strengthening your professional potential. (See Chapter 5 for time management tips for working students.) However, keep in mind that your primary goal is to get a degree. When making up your schedule, factor in time to study so you're not panicking before every test. Inform your instructors of your job commitments. If you are a diligent student and attend class regularly, they should be willing to take your work obligations into consideration.

Building Your Resume While in College

If you're worried that your resume looks a little skimpy, don't panic. Every person in the work force started somewhere. One way to bolster your qualifications is volunteering. Habitat for Humanity, Boys and Girls Clubs, the Red Cross, senior citizen centers, schools, and animal shelters are all excellent places to acquire work experience and new skills while giving back to your community.

You also can become an intern. Although typically unpaid, internships provide opportunities for networking, education, and experience. Go online or connect with local professionals about formal programs that may offer college credit. Even if it's just for a brief period, nothing can beat on-the-job experience in your chosen field—and it may lead to employment down the road.

A cautionary note: The process of competing for prized internships can be extremely stressful, as can living up to performance expectations. Adding a demanding internship to school, homework, friends, family, and socializing can feel overwhelming. If you find yourself in this situation, continue to practice effective time management in all areas of your life. Evaluate all of the short and long-term pros and cons of an internship. Be realistic with yourself and those around you. Keep open lines of communication with your internship supervisor.

Use Facebook and Twitter to share your professional interests and skills. Consider writing a blog to put your ideas and occupation-related information out into the world. Other networking sites, such as LinkedIn, can boost your online presence and showcase all that you have to offer.

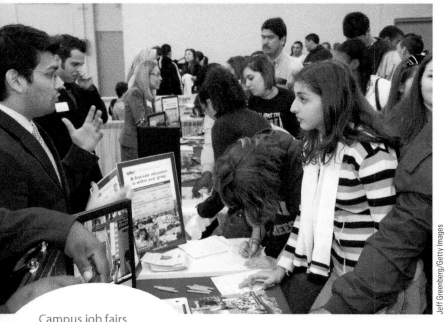

Campus job fairs offer a chance to learn more about potential careers and employers.

Jeff Greenberg/Getty Images

you most. Think of possible jobs based on items from the lists you have made. They could be jobs you've heard about or ones you formulate based on your interests. Perhaps you'd like to be a part of a start-up, care for animals, design sports gear, or launch a go-green initiative.

Continue to add to and edit your ideas in as much detail as possible.

✔ **Check-in:** How does the online world see you?

Look at your Facebook, Twitter, Instagram, and other social media platforms. What might a potential employer think of the images or links on your feed? Are you presenting yourself as responsible, mature, and capable?

Choosing a Career

"Choose a job you love," according to an anonymous sage, "and you will never have to work a day in your life." Not everyone is so fortunate or far-sighted. Perhaps you already have a clear idea of which profession interests you, but you also may not have a clue. Most college campuses have career development and job training centers meant specifically to prepare you for the professional world. Take full advantage of them.

Online tools also can guide you through the process of self-discovery. Questions, quizzes, and personality assessments can't tell you what your perfect job would be, but they can help you identify what's important to you in a career, what you enjoy doing, and where you excel.

🔧 **Stress Reliever:** Brainstorm Your Future

Make a list of things you are interested in and the classes that have engaged

Once you have identified some specific careers, gather information online on everything from job descriptions to average salaries and estimated future growth. This will also help you figure out the practical priorities: How stable is the field you are considering? Are you comfortable with the amount of risk? Is the salary range acceptable to you? Will you have to relocate for training or better job opportunities? How will this affect your family?

Finding a Job

Whether it's for the summer, the semester, or after graduation, you will need a job. Will potential employers need you? Your challenge is to convince them that they do. Start by identifying the skills you have and the skills you need. Remember, you're not completely starting from scratch. In your life to date, you've acquired *transferable skills* that can be applied to almost any field, such as technology/internet/programming expertise, a foreign language, research (both laboratory and library), and leadership (team leader and camp counselor, for instance). Attending a workshop or participating in a webinar in resume preparation can boost applicants' confidence—and their success in finding employment.[1]

Your resume is your foot in the door. It should show an employer how and why you are qualified for the job so you want to present your skills and experience in a way that will have the most chance of getting an interview.

The different formats for resumes include chronological (listing jobs/experiences according to dates, with the most recent first), functional (focused on skills), and combination (including work history and skills). Experiment with different types and get feedback from classmates and counselors. You can download templates from sites such as ResumeHelp.Com or jobsearch.about.com.

Networking

Networking simply means getting to know people—something you do every day and everywhere you go. You are networking when you strike up a conversation with the person next to you in line, introduce yourself to a stranger at a party, or meet a friend of a friend. When you're considering a major or a career, use your network of friends, acquaintances, instructor, and advisors to meet people in the field. They can provide a real sense of what type of work you will actually be doing. If possible, ask if you can "shadow" them for a day to gain more insight into your prospective field.

When it comes time to search for a job, networking may produce the best leads. Adopting a networking lifestyle—a lifestyle of connecting and helping others in good times and bad—will help you find potential openings as well as forge valuable connections and stay focused and motivated during your job search.

Preparing for a Job Interview

Certain experiences are, by their very nature, stressful. Interviewing for a job, especially one you dearly want, is one of them. As you've learned, a little stress will sharpen your mind and quicken your reflexes. However, too much stress can make you trip over your tongue or look frazzled rather than confident. Preparation can make all the difference—so can practice.

Go on as many interviews as possible, even if a job doesn't sound perfect. You never know when an interview for a "not-quite-right" job will lead to a surprising match, a referral to another opening, or an entirely new position tailored to fit your unique experience and abilities. By putting yourself out there and interviewing, you'll also learn about new trends and opportunities and meet people to add to your network.

Here are some steps that can help you make the most of an interview:

- When an interviewer says, "Tell me about yourself," make sure you're ready. A compelling job interview story should incorporate your experiences, achievements, and ambitions. Think about major events and turning points that shaped who you are. Make notes about what you learned and accomplished. Organize your narrative by time periods or jobs. Include "aha" moments or crucial experiences that sparked your passion for your field. Explain why you made certain decisions, such as changing your major, or what you gained from experiences such as studying abroad. Talk about your career goals and how they've evolved. Preparing your story

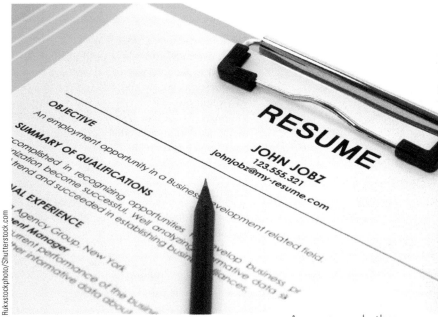

Rukastockphoto/Shutterstock.com

takes a lot of work and practice. However, the benefits to you and to your career can be enormous.

- What is it that would qualify you to be an outstanding teacher, salesperson, trainer, physician assistant? Give examples of your strengths. Was there a crisis that you responded to well? Was there a time when you learned valuable lessons from dealing with stress? Did you ever provide successful leadership? How did you overcome a failure or setback? Practice your replies until they flow

A resume—whether on paper or online—provides a potential employer with a first impression of your experience and skills.

Preparation and practice can make a job interview less stressful and more successful.

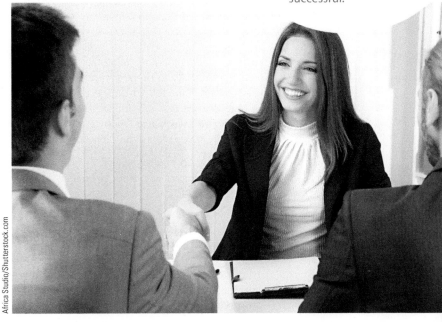

Africa Studio/Shutterstock.com

easily and work on adapting them to different types of questions.

- Record or videotape your story. Listen and watch carefully, and edit several times. Put yourself in the interviewer's shoes and pose the questions you would ask and the answers you might give. Don't rely on your ability to think on your feet. You want to make a memorable impression that demonstrates competency and ability.

Handling Interview Stress

Interviews can range from a few minutes of chit-chat at a job fair booth to a series of in-depth formal meetings, sometimes with more than one interviewer. The better prepared you are, the more relaxed and comfortable you will be when the questions start coming your way.

Before the Interview

- Do your research. Gather information about the company and the position available. Try to specifically relate your experience to the duties the job opportunity entails.

- Stay in touch with your references. Make sure that they know when and where you're interviewing, so they can anticipate an email or call.

- Practice interviewing with a friend or classmate. Eliminate verbal fillers like "uh" and "um."

- Anticipate likely questions. Interviewers may ask how you would handle situations such as getting along with a difficult coworker or the pressure of tight deadlines. Practice answering the interview questions and follow-up questions with several detailed examples or stories.

- The day before the interview, get your clothes and resume ready. Make sure you have directions. Double-check the time and the name of your interviewer.

During the Interview

- Be sure to take a bathroom break before the interview. And double check to make sure your phone and any other electronic devices are turned off (not just set on vibrate).

- Pay attention to body language (see Chapter 6) to signal confidence, even when you're not feeling it. Instead of tentatively entering an interview with your head down and eyes averted, stand tall with your shoulders back, smile. Maintain eye contact, and deliver a firm handshake.

- Don't ramble. By the time you reach the interviewing stage, you should be clear about what you want and what you offer to the company. Try to be thoughtful and self-reflective in both your interview questions and your answers. Show the interviewer you know yourself—your strengths and your weaknesses. Be prepared to talk about which areas would present challenges and how you would address them. Admitting true areas of weakness is much more convincing than claiming: "I have what you need and I can do anything I put my mind to."

- Ask questions. You can't just be an effective responder. You need to assert yourself, too. For example, you might ask about the attributes of the people who do well at the company or what specific challenges you could anticipate in the first six months.

On the Job

You will spend much of your life working. Your jobs may be frustrating, challenging, inspiring, boring, mundane, creative, exhausting, or exhilarating. Sooner or later, they will also be stressful. The key is learning which specific stressors in the work environment you are particularly sensitive to and recognizing the signs in your own body and mind that signal stress overload. As always, how you respond to stressors will determine whether you experience positive eustress as you learn and grow or chronic distress that can undermine your physical and psychological well-being.

What Kind of Worker Are You?

Workers in every field vary in their on-the-job experiences—and in the ways they respond to occupational demands. In a recent analysis, researchers categorized employees as:

- **Engaged or enthusiastic workers,** the happiest in their jobs. They take pleasure in and are challenged by jobs where they can use their skills and energy. They identify with their work and the organization they work for. Those scoring high in "work engagement" exhibit:
  - a persistent, positive "state of fulfillment."
  - vigor (high levels of energy and mental resilience while working).
  - dedication (being strongly involved in their work).
  - absorption (highly engrossed in their work).

- **Relaxed or 9-to-5 workers,** who seem content with their jobs but show little drive to excel. Although they do not feel bad at work and see themselves as competent, they lack enthusiasm and do not feel that their jobs are challenging.

- **Workaholics,** who labor excessively hard and compulsively. They feel competent and energetic and identify with their jobs, but they do not take pleasure in their work.

- **Fatigued workers,** who do not identify with their positions, do not feel competent, do not have enough energy to do their work properly, and seem exhausted and cynical.

- **Burned-out workers,** who report the lowest levels of energy, pleasure, skills, and challenge.[2] (Burnout is discussed later in this chapter)

✔ **Check-in:** If you have a job, which category best describes you?

Time and Task Management

In work, as in school, making the most of your time and energy is crucial. The management techniques in Chapter 5 provide a good beginning, but you may have to modify them to your new job.

Managing Your Time

- **Create a balanced schedule.** Analyze your schedule, responsibilities, and daily tasks. Try to find a balance between work and family life, social activities and solitary pursuits, daily responsibilities and downtime.

- **Don't over-commit yourself.** Avoid scheduling things back-to-back or trying to fit too much into one day. All too often, we underestimate how long things will take. If you've got too much on your plate, distinguish between the "shoulds" and the "musts." Drop tasks that aren't truly necessary to the bottom of your priority list or eliminate them entirely.

- **Get to work a bit early.** Even ten minutes can make the difference between frantically rushing and having time to ease into your day. Don't add to your stress levels by running late.

- **Plan regular breaks.** Make sure to take short breaks throughout the day to take a walk or sit back and clear your mind. Also try to get away from your desk or work station for lunch. Stepping away from work to relax and recharge will help you be more, not less, productive.

- **Take advantage of time off.** Long vacations (two weeks or more) that provide rest, relaxation, and pleasure boost health and well-being during time off and for a brief period afterward.[3] Even short vacations of four to five days can make a difference, although their beneficial effects don't last as long.[4]

Managing Your Tasks

- **Make a to-do list.** Using pen and paper or a note-taking or time-management app, list all the tasks that you need to complete. If they're complex, break out the first action step, and write this down under the larger task.

- **Prioritize.** Run through your list of tasks and allocate priorities from A (very important or very urgent) to F (unimportant or not at all urgent). Work your way through it in order, dealing with the A priority tasks first, then the Bs, then the Cs, and so on. As you complete tasks, tick them off or strike them through. If you have something particularly unpleasant to do, get it over with early. You'll feel better the rest of the day.

- **Delegate responsibility.** You don't have to do everything yourself. If coworkers or team members can take care of a task, let go of the desire to control or oversee every little step. You'll be letting go of unnecessary stress in the process.

- **Be willing to compromise.** When you ask someone to contribute differently to a task, revise a deadline, or change their behavior at work, be willing to do the same. Sometimes if you can both bend a little, you'll be able to find a happy middle ground that reduces the stress levels for everyone.

 Stress Reliever: Energy Burst

If you can feel your body tensing up, go to a private place. Pretend you're a boxer, and throw punches into the air. Try some karate kicks forward, backward, and to each side. If you're out of hearing distance, grunting intensifies the feeling of relief.

Emotional Intelligence at Work

As you learned in Chapter 8, emotional intelligence helps you manage and use your emotions in positive and constructive ways. When it comes to satisfaction and success at work, emotional intelligence matters just as much as intellectual ability. It can draw people to you, overcome differences, repair wounded feelings, and defuse tension and stress. Its major components include:

- **Self-awareness.** Recognize your particular fight-or-flight stress response, and become familiar with techniques that can rapidly calm and energize you. (See "Technique" in the Personal Stress Management Toolbox on page 230.)

- **Self-management.** Your moment-to-moment emotions influence your thoughts and actions, so pay attention to your feelings and factor them into your decision-making.

- **Body language.** Your nonverbal messages can either generate trust and cooperation or distrust and stress. You also need to accurately read and respond to the nonverbal cues that other people send at work.

- **Relationship management.** Resolving conflict in healthy, constructive ways can strengthen trust between people and relieve workplace stress and tension. Review the communication skills discussed in Chapter 6.

> **Stress Reliever:** Put a Workplace Problem in Perspective
>
> Ask yourself:
>
> Is it really worth getting upset over?
>
> Is it worth upsetting others?
>
> Is it that important?
>
> Is it that bad?
>
> Is the situation irreparable?
>
> Is it really your problem?

What if you're stuck in a job you hate? Reframe the experience. For instance, stocking warehouse shelves is undeniably tedious, but you can think of how you're contributing to an organization or helping get needed products to customers. Focus on the aspects of the job that you do enjoy—even if it's just hanging out with your coworkers in the break room.

You also can find meaning and satisfaction in your family, hobbies, or studies. Try to be grateful for having work that pays the bills. Plan an inexpensive fun activity for the weekend. If you have time, volunteer outside of work, which, as noted in Chapter 10, can lift your spirits, sharpen your skills, and introduce you to new people.

occupational stress Refers to distress related to any aspect of a job that can take a physical and psychological toll.

Occupational Stress

Occupational stress refers to distress related to any aspect of a job. Its economic costs may be as high as $300 billion a year. Its personal costs include digestive ailments, cardiovascular disease, and other health problem as well as anxiety, depression, and other psychological conditions.[5] Both life stress and job stress are higher when one or the other is present.[6]

According to a recent study, work stress may actually shorten Americans' life spans by nearly three years.[7] People with less education are much more likely to end up in jobs with more unhealthy workplace practices that cut down on life expectancy. Those with the highest educational attainment are less affected by workplace stress than individuals with the least education. Blacks and Hispanics lose more years of life because of work than whites, and women generally fare better than their male counterparts. Across all groups, unemployment, layoffs, and a lack of health insurance are the factors that exert the biggest influence. Low job control was the next biggest factor for both men and women, followed by job insecurity in men and shift work in women.[8]

Causes of Occupational Stress

Among the factors that contribute to occupational stress are the following:

- **A sense of powerlessness.** Secretaries, waiters and waitresses, middle managers, police officers, editors, and medical interns rank among the most highly stressed workers because they must constantly respond to others' demands and deadlines yet have little control over the situation. Psychological demands combined with low control or decision-making ability over one's job lead to job strain and health problem such as high blood pressure.[9]

- **Workaholism.** People obsessed by their work and careers can become so caught up in racing toward the top that they forget what they're racing toward and why. In some cases they throw themselves into their work to mask or avoid painful feelings or difficulties in their own lives.

- **Aggressive or demeaning treatment.** Despite stricter policies banning sexual harassment and discrimination, some companies tolerate comments and jokes that range from insensitive to upsetting. Harassment and intimidation have been shown to trigger the stress response and its harmful consequences.[10]

- **"Stress overload."** Health professionals, social workers, and other caregivers may become overwhelmed or drained by interactions with individuals who are sick, disabled, or in great need. In other fields, it can be the result of pressure to perform to meet rising expectations but with no increase in job satisfaction.

- **Long hours.** Employees who work 60 or more hours report less sleep and exercise, more work-family conflict, and more difficulty in trying to maintain their households.[11]

See Figure 11.1 for some environmental causes of workplace stress.

Coping with Occupational Stress

Keep in mind that many things at work are beyond your control—particularly the behavior of other people. The same stress management skills that you use in building relationships, such as active listening and using "I" statements (see Chapter 6), can also be effective in the workplace:

- Focus on the things you can control, such as the way you choose to react to problems.

- Resist the urge to control the uncontrollable or to strive for the impossible. Trying to attain perfection will simply add unnecessary stress to your day.

- Aim to do your best, no one can ask for more. When you set unrealistic goals for yourself or try to do too much, you're setting yourself up to fall short.

- Exercise regularly. Get enough sleep. Eat a healthy diet rich in fruits and vegetables rather than fast food and vending machine snacks.[12]

Burnout

✔ **Check-in:** Are you burned out?

You may be if:

Every day is a bad day.

You're exhausted all the time.

The majority of your day is spent on tasks you find either mind-numbingly dull or overwhelming.

You feel like nothing you do makes a difference or is appreciated.

You have frequent headaches, back and muscle pain, and other symptoms.

You feel increasingly negative, cynical, helpless, trapped, defeated, or detached.

You begin to isolate yourself from others.

If you have a job, does your workplace have any of these stressors?

- **Poor lighting.**
- **Loud background noise, such as music, traffic noise, or conversation.**
- **Chairs or desks that cause discomfort or repetitive strain injuries.**
- **Unhealthy air, including pollution, smoke, or unpleasant smells.**
- **Overcrowding or workstations in close proximity to others.**
- **Uncomfortable climate conditions, such as an office that is too hot, too cold, too humid, or too dry.**
- **An unclean or cluttered office space.**

Monkey Business Images/Shutterstock.com

FIGURE 11.1 Stressors in the workplace. Are there any steps you can take to make your workspace less stressful? If you don't have the authority to do so, how can you inform those in charge of the problem?

You procrastinate, skip work, avoid responsibilities.

You turn to food, drugs, or alcohol to cope.

Burnout may be the result of unrelenting stress, but it isn't the same as too much stress. Stress, by and large, involves *too much:* too many pressures that demand too much of you physically and psychologically. Stressed people can still imagine, though, that if they could just get everything under control, they would feel better.

Burnout, on the other hand, is about *not enough*. Being burned out means feeling empty, devoid of motivation, and beyond caring. People experiencing burnout often don't see any hope of positive change in their situations. If excessive stress is like drowning in responsibilities, burnout is being all dried up. While you're usually aware of being under a lot of stress, you don't always notice burnout when it happens.

Anyone who feels overworked and undervalued is at risk for burnout. This state of physical, emotional, and mental exhaustion occurs when workers or caregivers feel overwhelmed and unable to meet constant demands. Mothers and managers, firefighters and flight attendants, teachers and telemarketers may feel the flames of too much stress and not enough satisfaction. Many people, especially those caring for others at work or at home, get to a point where there's an imbalance between their own feelings and dealing with difficult, distressful issues on a day-to-day basis. The result has been called compassion fatigue. If they don't recognize what's going on and make some changes, their health and the quality of their work suffer.

burnout A state of physical, emotional, and mental exhaustion that occurs when workers or caregivers feel overwhelmed and unable to meet constant demands.

TABLE 11.1 Is It Stress or Burnout?

Stress vs. Burnout	
Stress	**Burnout**
Characterized by overengagement	Characterized by disengagement
Emotions are overreactive	Emotions are blunted
Produces urgency and hyperactivity	Produces helplessness and hopelessness
Loss of energy	Loss of motivation, ideals, and hope
Leads to anxiety disorders	Leads to detachment and depression
Primary damage is physical	Primary damage is emotional

Causes of Burnout

Burnout rarely stems from any one cause, but from a variety of conditions. A line cook may seem to have little in common with an air traffic controller—other than risk factors for burn-out. These include:

- Little or no control over responsibilities, rewards, or working conditions.
- Lack of recognition and compensation for good work.
- Unclear or overly demanding job expectations.
- Monotonous or unchallenging work.
- A chaotic or high-pressured environment.
- Long hours or shifts.

The psychological issues that increase the risk of burnout include:

- A desire for perfection.
- A sense that nothing is ever good enough.
- Negative or pessimistic outlook.
- A need for control, reluctance to delegate to others.
- A driven, high-achieving, Type A personality.

Lifestyle factors also influence the likelihood of burnout:

- Little or no time for relaxing and socializing.
- Lack of sleep.
- A sense of having to be too many things to too many people.
- Multiple responsibilities with little or no help from others.
- Lack of supportive relationships.

The Stages of Burnout

If you've been feeling a lot of pressure, check yourself for early signs of burnout (Figure 11.2).

If you recognize any of them in yourself, stop and reflect on ways to get your life back into balance. Cut back whatever commitments and activities you can.

If you don't make changes, burnout may intensify as you progress through its typical sequence of stages:

Stage 1: Physical, Mental, and Emotional Exhaustion

Workers take on greater responsibility without authority to make or enforce changes. They may struggle to juggle an unmanageable schedule or to accomplish more with fewer resources. Gradually their energy and optimism fade.

Stage 2: Shame and Doubt

Employees lose confidence and feel increasingly vulnerable and insecure. They may have difficulty sleeping. Some turn to alcohol or drugs.

Stage 3: Cynicism and Callousness

Workers' attitudes become more negative. Convinced that they have to watch out for themselves, they suspect others' motives and make compromises just to get along. Their behavior may seem insensitive or indifferent.

Stage 4: Failure, Helplessness, and Crisis

At this stage, employees are worn down. They withdraw emotionally, feeling indifferent and disengaged. Their moods may swing, and they begin to complain of physical symptoms that become more disabling.

Stage 5: Collapse

In the end-stage of burnout, workers may at risk of losing their jobs because of their poor performance. They also may develop severe, even life-threatening physical or psychological problems.

FIGURE 11.2 Early signs of burnout.

- **Physical and psychological fatigue and exhaustion**
- **Disengagement and cynicism toward work**
- **Irritability**
- **Sleep problems or nightmares**[13]
- **Increased anxiety or nervousness**
- **Muscular tension (headaches, backaches, and the like)**
- **Increased use of alcohol or medication**
- **Digestive problems (such as nausea, vomiting, or diarrhea)**

- **Loss of interest in sex**
- **Frequent body aches or pain**
- **Quarrels with family or friends**
- **Negative feelings about everything**
- **Problems concentrating**
- **Job mistakes and accidents**
- **Feelings of depression, hopelessness, or helplessness**[14]

Stock-Asso/Shutterstock.com

Job Loss and Unemployment

Our jobs are much more than just the way we make a living. They influence how we see ourselves as well as the way others see us and give our daily lives structure, purpose, and meaning. That's why job loss and unemployment are so stressful.

Job insecurity, such as uncertainty about whether you'll be let go in a pending round of layoffs, increase stress hormones and take a toll on health.[15] Workers who have been fired or laid off must deal with multiple losses: the loss of a paid position, a daily routine, and the camaraderie of coworkers, as well as the possible loss of the ability to support themselves and their families. They experience higher rates of depression and report significantly more anxiety, health complaints, and reduced life satisfaction.[16]

Losing a job forces you to make rapid changes. It's normal to feel angry, hurt, panicky, and scared. You have every right to be upset, so accept your feelings and practice self-compassion (see Chapter 8). Many, if not most, successful people have experienced major failures in their careers. But they've turned those failures around by picking themselves up, learning from the experience, and trying again. When bad things happen to you—like experiencing unemployment—you can grow stronger and more resilient in the process of overcoming them.

Here are some other ways to cope when you find yourself out of work:

- **Write about your feelings.** Express your feelings about being laid off or unemployed, including things you wish you had said (or hadn't said) to your former boss. This is especially cathartic if your layoff or termination was handled in an insensitive way.

- **Reach out.** Share your feelings and fears with trusted friends or family members. Surround yourself with positive, supportive people. Keep building your network of personal and professional acquaintances.

- **Accept reality.** Rather than dwelling on your job loss—how unfair it is; how poorly it was handled; how you could have prevented it; how much better life would be if it hadn't happened—try to accept the situation. The sooner you do, the sooner you can get on with the next phase in your life.

- **Don't beat yourself up.** It's easy to start criticizing or blaming yourself when you've lost your job and are unemployed. Arm yourself with positive affirmations; cultivate positive experiences.[17] But you'll need your self-confidence intact as you're looking for a new job.

- **Challenge negative thoughts.** If you start to think, "I'm a loser," reword your self-talk to say, "I lost my job because of the recession, not because I didn't do a good job."

- **Look for the silver lining.** What can you learn from the experience? Maybe your job loss and unemployment has given you a chance to reflect on what you want out of life and rethink your career priorities. Maybe it's made you stronger. If you look, you're sure to find something of value.

- **Keep a regular daily routine.** When you no longer have a job to report to every day, you can easily lose motivation. Treat your job search like a regular job, with a daily "start" and "end" time. Following a set schedule will help you be more efficient and productive while you're unemployed.

- **Create a job search plan.** Avoid getting overwhelmed by breaking big goals into small, manageable steps. Instead of trying to do everything at once, set priorities. If you're not having luck in your job search, take some time to rethink your goals.

- **List your positives.** Make a list of all the things you like about yourself, including skills, personality traits, accomplishments, and successes. Write down projects you're proud of, situations where you excelled, and things you're good at. Revisit this list often to remind yourself of your strengths.

- **Focus on the things you can control.** Rather than wasting your precious energy on things that are out of your hands—like whether you get a follow-up interview—turn your attention to things you can control, such as writing a great cover letter or setting up meetings with your networking contacts.

ecosystem
A community of organisms sharing a physical and chemical environment and interacting with each other.

Environmental Stress

Our beautiful planet faces growing stresses from climate change and global warming.

Ours is a planet under stress. Glaciers are melting; sea levels are rising; forests are being destroyed; droughts have become more frequent and more intense. Heat waves have killed tens of thousands of people; hurricanes and floods have ravaged cities. Millions have died from the effects of air pollution and contaminated water.

The planet Earth—once taken for granted as a ball of rock and water that existed for our use for all time—is a single, fragile **ecosystem** (a community of organisms that share a physical and chemical environment).

Increasingly, we're realizing just how important the health of this ecosystem is to our own well-being and survival. For good or for ill, we cannot separate our individual health from that of the environment in which we live. This, too, can be a source of stress. But while environmental issues may seem overwhelming, the lifestyle choices you make, the products you use, and the efforts you undertake to clean up a beach or save wetlands can make a difference.

✔ **Check-in:** What are your environmental values?

On a scale of 0 to 10, how important are each of the following to you?

Environmental issues	Importance	Degree of involvement
Slowing or stopping global warming	_____	_____
Improving air quality	_____	_____
Reducing pollution	_____	_____
Lowering ozone levels	_____	_____
Saving endangered forests and species	_____	_____
Limiting the need for more landfill	_____	_____
Reducing dependence on carbon fuels such as gasoline	_____	_____
Improving the quality of drinking water	_____	_____
Cleaning lakes, rivers, and seas	_____	_____
Lowering exposure to pesticides and toxic chemicals	_____	_____
Protecting natural wilderness and forests	_____	_____

Beside each of the same items, record a second number on a scale of 0 to 10 for how involved you currently are in taking action on each of the above items, with 0 representing not

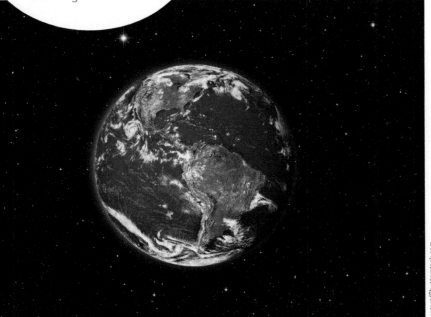

Muratart/Shutterstock.com

involved at all and 10 representing completely, totally, absolutely involved in taking action.

Reflect on your scores and how you see your role and responsibility as a citizen of Planet Earth. Make note of your current level of action regarding each item. Identify at least one step you might take to support your top environmental values.

Climate Change

After years of doubt and debate, leading experts agree that the buildup of greenhouse gases is changing climate and weather patterns in new and potentially dangerous ways. Climate change can imperil health directly—for example, as a result of floods or heat waves—and indirectly—by changing the patterns of infectious diseases, supplies of fresh water, and food availability. As the planet continues to warm, infectious diseases—particularly mosquito-borne illnesses such as malaria, dengue fever, yellow fever, and the zika virus—may spread to more regions.

Why is our planet getting warmer? Figure 11.3 shows the normal greenhouse effect: Certain gases in Earth's atmosphere trap energy from the sun and retain heat somewhat like the glass panels of a greenhouse. Greenhouse gases include carbon dioxide, methane, and nitrous oxide, produced by human activities, livestock, the decomposition of organic wastes, and agricultural and industrial processes. These emissions enhance the normal greenhouse effect, trapping more heat and raising the temperature of the atmosphere and Earth's surface.

✔ **Check-in:** How concerned are you about climate change as a threat to your health? To others on the planet? To the next generation?

Pollution

Any change in the air, water, or soil that could reduce its ability to support life is a form of **pollution**, a potentially deadly hazard. Among the health problems—and stressors—that have been linked with pollution are the following:

- Headaches and dizziness
- Decline in cognitive functioning

pollution Any change in the air, water, or soil that could reduce its ability to support life.

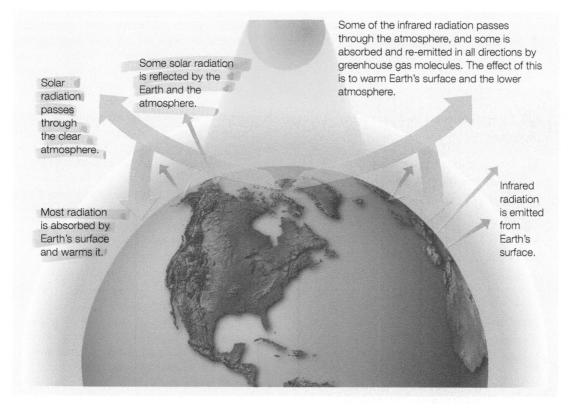

FIGURE 11.3 Greenhouse effect.

- Eye irritation and impaired vision
- Nasal discharge
- Cough, shortness of breath, and sore throat
- Constricted airways
- Constriction of blood vessels and increased risk of heart disease
- Increased risk of stroke and of dying from a stroke
- Chest pains and aggravation of the symptoms of colds, pneumonia, bronchial asthma, emphysema, chronic bronchitis, lung cancer, and other respiratory problems
- Birth defects and reproductive problems including lower success with in-vitro fertilization
- Nausea, vomiting, and stomach cancer
- Allergies and asthma from diesel fumes in polluted air

Remember the last time you stood at a busy intersection and had a bus or truck spew brownish fumes in your face? Maybe your eyes stung or your throat burned. Breathing polluted air can do more than irritate: Health problems linked with pollution include heart disease;[16] headaches and dizziness; decline in cognitive functioning;[17] eye irritation and impaired vision; nasal discharge; cough; shortness of breath; sore throat; aggravation of the symptoms of colds, pneumonia, bronchial asthma, emphysema, chronic bronchitis, and other respiratory problems; nausea; vomiting; and increased risk of cancer.

> **Stress Reliever:** Do Your Part to Reduce Environmental Stress
>
> Buy furniture and household items secondhand, or recycle your parents' things. If you can't find everything you need in the attic or basement, try a website such as www.freecycle.com, where you can barter your way to greener furnishings.
>
> Choose recycled notebooks and printer paper and eco-friendly shampoos, conditioners, and lotions.
>
> Buy a stainless steel or coated aluminum water bottle instead of using disposable ones.
>
> Use green cleaning products like vinegar and baking soda instead of expensive and potentially harmful chemicals.
>
> Tote books and groceries in canvas bags rather than paper or plastic ones.
>
> Don't throw anything out before asking yourself if it can be recycled, donated, or simply used in another way.

Noise

Although you may not think of it in the same way as polluted air or water, noise is a common environmental stressor—and one that may well affect you on a daily basis. The healthy human ear can hear sounds within a wide range of frequencies (measured in hertz), from the low-frequency rumble of thunder at 50 hertz to the high-frequency overtones of a piccolo at nearly 20,000 hertz. High-frequency noise damages the delicate hair cells that serve as sound receptors in the inner ear. Damage first begins as a diminished sensitivity to frequencies around 4,000 hertz, the highest notes of a piano (see Figure 11.4).

Although there is limited research, audiologists (who specialize in hearing problems) report seeing more cases of noise-induced hearing loss in young people. As many as one-quarter of college students may suffer mild hearing loss, including some who believe their hearing was normal. This loss could be the result of use of personal music devices such as MP3 players and extended use of earbuds, the tiny earphones that deliver sound extremely close to the eardrum. Regular use of over-the-counter painkillers also can lead to hearing loss, especially in younger men. Prolonged exposure to loud sounds (the equivalent of a power mower or food blender) or brief exposure to louder sounds, like rock concerts (which can be as loud as an air raid siren) can harm hearing.

✔ **Check-in:** How would you rate your hearing?

The dangers to your hearing depend on how loud the music is and how long you listen. Because personal music players have long-lasting rechargeable batteries, people—especially young ones—both listen for long periods and turn up the volume because they feel "low personal vulnerability" to hearing loss. As long as the sound level is within safety levels you can listen as long as you'd like. If you listen to music so loud that someone else can hear it two or three feet away, it's too loud.

For safe listening, limit listening to a portable music player with earphones or earbuds at 60 percent of its potential volume to one hour a day. At the very least, take a five-minute break after an hour of listening and keep the volume low.

Early symptoms of hearing loss include difficulty understanding speech and *tinnitus* (ringing in the ears). Brief, very loud sounds, such as an explosion or gunfire, can produce immediate, severe, and permanent hearing loss. Longer exposure to less intense but still hazardous sounds, such as those common at work or in public places, can gradually impair hearing, often without the individual's awareness.[18]

🔧 Stress Reliever: How to Protect Your Ears

If you must live or work in a noisy area, wear hearing protectors to prevent exposure to blasts of very loud noise. Don't think cotton or facial tissue stuck in your ears can protect you; foam or soft plastic earplugs are more effective. Wear them when operating lawn mowers, weed trimmers, or power tools.

Give your ears some quiet time. Rather than turning up the volume on your personal music player to blot out noise, look for truly quiet environments, such as the library, where you can rest your ears and focus your mind.

Beware of large doses of aspirin. Researchers have found that eight aspirin tablets a day can aggravate the damage caused by loud noise; twelve a day can cause ringing in the ears (tinnitus).

Don't drink in noisy environments. Alcohol intensifies the impact of noise and increases the risk of lifelong hearing damage.

When you hear a sudden loud noise, press your fingers against your ears. Limit your exposure to loud noise. Several brief periods of noise seem less damaging than one long exposure.

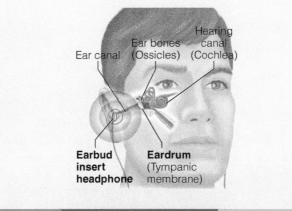

Decibels	Example	Zone
0	The softest sound a typical ear can hear	Safe
10 dB	Just audible	
20 dB	Watch ticking; leaves rustling	
30 dB	Soft whisper at 16 feet	
40 dB	Quiet office; suburban street (no traffic)	
50 dB	Interior of typical urban home; rushing stream	1,000 times louder than 20 dB
60 dB	Normal conversation; busy office	
70 dB	Vacuum cleaner at 10 feet; hair dryer	
80 dB	Alarm clock at 2 feet; loud music; average daily traffic	1,000 times louder than 50 dB
90 dB*	Motorcycle at 25 feet; jet 4 miles after takeoff	Risk of injury
100 dB*	Video arcade; loud factory; subway train	
110 dB*	Car horn at 3 feet; symphony orchestra; chain saw	1,000 times louder than 80 dB
120 dB	Jackhammer at 3 feet; boom box; nearby thunderclap	Injury
130 dB	Rock concert; jet engine at 100 feet	
140 dB	Jet engine nearby; amplified car stereo; firearms	1,000 times louder than 110 dB

FIGURE 11.4 Louder and louder.

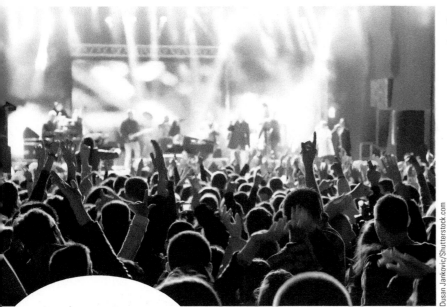

A rock concert can produce sounds louder than a jackhammer or thunder clap.

Dusan Jankovic/Shutterstock.com

Cell Phones

✔ **Check-in:** How much time do you spend on your phone every day?

Since cellular phone service was introduced in the United States in 1984, mobile and handheld phones have become ubiquitous, and concern has grown about their possible health risks. The federal government sets upper exposure limits for exposure to electromagnetic energy from cell phones, known as the specific absorption rate (SAR). A phone emits the most radiation during a call, but it also emits small amounts periodically whenever it's turned on.

More than 70 research papers on the potentially harmful effects of cell phone use have raised concerns about cancer, neurological disorders, sleep problems, or headaches; other studies have shown no association or have been inconclusive. Adverse effects of cell phone use include changes in brain activity, reaction times, and sleep patterns. Drivers using cell phones, whether handheld or hands-free, have a three- to four-times greater chance of an accident because of the distraction. Many states have banned or restricted cell phone use for texting or talking while driving. If you're caught, you could get a citation and a steep fine—additional sources of personal stress.

Researchers have found that a one-hour cell phone conversation stimulates the areas of the brain closest to the phone's antenna, but they do not know if these effects pose any long-term risk. The Food and Drug Administration (FDA) and Federal Communications Commission (FCC) have stated that "the available scientific evidence does not show that any health problems are associated with using wireless phones. There is no proof, however, that wireless phones are absolutely safe." Additional studies are under way.[21]

Chapter Summary

- The time to start developing tools to navigate the work world is sooner rather than later. You need to create a professional-quality resume and master certain skills, such as writing introductory e-mails, preparing for interviews, and making a positive impression on potential employers.

- An estimated 60 percent of college students have jobs. Despite the extra demands on time and energy, earning money while in school pays off in more than dollars and cents.

- Internships not only provide education and experience in a field but also may lead to future opportunities.

- Interview as much as possible, even if the job doesn't sound perfect. Be sure to do your research, practice, give examples of your strengths, and anticipate likely questions.

- Types of employees include engaged or enthusiastic workers; relaxed or 9-to-5 workers; tense or workaholic workers; fatigued workers; and burned-out workers.

- To manage time effectively on a job, create a balanced schedule, don't over-commit yourself, plan regular breaks, and take advantage of time off. To manage your tasks, make a to-do list, prioritize tasks, delegate responsibility, and be willing to compromise.

- Emotional intelligence on the job can draw people to you, overcome differences, repair wounded feelings, and defuse tension and stress. Its major components include

- self-awareness, self-management, body language, and relationship management.

- Occupational stress refers to distress related to any aspect of a job that can take a physical and psychological toll.

- Among the causes of occupational stress is a sense of powerlessness, felt by workers who must constantly respond to others' demands and deadlines with little control over events.

- Workaholics are so caught up in racing toward the top that they forget what they're racing toward and why.

- Employees who care for others—such as health professionals and social worker—may suffer "stress overload," the result of feeling overwhelmed or drained by interactions with others.

- Despite stricter policies banning sexual harassment and discrimination, some companies still tolerate comments and jokes that range from insensitive to upsetting.

- A stressful work place may shorten Americans' lives by up to nearly three years. People with less education are much more likely to end up in jobs with unhealthy workplace practices that cut down on life expectancy.

- Burnout is an extreme state of physical, emotional, and mental exhaustion that occurs when workers or caregivers feel overwhelmed and unable to meet constant demands. It progresses through various stages, from exhaustion to shame and doubt to cynicism and callousness, to failure and crisis, and collapse.

- Workers who have been fired or laid off must deal with the loss of a paid position, a daily routine, and the camaraderie of coworkers as well as the possible loss of the ability to support themselves and their possibilities.

- We cannot separate our individual health from that of the environment in which we live. But while environmental issues may seem overwhelming, individuals can make a difference.

- Noise is a common environmental stressor that can result in hearing loss. Among the dangers to young people are prolonged use of earbuds to listen to music and extremely loud rock music concerts.

- The potentially harmful effects of cell phone use include changes in brain activity, reaction times, and sleep patterns. While the available scientific evidence does not confirm any health problems associated with wireless phones, there is no proof that they are safe.

🔧 STRESS RELIEVERS

Energy Burst
If you can feel your body tensing up, go to a private place. Pretend you're a boxer, and throw punches into the air. Try some karate kicks forward, backward, and to each side. If you're out of hearing distance, grunting intensifies the feeling of relief.

Put a Workplace Problem in Perspective
Ask yourself:

_____ Is it really worth getting upset over?
_____ Is it worth upsetting others?
_____ Is it that important?
_____ Is it that bad?
_____ Is the situation irreparable?
_____ Is it really your problem?

Do Your Part to Reduce Environmental Stress

- Buy furniture and household items secondhand, or recycle your parents' things. If you can't find everything you need in the attic or basement, try a website such as www.freecycle.com, where you can barter your way to greener furnishings.

- Choose recycled notebooks and printer paper and eco-friendly shampoos, conditioners, and lotions.

- Buy a stainless steel or coated aluminum water bottle instead of using disposable ones.

- Use green cleaning products like vinegar and baking soda instead of expensive and potentially harmful chemicals.

- Tote books and groceries in canvas bags rather than paper or plastic ones.

- Don't throw anything out before asking yourself if it can be recycled, donated, or simply used in another way.

How to Protect Your Ears

- **If you must live or work in a noisy area, wear hearing protectors to prevent exposure to blasts of very loud noise.** Don't think cotton or facial tissue stuck in your ears can protect you; foam or soft plastic earplugs are more effective. Wear them when operating lawn mowers, weed trimmers, or power tools.

- **Give your ears some quiet time.** Rather than turning up the volume on your personal music player to blot out noise, look for truly quiet environments, such as the library, where you can rest your ears and focus your mind.

- **Beware of large doses of aspirin.** Researchers have found that eight aspirin tablets a day can aggravate the damage caused by loud noise; twelve a day can cause ringing in the ears (tinnitus).

- **Don't drink in noisy environments.** Alcohol intensifies the impact of noise and increases the risk of lifelong hearing damage.

- **When you hear a sudden loud noise, press your fingers against your ears.** Limit your exposure to loud noise. Several brief periods of noise seem less damaging than one long exposure.

⊜ YOUR PERSONAL STRESS MANAGEMENT TOOLKIT

REFLECTION: How Green Is Your Lifestyle?

Check each of the following things that you do on a regular basis:

_____ I buy products packaged simply in recycled or recyclable materials.

_____ I recycle all paper, aluminum, and plastic products by putting them in the appropriate bins.

_____ I bring my own tote bag when I go to a grocery.

_____ I reuse paper or plastic bags.

_____ I turn off all electrical appliances (TVs, CD and MP3 players, iPods, lights, printers, etc.). when I am not in the room or paying attention to them.

_____ I limit use of disposables such as paper napkins and plastic utensils.

_____ I donate discarded computers, cell phones, and other electronic devices to schools or a charitable organization.

_____ I wash my laundry in cold or warm, not hot water.

_____ I drink tap water rather than bottled water.

_____ I conserve water by turning off the tap while shampooing or brushing my teeth.

_____ I use typing and copy paper on both sides.

_____ I refill or recycle ink cartridges for a printer rather than buying new ones.

_____ I don't use aerosol or spray containers for deodorants, hairspray, and so on.

_____ I use a glass or mug rather than Styrofoam or plastic containers for beverages.

_____ I turn down the thermostat to use less fuel for heat in the winter and turn it up in the summer.

_____ I walk, bike, carpool, or take public or campus transportation rather than drive whenever possible.

_____ I drive a car with high mileage and fuel efficiency and keep it well maintained to reduce emissions.

_____ I turn off the engine if stopped for more than a minute.

_____ I pay attention to local environmental issues and vote, sign petitions, or e-mail or write legislators in support of measures to protect or clean up the environment.

Review your responses. Which behaviors could you improve?

TECHNIQUE: Instant Stress Relievers to Go

Wherever you go—to work, to class, to hike or bike or drive—you can find stress. That's why it's good to have some take-anywhere stress relievers to provide stress relief when you need it most. Try some of the following:

In a classroom, office, or meeting:

- During stressful moments, focus on your breath. Inhale deeply, and exhale slowly.

- Massage the tips of your fingers with your thumbs.

- Wiggle your toes.

- Check your posture. Straighten your spine. Lift your chin. Drop your shoulders.

- Sit near a window if you can, and periodically gaze at the view.

- Give yourself a quick hand massage.

On the phone:

- Pace back and forth to burn off excess energy.

- Conduct private conversations in solitary places—preferably outside or with a view you can look at.

- Inhale an energizing scent (that you carry with you in a small packet or vial) such as lemon, ginger, peppermint, or coffee.

- Rub your fingers over something soft and comforting: a silky scarf, a soft blanket, a furry pet, a stuffed animal.

At the computer:

- Try standing at an elevated table or desk.

- Every 10 minutes, do some knee bends, toe lifts, ankle circles, shoulder shrugs.

- Suck on a peppermint or chew sugarless gum (unless you have TMJ) to release tension in your jaw.

- Display images of people and places you love as your screen saver.

- Squeeze a rubbery ball to relieve tension and prevent strain.

In your room:

- Bring the outside indoors with a plant or fresh flowers.

- Surround yourself with colors that lift your spirits.

- Sing or hum a favorite tune.

- Use a white noise app to block out noisy neighbors or street sounds.

- Light a scented candle or use a scent infuser.

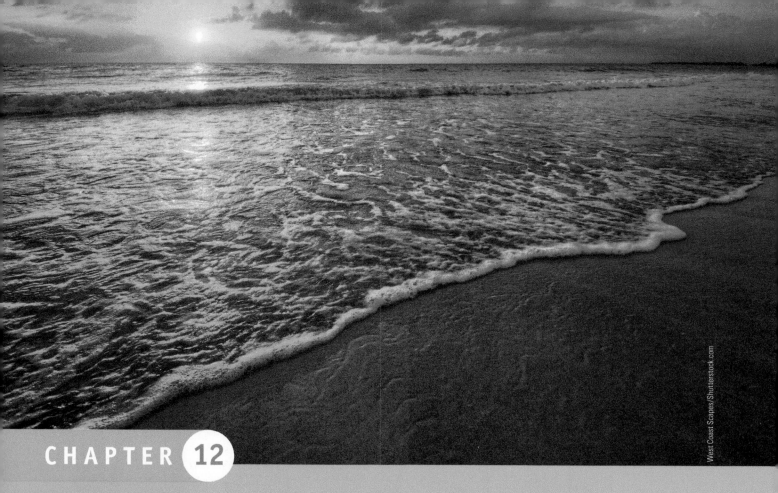

CHAPTER 12

Breathing, Relaxation, and Guided Imagery

After reading this chapter, you should be able to:

12.1 Describe the impact of breathing on stress.

12.2 Discuss the use of guided imagery as a strategy to reduce stress.

12.3 Evaluate the relationship between relaxation and stress relief.

_____ Breathe as you usually do, but place one hand on your chest and the other on your abdomen.

_____ After a few moments, direct attention to the feeling of the air as it enters and leaves your body. Notice how it feels in your nose or mouth.

_____ Direct attention to your hands while continuing to breathe as you normally do. Notice where your body expands with each inhalation of air.

If you feel your chest expand, your default mode of breathing is chest breathing. If you feel your stomach area expand, it is diaphragmatic or abdominal breathing. This chapter explains the differences between the two and the importance of breathing for stress reduction.

Life begins with a breath. The simple act of inhaling and exhaling air accompanies every minute of our time on Earth. As we breathe in, oxygen fills our lungs and travels through the blood vessels to energize our bodies. As we breathe out, we cleanse ourselves of the waste product carbon dioxide.

Breathing can do more than keep you alive. By monitoring, controlling, and directing the flow of air into and out of your lungs, you can progress from a state of stress to its physiological opposite—deep relaxation. Since it is impossible to be both relaxed and stressed at the same time, relaxation is a powerful tool for countering the wear and tear of daily life. Rather than gearing up for fight or flight, the relaxed body grows calmer and works more smoothly.[1] Adding vivid guided imagery takes relaxation to another dimension by enabling the mind to shift its focus from ceaseless fretting.

Breathing, relaxation, and imagery have proven effective in easing stress, depression, and anxiety and in enhancing overall well-being.[2] If you are tense or tired, worried or weary, the exercises in this chapter will release residual tension you may carry without even realizing and renew your spirit. We urge you to try several techniques. You may find one that helps you most, or you may prefer to incorporate a variety into your daily routine.

✔ **Check-in:** Just breathe.

Without changing anything about your breathing, notice which parts of your body move with each inhale and exhale. Focus on each inhale and exhale for several breaths. When your mind wanders, return to monitoring your breath and your body.

Breathing

Breathing, the process of transporting and exchanging oxygen and carbon dioxide, is essential to sustain life. You don't need to think about breathing. Just as your heart beats even when you're asleep or unconscious, your body breathes for you. But unlike your heartbeat, you can control your breathing, making it voluntary rather than automatic. This section describes various approaches to controlling your breathing in ways that enhance the flow of gases to and from your body and relieve many stress-related symptoms.

Understanding Breathing

A breath begins in the nose, which draws in air, warms it to body temperature, humidifies, and partially cleanses it. Air then travels down the trachea to the lungs. Like a tree, each lung has many branches, called bronchial tubes, that carry air to the **alveoli**, elastic air sacs that expand when air is inhaled and contract when it is exhaled. (See Figure 12.1.)

The small blood vessels called **capillaries** that surround the alveoli receive oxygen and carry it to the heart, which pumps oxygenated blood to all parts of the body. Blood cells receive oxygen and release carbon dioxide, which travels back to the heart and lungs. The **diaphragm**, the muscle that separates the lungs and the abdomen, contracts and relaxes as you breathe in and out.

The two major types of breathing patterns are **chest or thoracic breathing** and **diaphragmatic or abdominal breathing** (sometimes called "belly breathing"). Although you don't

alveoli Elastic air sacs in the lungs that expand when air is inhaled and contract when it is exhaled.

capillaries Small blood vessels surrounding the alveoli that receive oxygen and carry it to the heart.

diaphragm The muscle separating the lungs and the abdomen that contracts and relaxes as you breathe in and out.

chest or thoracic breathing A shallow breathing pattern, in which the chest expands and the shoulders rise with every inhalation, that delivers less oxygen to the heart and lungs.

diaphragmatic or abdominal breathing A breathing pattern that draws air deep into the lungs as the abdominal cavity expands and the diaphragm contracts downward. Deeper and slower than chest breathing, it enhances the flow of energizing oxygen.

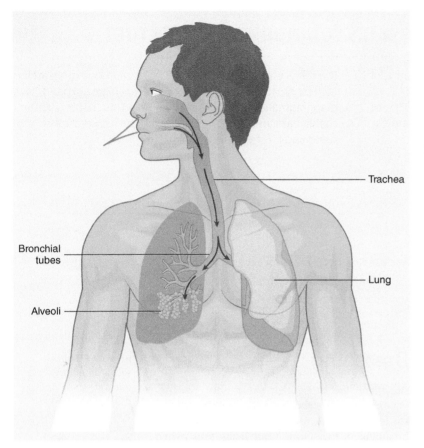

FIGURE 12.1 The anatomy of a breath. Each breath carries oxygen through the nose and trachea into the lungs.

Athletes practice deep diaphragmatic breathing to increase stamina and enhance performance.

actually breathe in your abdomen, its movements are a key to releasing your diaphragm.

In thoracic breathing, the chest expands and the shoulders rise with every inhalation. Because chest breathing is shallow, the body receives less

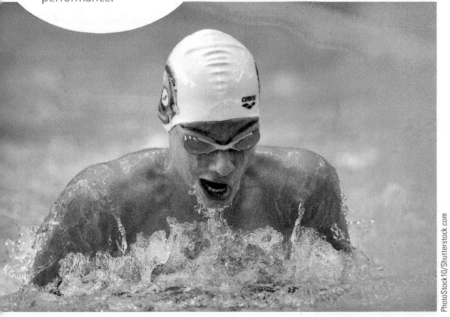

oxygen, and carbon dioxide builds up, causing feelings of fatigue. During the stress response (see Chapter 2), rapid, irregular chest breathing can produce symptoms such as light-headedness, shortness of breath, heart palpitations, weakness, numbness, tingling, and **hyperventilation** (extremely rapid and shallow breathing).

Diaphragmatic breathing draws air deep into the lungs as the abdominal cavity expands and the diaphragm contracts downward. When exhaling, the diaphragm relaxes, pushing up into the lungs and expelling air. This breathing pattern, deeper and slower than chest breathing, enhances the respiratory system's ability to do its job of producing energy from oxygen and removing carbon dioxide.

As breathing becomes more rhythmic, the number of inhalations and exhalations per minute decreases. Diaphragmatic breathing also reduces the activity of the sympathetic nervous system, the branch of the autonomic nervous system responsible for initiating the fight-or-flight response.

We automatically engage in abdominal breathing when we sleep. Athletes, singers, and dancers consciously practice abdominal breathing to maintain stamina and perform at their best.

Stress Reliever: How to "Belly Breathe"

Close your eyes, lean back in your seat or lie down, and place one hand on your stomach area.

Take a deep breath in through your nose and slowly exhale through your mouth.

As you inhale, visualize that you are filling a balloon in your belly.

With each exhale, notice how your diaphragm contracts. Visualize yourself exhaling stress and/or tension along with your breath. Pay attention to how your diaphragm contracts to expel these things.

The Benefits of Diaphragmatic Breathing

Diaphragmatic breathing is a relaxation technique in itself as well as a key component of practices such as progressive muscle relaxation (PMR), discussed later in this chapter, and autogenics, discussed in Chapter 14 (see Figure 12.2). Deep rhythmic breathing, used along with other

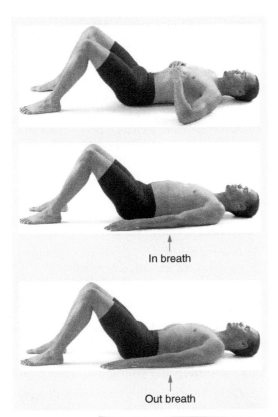

In breath

Out breath

FIGURE 12.2 Diaphragmatic or belly breathing. Begin by exhaling forcefully. As you inhale through your nose, feel your abdominal cavity expand with air. Exhale slowly through your mouth. Repeat.

techniques, has proven effective in relieving a variety of psychological and physical problems. Its benefits include:

- Cooling off anger
- Lifting feelings of depression
- Lowering anxiety in people with generalized anxiety or panic attacks[3]
- Improving sleep
- Relieving muscle tension and pain

What You Need to Know

You will need a quiet and private place for your breathing exercises. If you share a room or an apartment, you might work around your roommates' schedules or ask them to respect your need for quiet, uninterrupted time alone. If you live at home, explain your assignment to your family so they won't interrupt.

As you practice diaphragmatic breathing, you can incorporate other stress-relieving strategies, such as mental imagery, positive self-talk, or mantras. Here are some exercises for you to try:

Introductory Breathing Exercise

Listen to the audio instructions on MindTap, record yourself reading them, or pair up with a classmate and take turns leading each other through this exercise.

1. Choose a time and place where you will not be disturbed. Turn off cell phones, laptops, or any other device that may interrupt this calming exercise.

2. Sit comfortably, with your eyes closed and your spine reasonably straight. Place one hand gently on your abdomen.

3. Bring your attention to your breathing. Press your hand down on your abdomen as you exhale forcefully.

4. Let your abdomen push up against your hand as your inhale.

5. As you slowly inhale and exhale, pay close attention as each inhalation brings air first into your abdomen, then your middle chest, and finally your upper chest. Imagine filling a glass with water from bottom to top as you inhale.

6. Once you establish a pattern of smooth deep breaths, you can slow your breath even more. Inhale through your nostrils and exhale through your mouth as if you were breathing out through a straw. With each breath, feel your abdomen lower and rise.

7. Focus on the sound of your breaths as you become increasingly relaxed.

8. If thoughts or feelings enter your consciousness, take note of their arrival and then return to focusing on your breathing.

9. Repeat this basic breathing exercise for about five or ten minutes once or twice a day. Gradually extend your time to fifteen and then twenty minutes.

Nasal Switching or Alternate-Nostril Breathing

In this exercise you use your breathing to access your whole brain—the right, or "feeling" hemisphere and the left, or "thinking" hemisphere. It also is an excellent preparatory step for meditation and mindfulness exercises.

1. Sit in a comfortable position, with your spine erect and shoulders relaxed.

2. You can simply close your right nostril by pressing your thumb against it, and inhale through your left nostril. Try a few shallow breaths that bring air into your chest. Then inhale as deeply as you can, slowly and soundlessly, through your left nostril. Exhale

hyperventilation
Extremely rapid and shallow breathing.

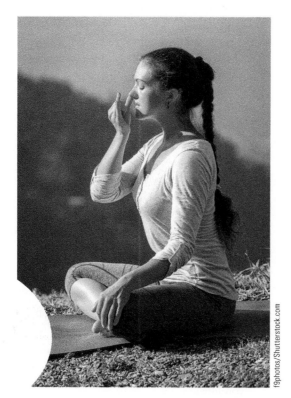

In nasal switching, you alternately block one nostril and breathe from the other.

f9photos/Shutterstock.com

as thoroughly as possible. Then switch, and block your left nostril as you inhale and exhale through your right nostril.

3. Yoga practitioners include alternate-nostril breathing in their breathing practices, discussed on page 235, but with a different hand position: Place the tip of your index finger and the middle finger of your right hand in between the eyebrows, the ring finger and little finger on the left nostril, and the thumb on the right nostril (see the following figure). Use the ring finger and little finger to close the left nostril and the thumb for the right nostril.

4. Press your thumb on the right nostril and breathe out gently through the left nostril.

5. After a few breaths, breathe in from the left nostril and then press the left nostril gently with the ring finger and little finger.

6. Remove your right thumb from your right nostril, and breathe out from the right.

7. Breathe in from the right nostril and exhale from the left. Continue inhaling and exhaling from alternate nostrils.

8. After every exhalation, remember to breathe in from the same nostril from which you exhaled.

9. Keep your eyes closed and continue taking long, deep, smooth breaths without any force or effort.

Controlled Breathing

1. Sit quietly in a room and focus on your breathing.

2. Take five slow, deep breaths, pulling air down into your lower abdomen. Concentrate on your breathing. If thoughts come into your mind, such as "I better check my messages," brush them aside and refocus on the rhythm of your breathing.

3. As you breathe in, let your belly rise, and picture yourself inhaling warm, soothing air.

4. As you breathe out, let your belly fall, and visualize yourself exhaling.

5. Imagine that you are gently rocking a baby as your belly extends and recedes.

6. Feel your diaphragm descend then lift as you count up to thirty.

Whenever stress builds, this technique can also serve as a quick antidote.

Diaphragmatic Breathing with Pelvic Tilt

1. Lie on your back on a firm but comfortable surface, such as a folded thick blanket on the floor. Bend your knees at a 90-degree angle. They should be slightly apart, about the same width as your hips.

2. Place your hands over your lower rib cage so your little fingers are just below your lowest rib. Rest your elbows on the floor.

3. Close your eyes.

4. Inhale, sending your breath under your hands. Feel your belly puff up toward the ceiling as you inhale and drop toward the floor as you exhale.

5. Take several deep controlled breaths. Your belly will puff out with each inhalation and drop toward the floor with each exhalation.

6. As you exhale, rock your pelvis so that the waistline part of your back drops toward the floor. Your lower back may even touch the floor as you complete your exhalation.

7. As you inhale, let your pelvis rock back to where it came from, and your lower back will arch slightly upwards, to its prior position.

8. Don't press into the floor with your feet in order to rock your pelvis. Let your legs rest, your feet relaxing into the floor. The muscle action that creates this movement is only in your abdomen. Your back, buttocks, and legs stay relaxed.

9. Continue this breath/movement, tipping your pelvis as you exhale so your lower

back descends toward the floor, and releasing this effort as you inhale so your pelvis untilts; that is, it returns to its "neutral" position, as does your back.

10. Continue for five to ten minutes. When your mind wanders to a thought, just bring it back to what you are doing.

11. To finish, end your control of your breath and return to autonomic, effortless breathing, noticing how this transition feels.

Counting or Bedtime Breathing

This form of diaphragmatic breathing uses counting to focus your mind. Although it can be performed at any time, it is especially useful in relaxing your body and clearing your mind before sleep.

1. Get into a comfortable position, and close your eyes.

2. Pay attention to your abdominal area as you take slow, deep, relaxing, diaphragmatic breaths. Continue to inhale and exhale while counting backwards from 100. Once you reach 0, pause, and slowly exhale.

3. Repeat this cycle. If your mind wanders, notice the thought but redirect your focus back to your breathing.

4. With each breath cycle, feel your body become more relaxed.

5. You also can experiment with counting during breaths: Inhale to a count of three, pause, then exhale to the count of three.

6. After a few breathing cycles, picture your body and mind beginning to relax. Inhale to the count of four, pause, and exhale to the count of four, picturing yourself relaxing more and more.

7. Repeat this cycle with increasing counts for each inhalation and exhalation. As you count to a bigger number, your average breaths per minute will decrease, and you will feel more relaxed and calm.

Breathing for Pain Relief

If you suffer from headaches, backaches, or other forms of chronic pain, use this exercise along with your doctor's prescribed treatments.

1. Close your eyes, and get comfortable.

2. Breathe deeply with your diaphragm to fill your abdominal area with air.

3. Visualize yourself gaining nourishment or strength with each inhalation.

4. Expel all the air from your body. As you do, imagine that you are exhaling your pain and stress.

5. To reinforce this image, add a mantra, such as "I am letting go" or "I am releasing my pain."

Yogic Breathing

Many people associate yoga with postures that stretch, strengthen, and relax the muscles (see Chapter 14 for a full description). However, another important component is **yogic breathing** (called **pranayama** in Sanskrit), which help energize the body, quiet the mind, and clarify perception.[4]

Yogic breathing practices include slowing your breaths, making inhalations and exhalations even, and holding your breath briefly during each cycle as a way of stopping mental turmoil. The best way to learn yogic breathing and postures is from a teacher. However, you can experiment with yogic breathing on your own. Keep these basic principles in mind:

- Don't strain or make an all-out effort. Breathe with ease—and precision.

- Stop if you feel dizzy or uncomfortable. Try again later or the next day.

- Keep some of your attention on relaxing, especially the muscles that aren't involved in breathing, such as your lower jaw, arms, shoulders, and legs.

- Don't hold your breath for more than a brief pause.

yogic breathing Breathing practices such as slowing down breathing, making inhalations and exhalations even, then holding the breath briefly during each cycle; used along with yoga postures. Also called **pranayama**.

pranayama The Sanskrit term for yogic breathing practices.

You can practice breathing exercises in any quiet, relaxing place.

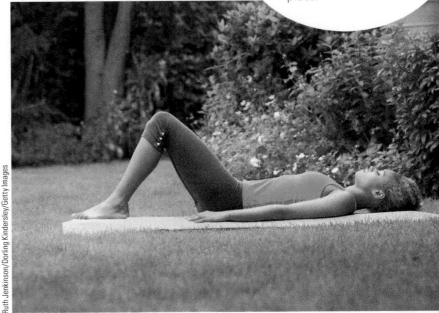
Ruth Jenkinson/Dorling Kindersley/Getty Images

The following breath awareness exercise is a good introduction to yogic breathing:

1. Lie on a firm yet comfortable surface, such as a thick blanket folded in half. You can bend your knees or straighten your legs. If bent, your knees and feet should be slightly apart, about the same as the width of your hips. If your legs are straight, they should be comfortable close together.

2. Rest your arms on the floor at your sides or bend your elbows a bit and rest your hands on your hips or upper thighs.

3. Close your eyes. Bring your attention to the sensations of heaviest where your body presses into the floor. Let the floor support your head, back, buttocks, legs, and arm.

4. After a few minutes, sift your attention to your breathing. Feel your belly, chest, and back moving in rhythm with your breath.

5. Continue this focus for a while and then explore the sensations made by your moving breath. Feel the rush of air past your nostrils, into your throat, down into your chest. Notice that the air is cool when entering your body and warm when leaving it. Feel the swelling of your belly as you inhale.

6. Notice the sensations in the muscles at the base of your ribs, in your mid-chest, in your back, in your shoulders and neck. Feel your muscles as you both inhale and exhale.

7. Even as you notice the feelings in other parts of your body, keep your attention on some sensation of breathing. If your mind wanders, gently guide your focus back to your breathing. This may happen over and over. That's fine; just keep doing back to your breath.

8. After five to ten minutes, take some purposeful deep breathes, stretch your arms and legs, and then roll onto your side. After a few seconds, slowly sit up.

Do not feel frustrated if you repeatedly lose focus. Return again and again to your breath, and notice that when you are really engrossed in a breath, your mind stops its usual chatter. Even though it may happen only for a second, this quieting slows your breathing and calms your mind.

Visualization Breathing

This is good preparation for the guided imagery exercises described on page 240–241.

1. Close your eyes, and get comfortable.

2. Breathe deeply in and out.

3. Choose a color you associate with strength or healing to represent the air coming into your body. Imagine this color nourishing and calming your body and mind.

4. Pause before exhaling, and visualize this color changing within your body as it energizes you and absorbs your stress.

5. As you slowly exhale, imagine the transformed color leaving your body and carrying with it your worries.

6. As you are expelling your stress, imagine your muscles loosening, and say to yourself "I am relaxed" or "I am at peace."

7. Repeat this cycle, visualizing the positive, healthful colored air entering your body, transforming into a different color as it heals you, and taking away bits of your stress with each exhalation.

✔ **Check-in:** Take a breath.

As you practice these breathing exercises, ask yourself:

What am I feeling?

Does the experience differ from what I expected? If so, how?

How would you describe what you feel to someone else?

Do different breathing exercises produce different sensations?

Guided Imagery

Imagine that you are holding an apple. How does it feel in your hand? What color is its skin? Is it shiny? Lift it to your mouth and take a bite. Can you hear the crunch? How does it taste? How do the sensations in your mouth change as you chew and swallow? Although you may not be aware of it, you probably salivated a bit as you added vivid details to your imaginary snack. The reason is that our bodies respond to mental images and sensations almost as if they were real.

This concept is fundamental to **visualization** and **guided imagery**. Although the terms are often used interchangeably, visualization, as its name implies, uses the imagination to "see" a place, person, or object in your mind. Guided imagery is a program of directed suggestions that involve all the senses—sounds, tastes, smells, textures, sights. Considered a relaxation technique, a meditation exercise, and a form of self-hypnosis,

visualization Use of the imagination to "see" a place, person, or object in your mind.

guided imagery A program of directed suggestions that involve all the senses—sounds, tastes, smells, textures, sights—to relax the body, promote healing, or improve performance.

guided imagery is especially effective in reducing stress because it involves body, mind, senses, and emotions.

Understanding Guided Imagery

Your mind constantly cues or directs your body to respond in certain ways. Think of a cherished pet, and you may smile. Hear a certain song, and you may get tears in your eyes as you remember listening to it with someone who is no longer in your life.

Guided imagery takes full advantage of this mind-body connection to transport you deep into the unconscious. It is most effective when you choose images that you find meaningful. If you listen to an audio of instructions, your imagination will automatically edit and change the script by conjuring images that are unique to your life experience.

Guided imagery changes your brain waves and biochemistry in ways that enhance intuition and creativity. Freed from the limits of logic, you can do things in this altered state that would be impossible in real life, such as soaring among the stars or floating on a cloud. As you concentrate fully on an imagined scene, you become less aware of your actual surroundings. You become calm and in control, a feeling that boosts self-esteem and optimism as it lowers anxiety and stress.

Even while sitting on a crowded bus, you can take yourself on an imaginary journey to a lush tropical island and relax. Because your unconscious doesn't know the difference between something real and something imagined, it responds physiologically as if you were really in that place. Your fellow passengers will never guess why you're smiling despite the bustle around you.

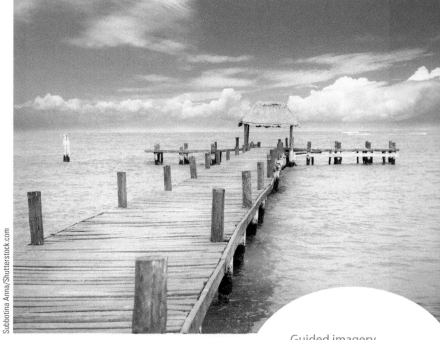

Subbotina Anna/Shutterstock.com

Guided imagery allows your mind to travel to beautiful, peaceful places where you can fully relax.

Sponge: Imagine that your body is a sponge in a pool of very warm water. As you breathe in, your body soaks up the warm water, and as you breathe out, the warm water saturates your body sponge. As you continue, your body becomes warmer and warmer and softer and softer.

 Stress Reliever: Soothing Images

Waves: With each inhalation, imagine a wave cresting just above your belly button, and with each exhalation imagine the wave washing away tension from every muscle in your body.

Colors: Imagine that you are breathing in air that is rich with a color that soothes you. With each exhalation, the air you breathe out is a little lighter. The soothing color fills your whole body, getting deeper and richer with each inhalation.

The Benefits of Guided Imagery

Guided imagery has proven helpful in the treatment of many medical problems, including headaches, asthma, and hypertension, and in promoting healing after surgery. In research studies, cancer patients who imagined their immune system devouring vulnerable cancer cells reported relief from the side-effects of chemotherapy, lower anxiety and pain, and a greater sense of control.[5] Imagery reduces blood loss during surgery, lowers blood pressure and cholesterol levels, and heightens short-term immune activity.

The simple act of imagining a peaceful place decreases arousal of the stimulating branch of the nervous system that triggers the stress response. By freeing your mind to think outside the box, imagery can lead to creative solutions to problems. Adding music to imaging sessions can enhance their positive impact on well-being, mood, and physical stress.[6] (See Chapter 15 for more on music therapy.)

Mental rehearsal, another imaging technique, lowers stress by improving confidence and positive thinking. A quarterback may pause for a second to visualize his pass soaring toward a receiver in the end zone. A ballerina may see every intricate gesture of a *pas de deux* as the curtain rises. Students who imagine themselves preparing for a test, sitting down, completing the exam with confidence, and getting a good grade report feeling calmer during a test and better able to remember the information they studied.

 Stress Reliever: Take a Screenshot

The next time you're about to engage in a situation that is stressful to you:

Conjure a snapshot image of it going the way you'd like it to turn out.

Take mental note of the parts of the situation that you have control over.

Encourage yourself through self-talk, such as "I'm going to ace this."

Imagine the result, such as going on line to check your grade and seeing an A.

Take a few minutes and write or share how you felt during this exercise and afterward.

What You Need to Know

All you really need to try this technique is imagination. Find a quiet place, make yourself comfortable in a sitting position, shut off any source of distraction, and block off as much time as your schedule allows. If you're dubious about this technique, just relax and give it a chance.

Free your imagination to conjure anything and everything, possible or impossible. There are no barriers or limits. Enjoy the experience; play with ideas and images; dare to imagine big, bold scenes; let symbols or pictures bubble up from your unconscious. Don't critique them or worry what others might think about them.

Images are most effective if they reflect your convictions and values. Add as many details and sensations as possible to make them come alive. Be sure to put yourself in the picture rather than observing as if you were watching a film or play. Tap into your feelings; if you become upset or sad, accept this emotional response as a sign that the images are working at a deep level of your unconscious mind.

Use the same posture—such as sitting with your head back and your hands in your lap—every time you practice guided imagery. This physical cue provides an anchor that signals your body to respond the way it has in previous sessions. If your mind wanders, don't worry. Simply make your way back to your imaginary place. You can combine guided imagery with other relaxation techniques, such as breathing or massage.

At the end of a session, give yourself time to travel back to the real world. Remain seated, and breathe deeply for several minutes.

Introductory Guided Imagery Exercise

Guided imagery is a skill that anyone can develop with practice. You can record the following basic steps and play back the instructions or team up with a partner and take turns reading them:

1. Close your eyes. Roll your eyeballs inward and upward as if you were trying to look at your own forehead (this practice in itself may alter brain wave activity).

2. Let an imaginary scene appear in your mind. Some people create a sandy beach on a perfect summer day; others walk through leafy forests, climb mountain peaks, or sail across a deep blue sea. Choose where you want to go in your mind.

3. If your imaginary scene is fuzzy or incomplete, concentrate more intently and ask, "What is this?" Keep focusing, and watch whatever appears in your imagination. The more details that you can include in your imagined scene, the easier it will be to relax.

4. You can fill in more details by asking questions such as: What is the temperature at the scene? What colors does it contain? What sounds are present? What movements are occurring?

5. Outline the images as if you were tracing them with a pencil. Concentrate on the colors. Are they vivid or muted? Is there a source of light? Where does it fall? Are there shadows? Is the wind blowing? What does the air smell like? If you are sitting or lying down, how does your body feel against the ground?

6. Think of yourself running your fingers over various objects and making note of how they feel to your touch.

7. From what perspective are you viewing the scene? Are you an outsider looking in? If so, shift your perspective so that you are looking at whatever you would view if you were in the scene. Rather than seeing

yourself floating on a tranquil pond, shift your perspective so that you are looking up at the sky and feeling the water buoying up your body.

8. If you're on a beach, feel the white sand beneath your toes; smell the salty air; lift your face to the warmth of the sun; listen to the water lapping the shore. Each time the breeze picks up, feel your muscles become more and more relaxed. Watch each wave as it rises and falls onto the shore.

9. As you inhabit this imaginary scene, let feelings of ease and happiness spread from head to toe. Feel your heart rate and breathing slow.

10. Relax for as long as your schedule allows. Gradually open your eyes. Take a deep breath. As you stretch and slowly stand, bask in the feeling of being at ease and in control.

As with other mind-based practices, your ability to create images get stronger with practice. Set aside time every day to imagine yourself in another place. If your shuttle bus gets caught in traffic, close your eyes and take yourself on a mini-vacation.

....
✔ **Check-in:** Pause and reflect.
....

As you finish your guided imagery exercise, take a moment to tune in to your feelings: Is your mind less cluttered? Do you feel more focused? How does your body feel? How would you rate the tension in your muscles? Do you feel differently than you did after the breathing exercises? If so, what is different?
....

Relaxation

Chill; lighten up; take five; calm down. Whatever the words and phrases, you've probably been told to relax. It's good advice, since your body and mind crave balance and calm. However, you can't achieve this degree of relaxation simply by streaming videos or playing computer games.

Relaxation, in the clinical sense, is a process of letting go of the residual stress that builds up, often without notice, in our muscles and our minds. With regular practice, relaxation techniques can prevent stress overload and help restore health and wholeness. Relaxation is an important component of many other stress-relieving practices, including meditation, massage, hypnosis, yoga, and t'ai chi.

Understanding Relaxation

The word "relax" comes from the Latin *relaxare*, meaning "to loosen." This is exactly what happens during relaxation. When you have a stressful thought, muscles in your body tense. This tension, in turn, increases anxiety. Relaxation exercises break this cycle of tension and stress.

Many people cannot consciously relax their muscles completely. However, when deliberately tensed in a step-by-step, systematic process, muscles become exhausted and automatically relax, which helps other internal organs relax and lowers your overall stress level. "Active" forms of relaxation involve muscle tensing followed by release; "passive" forms consist of focusing on a muscle or muscle group and simply letting go of any tension.

As described in Chapter 1, the stress response activates the sympathetic nervous system and increases epinephrine and norepinephrine, which speed oxygenated, nutrient-rich blood to the skeletal muscles. Relaxation targets the parasympathetic nervous system, which releases **acetylcholine**, a neurotransmitter (chemical messenger) that decreases metabolic activity and returns the body to homeostasis. While the sympathetic nervous system acts like a gas pedal pressed to the floor, revving your body for action during, the parasympathetic nervous system, responding to relaxation techniques, serves as a brake.

The Benefits of Relaxation

Relaxation counters the harmful effects of stress throughout the body.[7] See Figure 12.3. Stress speeds up your heart rate; relaxation slows it.

relaxation A process of letting go of the residual stress that builds up in our muscles and our minds.

acetylcholine A neurotransmitter that decreases metabolic activity and returns the body to homeostasis.

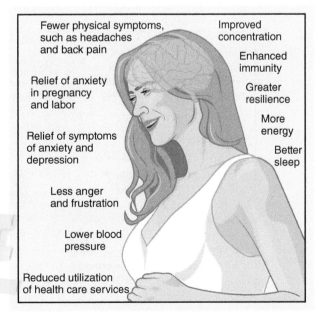

Fewer physical symptoms, such as headaches and back pain

Improved concentration

Enhanced immunity

Relief of anxiety in pregnancy and labor

Greater resilience

More energy

Relief of symptoms of anxiety and depression

Better sleep

Less anger and frustration

Lower blood pressure

Reduced utilization of health care services

FIGURE 12.3 Relaxation provides immediate and long term benefits for your mental and physical health.

Stress raises blood pressure; relaxation lowers it. Stress makes you breathe more rapidly; relaxation slows your breathing. Stress tightens muscles; relaxation releases them. The long-term practice of regular relaxation activities can also change the expression of genes that control the body's response to stress and trauma.[8]

Among the other health dividends of relaxation techniques:

- Fewer physical symptoms, such as headaches and back pain
- Relief of post-menopausal symptoms
- Relief of anxiety in pregnancy and labor[9]
- Less anger and frustration
- More energy
- Improved concentration
- Enhanced immunity
- Better sleep
- Lower blood pressure
- Relief of symptoms of anxiety and depression
- Greater resilience[10]
- Reduced utilization of healthcare services[11]

Among college students, even a shortened PMR exercise has proved beneficial in increasing physical and mental relaxation and lowering anxiety and levels of the stress hormone cortisol.[12]

What You Need to Know

Deliberate, systematic relaxation is a skill that anyone can master with regular practice. As you learn relaxation techniques, you'll become more aware of muscle tension and other physical sensations of stress. Once you recognize these feelings, you can make a conscious effort to employ a relaxation technique the moment your muscles start to tense. This can prevent stress from intensifying.

There are countless routes to relaxation, but most share certain common characteristics:

- A quiet environment
- A mental device to focus your attention
- A passive, accepting attitude
- A comfortable position

Caution: Some people, especially those with mental disorders or a history of being abused, may experience feelings of emotional discomfort during relaxation exercises. Although this is rare, if relaxation exercises produce distressing feelings, stop what you're doing. You may want to consider talking to a mental health professional about your reaction.

Progressive Muscle Relaxation (PMR)

Progressive or deep muscle relaxation (PMR) involves a physical component—usually the tensing and relaxing of various muscle groups in the body in a sequential pattern—and a mental component—focusing on the distinction between the feelings of tension and relaxation (see Figure 12.4). A physician named Edmund Jacobson developed PMR in the early 1920s to help patients relax their muscles before surgery so they would respond better and recover more quickly. Since muscle tension accompanies

progressive muscle relaxation (PMR) Alternate tensing and relaxing of various muscle groups in the body.

Progressive Muscle Relaxation

1. Tense **face muscles** including forehead, cheeks, mouth, upper neck. Release.

2. Gently **roll head** from side to side, with awareness of the tightening muscles. Release.

3. Tighten **shoulders**. Release.

4. Tense **right arm**, from shoulder to fingers without making a fist or lifting arm off of floor. Tense **left arm**. Release.

5. Gently tense **chest muscles** and abdomen without holding the breath. Release.

6. Tense **right hip and buttock**. Release.

7. Tense **right leg** down through feet and toes. Release.

8. Tense **left hip and buttock**. Release.

9. Tense **left leg** down through feet and toes. Release.

10. While no longer tensing any muscles, allow **attention** to drift back up through legs, abdomen, chest, arms, and back to the face.

FIGURE 12.4 Follow the steps to relieve tension and ease stress from head to toe.

anxiety, he theorized that learning how to relax the muscles could reduce anxiety. Jacobson spent more than seven decades documenting the effectiveness of PMR as a preventive measure to reduce stress and as part of the treatment for problems such as hypertension and insomnia. (See "Technique: Tense and Relax Exercise" on page 37 in Chapter 2.)

PMR teaches you to recognize what your body feels like when its muscles are very tense and when they are very relaxed. In active or overt PMR, you focus your attention on a specific muscle group such as the arm muscles and tense them tightly. After the tension builds for 20 to 30 seconds, you let go, and the tension flows away. In passive PMR, you quietly pay attention to a certain muscle or body part and let go of any tension you may feel. You do not have to do anything except allow the tension to flow away.

Here are guidelines for a basic active PMR exercise. Record and listen to the instructions below, or pair up with a classmate and take turns leading each other through this exercise:

1. Sit comfortably in a quiet place. Turn off your cell phone and all notifications and alerts.

2. Begin with your major muscle groups starting by clenching your fists as tightly as possible and then letting the tension go. Then move elsewhere as the instructions indicate.

3. When you tense your muscles, do so vigorously, but not so much that you develop a cramp. Hold the muscle in its tensed position for five to seven seconds, count "one thousand one, one thousand two, one thousand three," and so on, to time the contraction. Relax for 15 to 20 seconds.

4. Concentrate on what is happening. Feel the buildup of tension; notice the tightening of the muscles; feel the strain and then the release; relax and enjoy the sudden feeling of limpness.

5. You will be tensing and relaxing each muscle group twice. If any specific part of your body still feels tense after completing the exercises, go back and tense and relax those muscles again.

6. Keep all other muscles relaxed as you work on specific muscle groups. This is challenging at first, but you will soon become adept.

7. To begin, take three deep breaths, holding each one for five to seven seconds.

8. Clench your dominant fist (right, if you're right-handed; left, if left-handed). Hold and count for five to seven seconds; relax. Repeat.

9. Flex your dominant bicep. Tense, relax, tense, relax.

10. Clench the fist of your non-dominant hand; relax. Repeat. Proceed to the non-dominant bicep. Take a couple of deep breaths, and notice how relaxed and warm your arms feel. Enjoy the feeling.

11. Tense the muscles of your forehead by raising your eyebrows as far as you can. Hold for five seconds. Relax. Repeat. Let the wave of relaxation cover your face.

12. Close your eyes very tightly. Release and notice the relaxation. Repeat.

13. Clench your jaws very tightly. Make an exaggerated smile. Release and repeat.

14. Take a couple of deep breaths, and notice how relaxed the muscles of your arms and head feel.

15. Take a deep breath, and hold it for a few seconds. Release slowly. Repeat.

16. Try to touch your chin to your chest but use your neck muscles to keep it from touching. Release and repeat.

17. Try to touch your back with your head, but use your neck muscles to push the opposite way. Notice the tension building up. Release quickly. Repeat and let your neck become completely relaxed.

18. Push your shoulder blades back and try to make them touch. Notice the tension across your shoulders and chest. Relax and repeat.

19. Try to touch your shoulders by pushing them forward as far as you can. Hold, relax, and repeat.

20. Shrug your shoulders, trying to touch them to your ears. Hold, relax and repeat.

21. Take a very deep breath. Hold for several seconds, and release slowly. Do this again, noticing the wave of relaxation overtaking your body.

22. Tighten your stomach muscles and hold for several seconds. Release. Notice the relaxation in your abdomen. Repeat.

23. Tighten your buttocks. Hold, release, and repeat.

24. Tense your thighs, release quickly. Repeat.

25. Point your toes away from your body. Notice the tension. Return to a normal position. Repeat.

26. Point your toes toward your head; return to normal position. Repeat.

27. Point your feet outward, release quickly. Repeat.

28. Point your feet inward; hold. Relax and repeat.

29. Just let your body relax for a few minutes. Notice and enjoy the good feeling.

PMR exercises become more effective the more you use them, so you are able to relax more deeply in less time. Focusing your attention on this process becomes relaxing in itself. And there is an additional important benefit: You learn to recognize subtle tension that builds up during the day, and you can release it because you now know what complete relaxation feels like with simple exercises such as the following:

> **🔧 Stress Reliever:** Quick Muscle Relaxers
>
> ....
>
> Curl both of your hands into fists, tightening your biceps and forearms. Hold this pose for five to seven seconds and then relax for 15 to 30 seconds, noticing the contrast between the sensations of tension and relaxation.
>
> ....
>
> Roll your head on your neck in a complete circle, first clockwise then counterclockwise.
>
> ....
>
> Scrunch the muscles of your face—wrinkle your forehead, squeeze your eyes, clench your jaws. Relax.
>
> ....
>
> Straighten your legs and point your toes back toward your face, tightening your calves and thighs. Hold for five to second seconds and then relax. Straighten your legs and curl your toes as you tighten and release your calves, thighs, and buttocks.

The Relaxation Response

In the 1970s cardiologist Herbert Benson and his colleagues at Harvard Medical School documented physiological changes in regular practitioners of transcendental meditation (discussed in Chapter 13), including reduced heart and respiration rate, lower blood pressure, and altered brain activity. They dubbed this state of reduced arousal the "relaxation response," a period of rest and recovery that undoes the harmful effects of the stress response. As extensive research has documented, the relaxation response brings about long-term health benefits and counteracts the adverse effects of stress on hypertension, anxiety, diabetes and aging.[13]

Here are the basic instructions for inducing the Relaxation Response. Record and listen to the instructions below, or pair up with a classmate and take turns leading each other through this exercise.

1. Sit quietly and close your eyes.

2. Breathe through your nose. Become aware of your breathing. As you breathe out, say the word, "ONE", silently to yourself. For example, breathe IN ... OUT, "ONE", IN... OUT, "ONE", etc. Breathe easily and naturally.

3. Beginning at your toes, relax various muscle groups in your body: the feet, the shin, the thigh, the pelvic area, the lower back, the upper back, the shoulders, each arm and hand (including the fingers), the neck, the jaw, the forehead.

4. Continue for 10 to 20 minutes. You may open your eyes to check the time, but do not use an alarm.

5. When you finish, sit quietly for several minutes, at first with your eyes closed and then with your eyes open. Do not stand up for a few moments.

6. Do not worry about whether you are successful in achieving a deep level of relaxation. Maintain a passive attitude and permit relaxation to occur at its own pace.

7. Do not practice this technique within two hours after any meal, because the digestive processes seem to interfere with the elicitation of the Relaxation Response.

8. Do not rush. Complete each step, skipping none.

> **🔧 Stress Reliever:** The Faith Factor
>
> ....
>
> In his research, Benson found that repetitive prayer—"Hail, Mary" for Catholics, "Our Father" for other Christians, "Shalom" for Jews—can help evoke the relaxation response. If prayer or religion is an important part of your life, repeat a prayer or phrase from your faith as you breathe in and out.

ABC Relaxation

....

✔ **Check-in:** Have you ever experienced any of the following after a relaxation exercise?

....

_____ Sleepy

_____ Quiet

_____ At ease/at peace

_____ Energized

_____ Aware

_____ Joyous

_____ Thankful

_____ Prayerful

_____ In awe

_____ Filled with a sense of wonder, mystery, love, and boundless infinity[14]

_____ Other

....

According to the ABC theory, relaxation or "centering" consists of three stages:

- Attention (sustained focus on a single thing)

- Behavior (minimal purposeful activity)

- Cognition (passive observation rather than analysis, planning, and other thoughts)[15]

The ABC concept applies to any relaxation technique that involves sustained focus and minimal physical and mental activity.[16] In studies, volunteers who regularly practiced ABC forms of relaxation reported a range of feelings, including those listed above.[17]

As you experiment with relaxation techniques, continue to monitor yourself and take notes on your experiences. What matters more than how you feel immediately after a relaxation session is how you feel and function throughout the day. Do you feel more alert? Calmer? Better able to handle the unexpected? Whenever you feel tension build, remind yourself to do something vitally important: Breathe!

Chapter Summary

- The two major types of breathing patterns are chest or thoracic breathing, which is shallow and often rapid, and diaphragmatic or abdominal breathing (sometimes called "belly breathing"). Deeper and slower, it reduces the activity of the sympathetic nervous system, the branch of the autonomic nervous system responsible for initiating the fight-or-flight response.

- Diaphragmatic breathing has proven effective in relieving anger, depression, anxiety disorders (such as generalized anxiety and panic attacks), insomnia, muscle tension, and pain.

- Guided imagery is a program of directed suggestions that involve all the senses—sounds, tastes, smells, textures, movements. Considered a relaxation technique, a meditation exercise, and a form of self-hypnosis, it is especially effective in reducing stress because it involves body and mind, senses and emotions.

- Guided imagery has proven helpful in treating medical problems, including headaches, asthma, and hypertension; promoting healing after surgery; easing anxiety and pain in cancer patients; a helping performers and public speakers overcome stage fright; and enhancing athletic performance.

- Relaxation, the process of letting go of the residual stress that builds up in our muscles and our minds, is an important component of many other stress-relieving practices, including meditation, massage, hypnosis, yoga, and Tai chi.

- Relaxation slows the heart rate and breathing, lowers blood pressure, and releases muscle tension. Its benefits include fewer physical symptoms, such as headaches and back pain; more energy; improved concentration; enhanced immunity; better sleep; lower blood pressure; and less anxiety and depression.

- Relaxation techniques usually involve refocusing your attention to something calming and increasing awareness of your body. Progressive muscle relaxation consists of alternate tensing and relaxing of various muscle groups in the body.

- The Relaxation Response, developed by Dr. Herbert Benson of Harvard Medical School, involves a combination of breath-counting and relaxation of various muscle groups in the body.

- The ABC theory explains relaxation as consisting of three components: attention (focused on a single stimulus), behavior (minimal), and cognitive (observation rather than analysis or thinking).

STRESS RELIEVERS

How to "Belly Breathe"

- Close your eyes, lean back in your seat or lie down, and place one hand on your stomach area.

- Take a deep breath in through your nose and slowly exhale through your mouth.

- As you inhale, visualize that you are filling a balloon in your belly.

- With each exhale, notice how your diaphragm contracts. Visualize yourself exhaling stress and/or tension along with your breath. Pay attention to how your diaphragm contracts to expel these things.

Soothing Images

- Waves: With each inhalation, imagine a wave cresting just above your belly button, and with each exhalation imagine the wave washing away tension from every muscle in your body.

- Colors: Imagine that you are breathing in air that is rich with a color that soothes you. With each exhalation, the air you breathe out is a little lighter. The soothing color fills your whole body, getting deeper and richer with each inhalation.

- Sponge: Imagine that your body is a sponge in a pool of very warm water. As you breathe in, your body soaks up the warm water, and as you breathe out, the warm water saturates your body sponge. As you continue, your body becomes warmer and warmer and softer and softer.

Take a Screenshot

The next time you're about to engage in a situation that is stressful to you:

- Conjure a snapshot image of it going the way you'd like it to turn out.

- Take mental note of the parts of the situation that you have control over.

- Encourage yourself through self-talk, such as "I'm going to ace this."

- Imagine the result, such as going on line to check your grade and seeing an A.

Take a few minutes and write or share how you felt during this exercise and afterward.

Quick Muscle Relaxers

- Curl both of your hands into fists, tightening your biceps and forearms. Hold this pose for five to seven seconds and then relax for 15 to 30 seconds, noticing the contrast between the sensations of tension and relaxation.

- Roll your head on your neck in a complete circle, first clockwise then counterclockwise.

- Scrunch the muscles of your face—wrinkle your forehead, squeeze your eyes, clench your jaws. Relax.

- Straighten your legs and point your toes back toward your face, tightening your calves and thighs. Hold for five to second seconds and then relax. Straighten your legs and curl your toes as you tighten and release your calves, thighs, and buttocks.

The Faith Factor

In his research, Benson found that repetitive prayer—"Hail, Mary" for Catholics, "Our Father" for other Christians, "Shalom" for Jews—can help evoke the relaxation response. If prayer or religion is an important part of your life, repeat a prayer or phrase from your faith as you breathe in and out.

YOUR PERSONAL STRESS MANAGEMENT TOOLKIT

REFLECTION: What Are Your Tension Targets?

Answer the following questions:

- Do you feel short of breath when under stress?

- Does your heart race?

- Do your muscles tighten?

- Do your neck, shoulders, and upper back often feel tense?

- Do you have problems falling or staying asleep?

- Would you like to feel calmer?

The more "yes" answers that you give, the more you may gain by incorporating breathing and relaxation techniques into your life.

TECHNIQUE: Breathing for Tension Relief

- Once you are comfortable, inhale deep into your abdominal cavity, and say to yourself, "Breathe in."

- Pause and hold your breath for a moment.

- As you exhale, say to yourself, "Relax."

- Pause and then inhale. Pay attention to any parts of your body that feel tense.

- As you exhale, feel the tension leaving your body.

- With every exhalation, let go of more tension and feel your body becoming more relaxed.

- Gradually extend the length of this exercise from five to twenty minutes.

Gala Matorina/Shutterstock.com

CHAPTER 13

Mindfulness, Meditation, and Self-hypnosis

After reading this chapter, you should be able to:

13.1 Explain how meditation and mindfulness help achieve inner peace and increased awareness.

13.2 Define the process of meditation.

13.3 Discuss the relationship between hypnosis and relaxation.

Mindful Attention Awareness Scale

Day-to-Day Experiences

Below is a collection of statements about your everyday experience. Using the 1–6 scale below, please indicate how frequently or infrequently you currently have each experience. Please answer according to what really reflects your experience rather than what you think your experience should be. Please treat each item separately from every other item.

1	2	3	4	5	6
Almost Always	Very Frequently	Somewhat Frequently	Somewhat Infrequently	Very Infrequently	Almost Never

	1	2	3	4	5	6
I could be experiencing some emotion and not be conscious of it until sometime later.	1	2	3	4	5	6
I break or spill things because of carelessness, not paying attention, or thinking of something else.	1	2	3	4	5	6
I find it difficult to stay focused on what's happening in the present.	1	2	3	4	5	6
I tend to walk quickly to get where I'm going without paying attention to what I experience along the way.	1	2	3	4	5	6
I tend not to notice feelings of physical tension or discomfort until they really grab my attention.	1	2	3	4	5	6
I forget a person's name almost as soon as I've been told it for the first time.	1	2	3	4	5	6
It seems I am "running on automatic," without much awareness of what I'm doing.	1	2	3	4	5	6
I rush through activities without being really attentive to them.	1	2	3	4	5	6
I get so focused on the goal I want to achieve that I lose touch with what I'm doing right now to get there.	1	2	3	4	5	6
I do jobs or tasks automatically, without being aware of what I'm doing.	1	2	3	4	5	6
I find myself listening to someone with one ear, doing something else at the same time.	1	2	3	4	5	6
I drive places on 'automatic pilot' and then wonder why I went there.	1	2	3	4	5	6
I find myself preoccupied with the future or the past.	1	2	3	4	5	6
I find myself doing things without paying attention.	1	2	3	4	5	6
I snack without being aware that I'm eating.	1	2	3	4	5	6

To score the scale, compute a mean (average) of the 15 items. Add the scores and divide the total by 15. Higher scores reflect higher levels of mindfulness.[1]

Total score _____

Total score divided by 15 _____

Relaxation, as described in the previous chapter, allows body and mind to stop "doing" and just "be." Mindfulness, meditation, and hypnosis require some degree of physical relaxation but are active processes that engage and focus the mind. Each takes a somewhat different approach, but involves using the mind in ways that soothe and heal body and spirit.

Mind-based approaches have been used for decades to reduce stress and enhance well-being. Although there have been many anecdotal reports of their benefits, few large, controlled trials have tested and documented their effectiveness.[2] According to an analysis of the most scientifically rigorous studies, mindfulness and meditation generally yield "small to moderate reductions" in negative effects of stress, such as anxiety and depression, as well as in pain.[3] However, in some cases, the improvements are comparable to those produced by psychiatric drugs—without any side effects or safety issues.

To determine whether mindfulness, meditation, and hypnosis can benefit you, we recommend trying various practices, making notes on how you feel after each exercise, and choosing the one or ones that suit you best.

Mindfulness

Mindfulness, based on an ancient contemplative tradition of Tibetan Buddhism called *vipassana* or "seeing clearly," involves fully experiencing the physical and mental sensations of the present moment.[4] It can be defined as awareness that emerges from paying **attention** to the unfolding of experience in a particular way—on purpose, in the present moment, and nonjudgmentally.[5]

When you are mindful, you pay careful attention to what you're thinking, feeling, and sensing in the here and now, without analyzing or reacting to what you experience. By keeping your awareness in the present, mindfulness shuts off the stress response. By providing a distance from thoughts and feelings, it helps you work through difficult emotions rather than being overwhelmed by them.

Even a few moments of being fully aware of your senses can be relaxing and calming. As you come to appreciate more of what is happening right now, you live your life in a more fulfilling, appreciative, meaningful way. Mindfulness also triggers a "positive spiral"[6] of effects, with positive emotions countering negative ones[7] and taking a greater role in your life. (See Chapter 8 for more on positive emotions.)

....

✔ **Check-in:** How mindful are you?

....

What do you remember about walking to class today? What did you notice around you? What about right now? Close your eyes, and picture in your mind who is around you, what they are wearing, the color of the walls, the sounds from outside, and other details.

....

Understanding Mindfulness

More than a relaxation technique, mindfulness is a form of mental training that enhances your ability to experience the present through the senses without being judgmental or reactive. By maintaining awareness as life unfolds moment by moment, you become less vulnerable to the reactions that heighten emotional stress. By being mindful, you observe *what is* rather than thinking about *what if* or *if only*.[8] If you think of your mind as a blackboard covered with words, equations, drawings, and tables, mindfulness serves as your eraser to wipe it clean. Since a cluttered mind is a stressed mind, such mental cleansing brings a sense of order and tranquility.

Some practitioners describe the untrained mind as a "curious monkey" constantly flitting from one thing to the next and pulling all sorts of "monkey tricks."[9] Mindfulness tames this wild creature by developing:

- **Concentration**, the learned control of keeping one's awareness on a particular object or thought.

- Attention, focused observation of thoughts, feelings, and physical sensations as they occur. This requires turning off any and all chatter about the past or the future and noticing only what is happening now.

- A nonjudgmental attitude of openness and curiosity. In a state of mindfulness, you accept your thoughts and feelings without evaluating them, forming an opinion, or comparing them to any expectations.

mindfulness Fully experiencing the physical and mental sensations of the present moment without being judgmental or reactive.

attention Focused observation of thoughts, feelings, and physical sensations as they occur.

concentration The learned control of keeping one's awareness on a particular object or thought.

The Benefits of Mindfulness

Mindfulness is particularly helpful in reducing stress, which can occur only when we allow our minds to think or worry about things beyond what is happening in our current experience.[10] Mindfulness-based stress reduction has been shown in well-controlled studies to yield small to moderate improvements in anxiety, depression, pain, feelings of stress/distress, and health-related quality of life.[11] A recent review of 40 studies found that mindfulness meditation can decrease stress and anxiety in college students.[12] Other research has confirmed its benefits for dental and medical students.[13]

Among the other positive effects of mindfulness are:

Physical Benefits

Overall improved health[14]

Lower levels of the stress hormone cortisol[15]

Enhanced immunity[18]

Relief of chronic pain[19]

Relief of symptoms of fibromyalgia,[20] cancer, and other illnesses

Relief of digestive disorders such as ulcerative colitis[21] and irritable bowel disorder[22]

Help in smoking cessation[23]

Psychological Benefits[16]

More positive emotions and less depression[17]

Greater self-compassion

Decreased absent-mindedness

Greater resilience[18]

Less likelihood of burnout in high-risk professions[19]

Greater ability to regulate emotions[20]

Improved ability to handle the stresses of demanding professions and training[21]

Reduced worry, rumination, and perceived stress.[22]

Relief of psychological symptoms[23]

Reduced recurrences of major depression[24]

Less loneliness in the elderly[25]

Enhanced appreciation and enjoyment of pleasant daily-life activities[26]

Cognitive Benefits

Improved performance on tasks requiring sustained attention

Improved memory

May help in treatment of attention disorders[27]

May slow age-related cognitive decline[28]

What You Need to Know

You can practice mindfulness in all aspects of daily life simply by bringing your full awareness to your activities and experiences. When you

Mindfulness is similar to the intense concentration required for many intricate tasks.

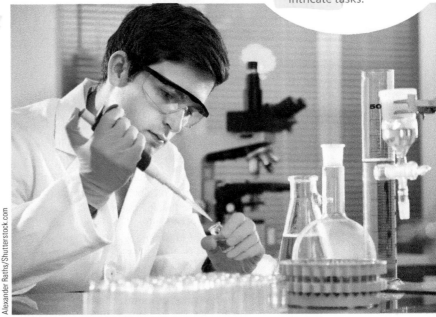

Alexander Raths/Shutterstock.com

become totally absorbed in the task at hand, you perform better—whether you're at bat in a softball game or troubleshooting a software glitch. As you become mindful in more circumstances and moments, you clear your mind of clutter and feel less pressure and stress. Here is how to begin:

- Get into a relaxed position. You might sit in a comfortable chair or on a cushion on the floor. Keep your back upright but not too rigid.

- Assure yourself some privacy. Close and lock the door to your room, if possible. If you share your living space, explain to your roommates that you need some quiet time or find a study cubicle or another quiet place on campus.

- Take a few minutes to notice and relax your body. Pay attention to its shape, its weight, the sensations it is experiencing, and how it feels against the chair or cushion. If you feel any areas of tension, let your muscles relax.

- Tune into the natural flow of your breath as you inhale and exhale. You don't need to do anything to your breath. Simply notice where you feel your breath in your body: In your nostrils? In your throat? In your chest? In your abdomen? Feel the sensations of your breath as it enters and leaves your body.

Mindfulness Skills

You can become mindful by developing a range of skills, sometimes categorized as "what" and "how" skills. The "what" skills include:

- **Observation.** This involves looking at and experiencing things as they are, free from thoughts, feelings, and judgments. You don't see a "sad" person but rather someone with a downcast look and tear-filled eyes.

- **Description.** Consciously find words for what you're experiencing, whether it's "my feet are sore" or "the room is cold." Pay attention to what you're experiencing with each of your senses, as well as the thoughts and judgments running through your head.

- **Participation.** Engage fully in each and every thing that you do. When you are eating, focus on the flavors, the texture, the scents, the process of eating. When washing your face, hear the water, feel its warmth, smell the soap.

The "how" skills include:

- **Being nonjudgmental.** Separate facts (the driver behind you is honking his horn) from judgments (the driver is angry with you).

- **Being single-minded.** Focus all your attention on what you are doing in the moment. When you eat, eat. When you drive, drive. When you are having a conversation, listen.

- **Acting effectively.** Rather than worrying about doing things the "right" way, concentrate on doing what will work in a given situation so you can achieve your goal.

Mindfulness-Based Stress Reduction (MBSR)

This therapeutic approach, which focuses on progressive development of mindful awareness, has proven beneficial for patients with a wide variety of medical problems as well as for healthy people coping with daily stress.[29] Mindfulness-Based Cognitive Therapy (MBCT) integrates this approach with cognitive therapy (discussed in Chapter 3 and Chapter 9).[30] These approaches are usually taught in programs lasting four to eight weeks and often targeting specific conditions, such as depression.

Mindlessness, the opposite of mindfulness, occurs when we tune out what is happening around us. Instead, we remember incidents from the past, wonder what others are thinking or doing, make plans, weave fantasies, or worry about the future. As a result, we lose touch with the only reality we know: the present moment.

 Stress Reliever: Are You Sleep-Walking?

Do you ever walk into a classroom and not realize how you got there? This is an example of being asleep with your eyes wide open rather than being fully awake, alive, present, and in the moment. The next time it happens, think of all you may be missing when you sleep-walk your life away:

What are you missing when you focus on your thoughts and feelings about yesterday or tomorrow?

What thoughts, feelings, or worries do you have about things that are in your past and can't be changed?

What thoughts, feelings, or worries do you have about things you think will take place in the future?

Identify three strategies you might use to focus on the here and now rather than what was or what will be.

Mindfulness Practices

Some of the most useful mindfulness practices include:

Mindful Breathing

Mindful breathing gives you an anchor—your breath—on which you can focus when a stressful thought enters your mind. By concentrating on your breathing, you can stay "present" in the moment rather than being distracted by regrets from the past or worries about the future.

The primary goal of mindful breathing is calm, non-judging awareness, allowing thoughts and feelings to come and go without getting caught up in them. It's natural for thoughts to enter into your awareness and for your attention to follow them. When you notice this happening, just keep bringing your attention back to your breathing.

Listen to the Mindful Breathing audio instructions in MindTap, record your own, or pair up with a classmate and take turns leading each other through this exercise.

1. Sit comfortably, with your eyes closed and your spine reasonably straight.

2. Bring your attention to your breathing. Take a deep breath in through your nostrils. Hold the breath inside. Then slowly exhale through your mouth.

3. Imagine that you have a balloon in your stomach. Every time you breathe in, the balloon inflates. Each time you breathe out, the balloon deflates.

4. Notice the sensations in your abdomen as your inner balloon inflates and then deflates. Be mindful of your abdomen rising with the in-breath, the fullness within you as you hold the breath, and the experience of release with the out-breath.

5. Thoughts will come into your mind because that's what the human mind does. Simply notice these thoughts and bring your attention back to your breathing.

6. You may notice sounds, physical feelings, emotions. Again, just bring your attention back to your breathing.

7. Be mindful of the rhythm you create as you take deep inhalations through your nose and slowly exhale through your mouth.

8. You don't have to follow thoughts or feelings the pop into your mind, don't judge yourself for having them, or analyze them in any way. It's okay for the thoughts to be there. Just notice these thoughts, and let them drift on by.

9. Whenever you notice that your attention has drifted off and is becoming caught up in thoughts or feelings, simply note that the attention has drifted, and then gently bring the attention back to your breathing.

10. Continue to fill your inner balloon with air, be aware of the oxygen filling your body, and be mindful of the slow release of your breath.

11. Open yourself to focus on all the sensations that enter your awareness.

Mindful Walking

Walking mindfulness uses the rhythm of walking and breathing to stay in the present moment. It is important to remember that you aren't walking to reach a destination or to get exercise, but rather to develop mindfulness.

1. Find a quiet path, about 10 to 20 feet in length, where you can walk back and forth.

2. Begin by focusing on the sensations of standing, feeling your weight and your feet—all the subtle movements involved in keeping you upright and balanced.

3. Begin to walk slowly, keeping your intention on the experience of walking.

4. Mentally notice when you are "lifting," "stepping," or "placing" your feet onto the pavement or ground.

5. Feel your arms swing.

6. Notice your breathing. Follow each breath as it enters and leaves your body.

7. Keep your mind focused on the present. If it wanders, simply say to yourself "wandering" or "thinking," and refocus on the physical sensations and movement of walking.

8. When you reach the end of the path, pause, pay attention to your posture, and reconnect with your breathing. When ready, turn and walk back along the path.

9. Repeat this pacing back and forth for 15 to 30 minutes. When you are ready to finish, focus on how your body feels and thank yourself for devoting time to your body, mind, and spirit.

Mindfulness on the Bus or Subway

1. If you can safely do so, close your eyes; otherwise, focus on an object several feet in front of you and soften your gaze.

2. Scan your body from head to toe, noting the slightest sensations and allowing whatever you experience—an itch, an ache, a feeling of warmth—to enter your awareness.

3. Notice your environment by tuning into the sounds around you and noticing the temperature. Are you hot or cold?

4. Focus specifically on your breathing, following your breath from start to finish. Is it shallow or deep, slow or fast?

5. Count one on each inhale and two on exhale to strengthen your awareness.

6. Whenever your mind wanders, gently bring your attention back to breathing.

7. If something distracts you, name it—door opening, passenger talking loudly—and return to your breathing. You don't have to block out noise or movements. Just keep bringing your attention back to your breathing in the present moment.

8. Do this for at least five to ten minutes during your commute. You can set a timer on your phone or watch, or you can begin the exercise at a certain stop on the route and end at another.

Mindfulness and Meditation Apps and Videos

Mindfulness apps, videos, audios, and programs are available to download to use whenever and wherever you choose. Although they have not been extensively studied, users have found them helpful in increasing positive emotions and easing negative feelings.[31] Mobile mindfulness exercises make it easier to incorporate meditation and mindfulness into your daily routine. Among those that have been well reviewed are:

- **Headspace (https://www.headspace.com):** This program offers a free introduction to the basics of meditation in 10-minute meditations for each of ten days, with an option to buy a paid version by the month or year. In a research study, participants completing the ten-day introduction reported more positive emotions and less depression (compared to another group of participants who used an app that was relatively neutral in content).

- **Calm (http://www.calm.com):** The Calm app features nature sounds and/or music paired with a variety of backgrounds (such as mountains, raindrops on leaves, clouds, beaches, and abstract shapes). Two guided meditations—one that focuses on calmness and one that is a "body scan" (focusing on each part of the body, one at a time)—are free. A "Seven Days of Calm" program helps start your meditation practice, and you can create an account to track your progress.

- **Omvana (http://www.omvana.com):** On Omvana, you can choose meditation "tracks"—some free, others priced under $5—for a variety of categories, such as sleep, energy, focus, and happiness. An introductory track focuses on making meditation accessible and emphasizes relaxing rather than trying to clear your mind completely.

You can also find instructional videos on line. Among those that offer good introductions are:

- 20 Minute Guided Mindfulness Exercise: https://www.youtube.com/watch?v=thYoV -MCVs0

- Mindfulness Meditation Breathing Exercise. https://www.youtube.com/watch?v =LSIlM4ZePWM

- Leaves on a stream mindfulness. https://www.youtube.com/watch?v=yMz _UagXkFk

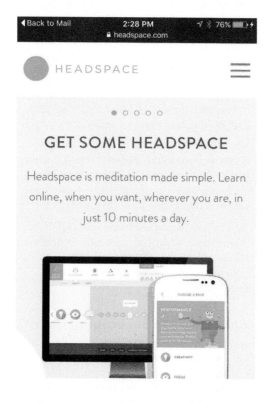

Users report that mindfulness apps help increase positive emotions and ease stress.

> **Stress Reliever:** Everyday Mindfulness
>
> You can apply mindfulness to every aspect of your daily life, including routines and chores:
>
> In the shower, mentally scan your body from head to toe, allowing the slightest

sensation to enter your awareness. Actively focus on and be mindful of the feel of the spray, the smells, the sounds, the taste in your mouth, the steam filling the room.

When washing dishes, focus on the water and soap, the shape of each dish, and how it looks and feels as you wash it.

If you're drinking water, be mindful of how your glass or water bottle feels in your hand, of its color, temperature, and texture, of how the water feels and tastes when you take a sip.

Meditation

Meditation is an intentional process of deepening attention and focus that has been practiced in many forms over the ages. The National Center for Complementary and Alternative Medicine defines meditation as a mind-body intervention in which a person focuses attention in a nonjudgmental way in order to achieve a state of greater calmness, physical relaxation, and psychological balance.[32]

The ancient Eastern religions of Hinduism, Buddhism, Taoism, and Confucianism use meditative techniques to help people clear the mind, transcend the body, and deepen their understanding of the sacred and mystical forces of life. Western religions, including Judaism, Christianity, Protestantism, and Islam, also incorporate meditative practices such as repetitive prayer and contemplative silence. Although part of many faith traditions, meditation is not a religious practice. Regular meditators, according to research, are less likely to believe in God and more likely to believe in "inner wisdom."[33]

Approximately 10 percent of Americans have some experience with meditation. People meditate for many different reasons, including:

- Health maintenance, healing, therapy, and relief of symptoms of illnesses and chronic medical conditions.

- Enhanced performance, creativity, problem-solving, and relationships.

- Creation of balance between mind, heart, and body.[34]

Many medical and educational centers offer courses in meditation to patients seeking alternative or additional methods to relieve symptoms or enhance health. Even children can learn and benefit from meditation and other mind-body practices.[35]

Understanding Meditation

Meditation encompasses various approaches that use quiet sitting, breathing techniques, and/or chanting or movement to relax, improve concentration, and reach a state of inner peace and harmony. Meditation involves choice: You choose to train your attention by focusing on something—a candle, a word, your own breath—or opening up your awareness to every stimulus around and within you. Like mindfulness, it helps regular practitioners gain control of their attention so they can choose what to focus upon rather than reacting to people, events, or intrusive thoughts.

Through meditation, you can transcend the kind of thinking in which you get lost or upset by your thoughts. It develops your ability to observe your thoughts as they enter and exit your mind, just as you observe other experiences.

The relaxed state induced by meditation is characterized by significant physiological changes, including:[36]

- Decreased metabolic rate and oxygen consumption, similar to what occurs during sleep or hibernation. However, meditators remain awake and alert as their bodies slow down and rest.

- Slowed heart rate. On average, heart rate decreases by an average of three beats per minute during meditation.

- Altered respiration. Meditators breathe more slowly and require less oxygen.

- Changes in brain activity: **Alpha waves** (slow, low-amplitude brain waves associated with a low-stress, resting state) become more frequent and intense. Meditation shifts brain activity from the left hemisphere to the more intuitive right hemisphere and allows both hemispheres to work together in unison.

The Benefits of Meditation

The altered state induced by meditation effectively cancels out the stress response by slowing body and mind; reducing negative emotions, thoughts, and behaviors; increasing positive emotions, thoughts, and behaviors; and altering relevant physiological processes. Some effects, such as calmness, can occur within seconds of beginning meditation. Others may occur over a period of weeks, months, or even years. Among lifelong practitioners, meditation may physically change the brain and body in ways that could potentially improve health and promote healthy behaviors.

meditation The intentional process of deepening attention and focus that has been practiced in many forms over the ages.

alpha waves Slow, low-amplitude brain waves associated with a low-stress, resting state.

Additional positive effects of meditation include:

Physical Benefits:

Symptom relief for patients with fibromyalgia, cancer, hypertension, and psoriasis.

Help in treatment of medical conditions worsened by stress, including allergies, asthma, atherosclerosis (narrowing of arteries), chronic headaches, heart disease, and sleep disorders.[37]

Lower blood pressure[38]

Enhanced immunity[39]

Relief of chronic pain[40]

Lower hospitalization and mortality rates

Help in recovery from eating disorders and alcohol or drug abuse.

Smoking reduction or cessation[41]

Slowing, stalling, or even reversing the aging process.[42]

Psychological Benefits:

Less anxiety[43]

Less depression

Helpful in treating other mental disorders[44]

Enhanced mood and self-esteem

Reduced worry, rumination, and perceived stress.[45]

Greater feelings of love, thankfulness, prayerfulness, and mental quiet[46]

Changes in regions of the brain that may bolster empathy and compassion in individuals with extensive experience in meditation (including lay practitioners as well as Tibetan monks). These alterations persist beyond periods of active meditation.[47]

Cognitive Benefits:

Improved memory

Greater creativity

Enhanced performance in school, sports, and careers.

Improved attention and cognition in older adults.

Faster processing of information, due to increased folds in the outer layer of the brain among long-term meditators[48]

What You Need to Know

Meditation is simple, inexpensive, and doesn't require any special equipment. With practice, you can induce a meditative state almost anywhere—whether you're in your room, out for a walk, riding the bus, doing the laundry, or waiting at the doctor's office.

Most forms of meditation have common components:

- A tranquil environment
- Sitting quietly for 15 to 20 minutes once or twice a day (you're likely to fall asleep if you lie down)
- Concentrating on a word or image
- Breathing slowly and rhythmically

If you decide to try meditation, it often helps to have someone guide you through your first sessions. You can listen to the Mediation audio file in MindTap or record your own voice, with or without music in the background. Listening to audio instructions frees you to concentrate on your goal of turning your attention within.

Try to meditate at the same time every day, such as immediately after you wake up or before dinner. (Avoid meditating after a meal when you may feel sluggish or sleepy.) Don't consume energizing drinks that contain caffeine or other stimulants before meditating since your goal is to relax, not rev up.

Be patient when you start meditation. It's common for the mind to wander, no matter how long you've been practicing. To bring yourself back to your focus, picture balloons floating away with your distracting thoughts, or imagine that they are pigeons and mentally clap your hands so they fly away.

The best indicator of a good meditation experience is not what happens during the session but how you feel afterward. The fact that your mind

With practice you can induce a meditative state almost anywhere, including classes like this.

Stefano Tinti/Shutterstock.com

repeatedly wanders does not matter as long as you continue to return to your focal point.

Meditation Practices

There are many types of meditation, and no one right way to meditate. Many people have discovered how to meditate on their own, without even knowing what it is they are doing. Prayer, whether in your own words or those of spiritual leaders, is the most widely practiced example of meditation. (See Chapter 10 for more on spirituality and stress.)

Among the many forms of meditation, most involve one of two approaches:

- Concentrating your attention and excluding all other thoughts (sometimes called exclusive meditation) or

- Opening up your attention to everything that is happening within and around you (inclusive meditation).

Exclusive, Concentration, or Focused Meditation

All forms of **exclusive, concentrated, or focused meditation** direct attention to a focal point that can be a thought, phrase, sound, image, or object. The goal is to push away distractions of every type. Purposefully or intentionally focusing on one thing clears the mind of other thoughts and allows it to focus inwards with increased awareness, reflection, and relaxation.

Mantra meditation involves focusing on a **mantra**, a phrase or name that you repeat silently or aloud. It doesn't matter which word you use, as long as it is easy to remember and repeat.

Stress Reliever: Choose a Mantra

Experiment with different words or phrases, such as:

Om, a Sanskrit word used in Hinduism, Buddhism, and other Eastern religions.

One, a word that suggests that your body and mind are one and that you feel at one with the universe.

A calming word such as "peace," "still," "tranquil," or "silent."

A sound such as "haa" or "aah" that you make with every exhalation.

A word in another language, such as "shalom" ("peace" in Hebrew).

Transcendental Meditation (TM) was introduced as a technique in the mid-20th century by Marharishi Mahesh Yogi, a physicist who spent years developing a simple form of meditation that could be easily taught and learned. His global educational campaign helped popularize meditation in Western cultures.

TM generally consists of a standardized program with regular classes over the course of several weeks or months. Students are expected to practice daily. TM uses a mantra, not solely as a focus for concentration, but as a vehicle to "automatic self-transcending," a process in which one attempts to reach a higher state of being through meditation.

In **Soto Zen meditation**, you focus on a visual mantra such as a **mandala**, a circular figure that represents wholeness (see Figure 13.1). With an intricate design and intense colors, a mandala serves as a cosmic diagram of a universe that exists both beyond and within our bodies and minds.

You can download images of mandalas as well as templates to color. To meditate, stare at the mandala as long as you can until you feel you have completely memorized its details. Then close your eyes and try to picture the object in your mind. If and when the image fades, open your eyes and stare at the object again, then continue to try and "see" it with your eyes closed.

Visual mantras can take other forms, such as a candle flame, a plant or flower, the ocean, or a favorite picture. As you focus your mind and attention, all other thoughts fade away.

exclusive, concentration, or focused meditation Focused meditation requiring concentration on a thought, phrase, sound, or object.

mantra meditation A type of meditation that focuses on a repeated word, sound, or phrase.

mantra A word or phrase repeated during a meditative state.

Transcendental Meditation (TM) A type of meditation that involves going into a meditative state by repeating a special, individualized mantra.

Soto Zen meditation A form of concentration meditation in which you stare at a visual mantra until you feel you have completely memorized the object and its details.

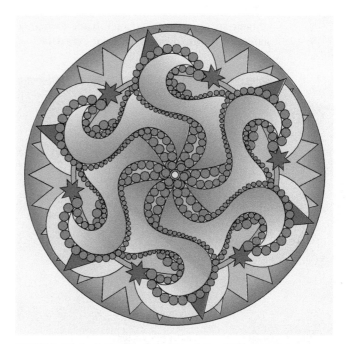

FIGURE 13.1 A Meditation Mandala. With intense colors and an intricate design, a mandala represents the unity of the cosmos.

You can also focus on a repeated sound, called **nadam**, that you imagine or listen to with an app or software download or an object, like a small stone or shell, that you hold and touch. Hindu yogis use a strand of beads (called a Mala) and repeatedly roll the beads one-by-one through their fingers while they meditate. Rosary beads, used in the Catholic religion, can provide a comparable focus of concentration.

One Zen meditation practice uses **koans**, unsolvable, illogical riddles that force the mind to focus on a concept that has no answer. Examples include: What is the sound of one hand clapping? Where would unicorns live? What color are their horns?

In **Lovingkindness Meditation**, you focus your attention on a sacred object or being, weaving feelings of love and gratitude into your thoughts. You can also close your eyes and use your imagination or gaze at representations of the object.

Open or Inclusive Meditation

Unlike concentration meditation, in which you push distractions aside to focus on one thought, **inclusive meditation** allows the mind to wander and to observe any and all thoughts with "detached observation"—that is, without emotion, judgment, consideration, or contemplation. In essence, you step outside yourself to observe your own thought processes.

Inclusive meditation encompasses certain types of Buddhist meditation, contemplative meditation, and centering prayer in which becoming an observer of yourself leads to higher states of consciousness. **Zazen meditation**

focuses on subjective states of consciousness and detachment from emotional thoughts.

When you try inclusive meditation, it can help to imagine being in a white room with nothing in it but doors on opposite sides. Thoughts enter through one door, and you acknowledge them but don't invite them to stay. You watch as they pass through and exit the opposite door without focusing on them.

Active Meditation

You can also reach a meditative state through repetitive motion, using physical repetition as the focus of thought. Sufi whirling dervishes constantly move, dance, and sway in order to achieve a trance-like state. Rhythmic activities such as swimming, walking, or running can also induce a meditative state sometimes referred to as "runner's high."

Meditation Exercises

In addition to the following practices, you can find other exercises starting on page 262 at the end of this chapter.

Mantra Meditation

Find a quiet environment where you won't be disturbed.

1. Sit comfortably in a chair, and begin smooth abdominal breathing.

2. Close your eyes, and begin repeating the mantra you have chosen in your mind. Do not say it out loud.

3. Attend only to your mind as it repeats your mantra. Don't try to change your thoughts in any way. Just allow yourself to keep whispering the word silently to yourself.

4. When you notice your mind wandering, gently bring your attention back to your breathing and your mantra. Do the same if you nod off and then awaken.

5. Don't set an alarm clock, but you can briefly open your eyes to check the time; then close them again and return to the mantra.

6. Take several minutes to return slowly to full consciousness.

7. Practice for ten to twenty minutes at least three or four times per week.

Walking Meditation

1. Choose a quiet path where you're not likely to be distracted. It doesn't have to be long; you can walk back and forth several times.

<div class="margin-glossary">

mandala A circular figure with intricate designs and intense colors that serves as the focus of concentration during meditation.

nadam A repeated sound that meditators imagine or listen to.

koans Unsolvable, illogical riddles that force the mind to focus on a concept that has no answer.

Lovingkindness meditation A form of concentration meditation in which you focus on a sacred object or being, weaving feelings of love and gratitude into your thoughts.

Active meditation combines the benefits of physical activity and mental concentration.

</div>

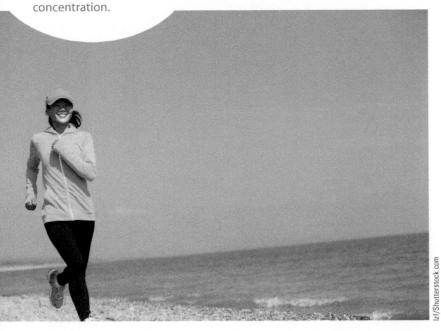

izf/Shutterstock.com

2. As you walk, focus on your body.

3. Be aware of your posture.

4. Feel your feet hit the pavement.

5. Feel your arms swing.

6. Note your breathing.

7. As you feel yourself relax, you can choose to repeat your mantra, recite a prayer, or play an uplifting song in our mind.

8. Continue for a least twenty minutes.

9. At the end of your walk, pause to take a few deep breaths and savor the way your body feels.

Self-Hypnosis

✔ **Check-in:** Have you ever entered a hypnotic state?

You have if you ever:

Got lost in a daydream.

Found yourself arriving at a destination without remembering the details of how you got there.

Became so caught up in a movie or book that you didn't notice what was happening around you.

"Zoned out" while walking, hiking, cycling or simply staring into space.

Derived from *ýpnos*, the Greek word for "sleep", **hypnosis** uses suggestions to induce an altered state of consciousness that is similar to sleep. However, unlike sleep, a hypnotized person never completely loses awareness. When hypnotized, you become deeply relaxed, block out distractions, concentrate intensely, and are more open to suggestions.

Understanding Hypnosis

Hypnosis is a state of concentration characterized by focused attention, deep relaxation, greater responsiveness to suggestions, more openness, and a suspension of belief and criticism. It seems to affect how the brain communicates with the body. While hypnotized, you willingly experience your thoughts and images as real, just as you do when immersed in a book or movie. Hypnosis can only take place with your voluntary and active participation.

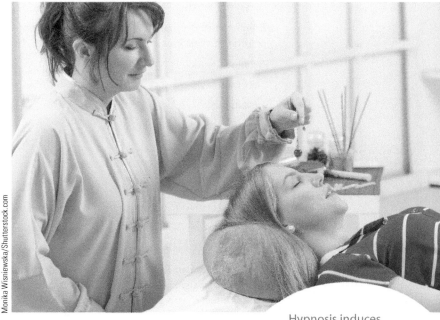

Monika Wisniewska/Shutterstock.com

When hypnotized, a person goes into an altered state of consciousness. The more critical and analytical conscious mind is temporarily subdued, so suggestions travel directly to the subconscious mind. Without the interference of the conscious mind, the subconscious simply does whatever it is told to do.

> 🔧 **Stress Reliever:** Hypnosis Videos
>
> Check out instructional videos on hypnosis, such as the following:
>
> Self-Hypnosis Anxiety Reduction: https://www.youtube.com/watch?v=cCJJwkbn-eY
>
> Self-Hypnosis Learning to Relax: https://www.youtube.com/watch?v=uvJ6vrdml7w
>
> Motivation Hypnosis: https://www.youtube.com/watch?v=0_FYo1Ss41w

The Benefits of Hypnosis

In itself hypnosis is not a form of therapy, but it can be used in therapeutic ways. Because hypnotized individuals are more suggestible, they are more receptive to breaking bad habits, such as smoking and overeating. Mental health professionals use hypnosis to treat various problems, including phobias, and it is remarkably effective in relieving pain from burns, arthritis, and other chronic conditions. Hypnosis also has proven useful in helping trauma victims work through upsetting memories of what happened to them.

Hypnosis induces a state of focused attention, deep relaxation, greater openness, and a suspension of belief.

open or inclusive meditation A form of meditation that allow the mind to wander and to observe any and all thoughts with "detached observation"— that is, without emotion, judgement, consideration, or contemplation.

Zazen meditation A form of open meditation that focuses on subjective states of consciousness and detaching yourself from emotional thoughts.

hypnosis A state of concentration characterized by focused attention, deep relaxation, greater responsiveness to suggestions, more openness, and a suspension of belief and criticism.

Other benefits include:

Enhanced performance in sports, entertainment, or other professions

Relief of headache

Less pain[49]

Less anxiety

Improvements in chronic fatigue

Better sleep

Relief of hot flashes[50]

Improvement in inflammatory bowel disorder[51]

Less pain, fatigue, and discomfort after surgery[52]

What You Need to Know

Self-hypnosis can be learned quickly and safely. However, individuals vary in their responsiveness. To test if you are a good candidate, try the following exercise:

1. Stretch your arms in front of you at shoulder level. Close your eyes and imagine a weight being tied to your right arm as you struggle to keep it up.

2. Imagine a second weight and then a third. Feel the strain on your arm as the weights get heavier, heavier, heavier.

3. Visualize a huge balloon being tied to your left arm and tugging your arm up into the air—higher, higher, higher.

4. Open your eyes and notice whether your arms have changed from their original position.

Most people see at least some movement. If you don't, try a few more times. If you still don't notice even a slight change in position, hypnosis may not be for you.

If you try self-hypnosis, allow at least twenty to thirty minutes to enter and deepen the hypnotic state.

Self-Hypnosis Exercise

Hypnosis relies on the power of **hypnotic suggestion**, usually a series of steps that narrow awareness and deepen relaxation. We recommend that you record the following suggestions and play the audio to guide you through the steps:

1. Sit in a comfortable chair that supports your arms, hands, neck, and head. Keep your feet on the floor. Rest your hands in your lap. Hypnosis usually is done with closed eyes.

2. Sum up your goal for using hypnosis in a few words, such as "relax" or "calm down."

Repeat this phrase as you close your eyes and begin self-induction.

3. Breathe deeply into your abdomen and feel a spreading sense of relaxation as you exhale.

4. Systematically relax your body. As you focus on your legs and arms, repeat the phrase "heavier and heavier, more and more relaxed." As you relax your forehead and cheeks, say, "letting go of tension, smooth and relaxed." As you move to your jaw and neck, say "loose and relaxed." As you shift attention to your chest, abdomen, and back, take deep breaths and repeat "calm and relaxed" with each exhalation.

5. Visualize a staircase or path that you descend step by step to enter a peaceful place. Count backward from ten to one. With each number, you take a step down and become more and more relaxed. You can repeat this process two or three times to achieve deeper relaxation.

6. Imagine yourself arriving at your destination—a special place of peace and tranquility, such as a quiet beach or a field of flowers. Look around and notice the shapes and colors; listen to the sounds; smell the fragrances. Notice the temperature; tune in to how your body feels.

7. Deepen your hypnotic state by repeating suggestions such as "drifting deeper and deeper," "feeling more and more drowsy," "drifting down, down, down," and "totally relaxed." Use creative images, such as imagining floating on a cloud, as you become more relaxed.

8. Once you've spent some time in deep relaxation, give yourself a post-hypnotic suggestion, such as "I will be calm and confident" or "I feel relaxed and refreshed." Repeat at least three times.

9. When it's time to end your hypnotic trance, count from one to ten. Pause between each number to tell yourself that are becoming "more and more alert and refreshed." As you reach number nine, tell yourself that your eyes are opening. As you say the number ten, tell yourself that you are totally alert and wide awake.

Like breathing and relaxation exercises, hypnosis becomes easier with practice. Don't worry about how you're doing. Remember to take deep breaths, and use adjectives such as "drowsy" and "peaceful" during self-induction. Repeat suggestions several times until they begin to take hold.

hypnotic suggestion
A statement that the mind believes is accurate or true and that is used to narrow awareness and deepen relaxation.

- Mindfulness, meditation, and self-hypnosis are active processes that engage and focus the mind. Each takes a somewhat different approach, but their goal is similar: to use your mind in ways that can soothe and heal your body and spirit.

- Mindfulness involves fully experiencing the physical and mental sensations of the present moment without being judgmental or reactive. By maintaining awareness in the present as it happens moment by moment, you become less vulnerable to the reactions that heighten emotional stress.

- Mindfulness has been linked with better health, lower anxiety, and greater resilience. Focusing on the present in mindfulness practices can lower levels of the stress hormone cortisol.

- Mindfulness also improves cognitive functions and, by providing a distance from thoughts and feelings, can help you work through difficult emotions rather than being overwhelmed by them.

- Mindfulness-Based Stress Reduction focuses on progressive acquisition of mindful awareness to help patients with medical problems as well as healthy people coping with daily stress.

- Meditation includes a group of approaches that use quiet sitting, breathing techniques, and/or chanting or movement to relax, improve concentration, and reach a state of inner peace and harmony.

- Meditation induces an altered state characterized by decreased metabolic rate and oxygen consumption, changes in brain activity, slowed heart rate, and decreased respiration.

- Meditation can help individuals with a variety of medical conditions worsened by stress, including major chronic diseases, sleep disorders, eating disorders, anxiety, phobias, and alcohol or drug abuse.

- Although there are many forms of meditation, most involve focusing your attention and excluding all other thoughts (sometimes called "exclusive" meditation) or opening your attention to everything that is happening within and around you (inclusive meditation).

- All forms of exclusive meditation require concentration on a focal point that can be a thought, phrase, sound, or object. Purposefully or intentionally focusing on one thing allows it to focus inwards with increased awareness, reflection, and relaxation.

- One of the most popular and well-known forms of concentration meditation is Transcendental Meditation (TM), in which you focus on a mantra, a sacred phrase or name that you repeat silently or aloud.

- In Soto Zen meditation, you focus on a visual mantra or mandala as long as you can until you feel you have completely memorized the object and its details. You then close your eyes and try to picture the object in your mind.

- In Lovingkindness Meditation, you focus your attention on a sacred object or being, weaving feelings of love and gratitude into your thoughts. You can also close your eyes and use your imagination or gaze at representations of the object.

- Inclusive Meditation allows the mind to wander and to observe any and all thoughts with "detached observation"—that is, without emotion, judgment, consideration, or contemplation.

- Active meditation produces a meditative state through repetitive motion, using physical repetition as the focus of thought and allowing the mind to hear and allow for meditation.

- Hypnosis uses suggestions to induce a state of concentration characterized by focused attention, greater responsiveness to suggestions, more openness, and a suspension of belief and criticism.

- Hypnosis can help in relieving headache, anxiety, chronic fatigue, tremors, and insomnia.

STRESS RELIEVERS

Your Hand

Focus on your non-dominant hand. Notice the length of the fingers and nails. Look closely at the whorls of flesh within your palm. Pay attention to the lines that crisscross it and the pad of flesh at the base of your thumb. Turn your hand around to observe the other side. How prominent are your knuckles? Can you trace the blood vessels just under your skin? Bend each finger. Touch your thumb to the tips of your index, middle, ring, and little finger. Spend a few minutes describing your hand in detail.

Once you finish, reflect on this experience of intense concentration. Did the time pass quickly? Were you aware of distractions? Did you feel any stress?

Are You Sleep-Walking?

Do you ever walk into a classroom and not realize how you got there? This is an example of being asleep with your eyes wide open rather than being fully awake, alive, present, and in the moment. The next time it happens, think of all you may be missing when you sleep-walk your life away:

- What are you missing when you focus on your thoughts and feelings about yesterday or tomorrow?

- What thoughts, feelings, or worries do you have about things that are in your past and can't be changed?

- What thoughts, feelings, or worries do you have about things you think will take place in the future?

Identify three strategies you might use to focus on the here and now rather than what was or what will be.

Everyday Mindfulness

You can apply mindfulness to every aspect of your daily life, including routines and chores:

- In the shower, mentally scan your body from head to toe, allowing the slightest sensation to enter your awareness. Actively focus on and be mindful of the feel of the spray, the smells, the sounds, the taste in your mouth, the steam filling the room.

- When washing dishes, focus on the water and soap, the shape of each dish, and how it looks and feels as you wash it.

- If you're drinking water, be mindful of how your glass or water bottle feels in your hand, of its color, temperature, and texture, of how the water feels and tastes when you take a sip.

Choose a Mantra

Experiment with different words or phrases, such as:

- "Om," a Sanskrit word used in Hinduism, Buddhism, and other Eastern religions.

- "One," a word that suggests that your body and mind are one and that you feel at one with the universe.

- A calming word such as "peace," "still," "tranquil," or "silent."

- A sound such as "haa" or "aah" that you make with every exhalation.

- A word in another language, such as "shalom" ("peace" in Hebrew).

Hypnosis Videos

Check out instructional videos on hypnosis, such as the following:

- Self-Hypnosis Anxiety Reduction: https://www.youtube.com/watch?v=cCJJwkbn-eY

- Self-Hypnosis Learning to Relax: https://www.youtube.com/watch?v=uvJ6vrdml7w

- Motivation Hypnosis: https://www.youtube.com/watch?v=O_FYo1Ss41w

---

⊜ YOUR PERSONAL STRESS MANAGEMENT TOOLKIT

REFLECTION: Are You Present?

Take a deep breath, inhaling air into your abdominal cavity and exhaling slowly and steadily.
Ask yourself:

- What am I thinking (daydreams, plans, worries)?

- What am I feeling (anxious, happy, annoyed)?

- What am I seeing? Hearing? Feeling? Tasting? Smelling?

- What am I experiencing in my body (hunger, fullness, tension)?

- Observe all of the sensations you are experiencing as you breathe steadily.

- Bring your focus back to the here and now.

TECHNIQUE: Sitting Meditation

Record yourself reading the following instructions or take turns with a classmate reading the directions aloud for each other.

- Turn off your phone, laptop, computer—anything that may disrupt your concentration.

- Sit upright in a comfortable chair, with your feet slightly in front of your knees and hands resting in your lap or one the arms of the chair. Do not lie down since you're more likely to fall asleep.

- Let your muscles relax without trying to force them to do so.

- Focus on your breathing. Pay attention to every inhalation and exhalation.

- Close your eyes.

- Repeat in your mind the word "one" as you inhale and the world "two" as you exhale. Do not try to control your breaths. Simply count them.

- When random thoughts pop into your brain (and they will), don't chastise yourself for doing something wrong. Simply inhale and once again focus on the word "one" as you breathe in and "two" as you breathe out.

- Continue for 20 minutes. (It's better not to set an alarm. You can check your watch or cellphone when you feel the time is up. This gets easier with practice.)

- Take a few moments to re-adapt. Open your eyes gradually, focusing one object at a time. Take several deep breaths. Stretch your arms while still seated. When you're ready, stand up slowly and stretch again.

- Repeat twice a day for a week. More often is better because every day brings new circumstances to your life. You may be hungry or tired or upset—all factors that influence your ability to engage in mind-based techniques. You also become more comfortable with each approach every time you perform an exercise.

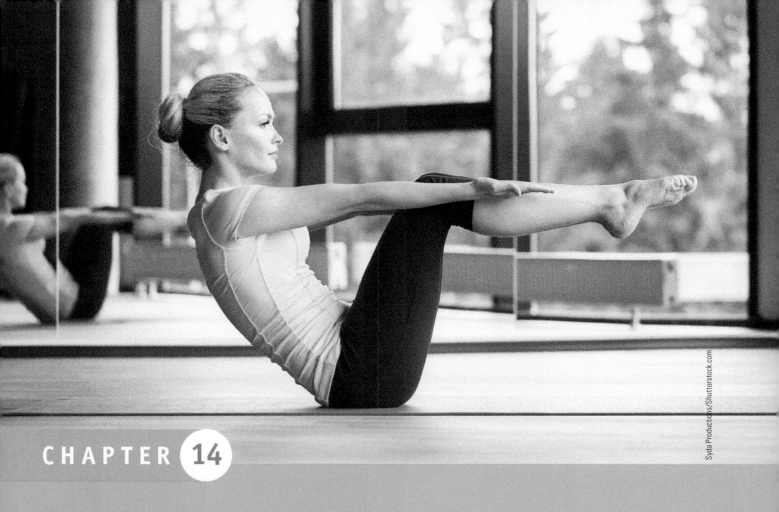

Syda Productions/Shutterstock.com

CHAPTER 14

Physical Techniques

After reading this chapter, you should be able to:

14.1 Describe the use of autogenics to attain deep levels of relaxation.

14.2 Summarize the relationship between biofeedback and stress reduction.

14.3 Explain the mental, physical, social and spiritual components of yoga.

14.4 Describe the ancient Chinese practice of t'ai chi and its benefits.

14.5 Discuss Pilates and its benefits.

14.6 Analyze the effectiveness of dance therapy in decreasing anxiety and boosting mood.

What is your experience with physical relaxation techniques?

_____ I wear yoga pants, but I've never tried it
_____ I've dropped in on a few Pilates classes
_____ I can do anything from downward dog to a headstand with ease

How fit are you?

_____ I get winded climbing a flight of stairs
_____ I exercise when I can and I'm generally healthy
_____ I am in great shape and can't imagine not working out every day

Do you prefer passive exercises that you can do lying down or intensely active ones?

_____ I'd rather not break a sweat
_____ I like a combination
_____ I like to push my limits in every workout

Are you interested in combining spirituality with physical movement?

_____ No, I go to the gym for my body, not my soul
_____ I'm open minded
_____ Yes, I like to bring together mind, body, and spirit whenever I can

What do you hope to gain from a mind-body practice?

_____ Relaxation
_____ Feeling balanced and centered
_____ Strength and confidence

There are no right or wrong answers to these questions, but keep your replies in mind as you read about the techniques presented in this chapter. Give some a try, and decide which ones you're most likely to enjoy.

Your body is constantly changing. Your temperature rises and falls; your heart speeds up and slows down; the pattern of your brain waves differs when you're awake or asleep, stressed or relaxed. You may think these fluctuations are beyond your conscious control, but in fact the mind has great power to influence the way the body works.

Ancient disciplines such as yoga and tai chi tap into this power, as do approaches like autogenics and biofeedback. By sampling a variety of techniques that engage body and mind to lessen, manage, and recover from excess stress, you can see—and feel—for yourself which may help you most.

Autogenics

Derived from the Greek words *autos* (self) and *genos* (origin), **autogenics** is a self-directed relaxation technique based on the power of suggestion.

Decades of use and study have established autogenics as an effective means of relaxing the body and reducing stress-related symptoms.

Understanding Autogenics

This technique uses both visual imagery and body awareness to reduce stress as you mentally repeat words or suggestions to help you relax

autogenics or autogenic relaxation
A technique that uses both visual imagery and body awareness to reduce stress.

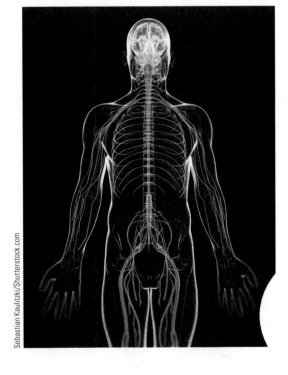

Sebastian Kaulitzki/Shutterstock.com

Autogenics combines visual imagery, body awareness, and the power of suggestion to reduce stress.

and reduce muscle tension. For instance, you may imagine a peaceful place and then focus on controlled breathing, slowing your heart rate, or relaxing your arms and legs.

Autogenics was developed in the early 20th century. While investigating hypnosis (discussed in Chapter 13), physiologist Oskar Vogt observed that individuals in a hypnotic state reported less tension, fatigue, and headaches. Building on this research, psychiatrist Johannes Schultz observed that deep hypnosis often produced pleasant physical sensations of warmth and pressure. The reason is that, in response to **hypnotic suggestion**, the parasympathetic nervous system, which returns the body to homeostasis after activation of the stress response, causes blood vessels to dilate, or increase in diameter, so more blood flows to the extremities. This creates a sensation of warmth. The relaxation of tense muscles induces the sense of heaviness.

With practice in autogenic training, people are able to attain levels of relaxation as deep as those achieved with hypnosis or meditation.

 Stress Reliever: Autogenic Videos

Check out instructional videos, such as the following:

Autogenic Training I: https://www.youtube.com/watch?v=E_sdaDwa2Ek

Autogenic Relaxation: https://www.youtube.com/watch?v=5Lzi4T6muOU

An autogenic exercise for sleep: https://www.youtube.com/watch?v=74aXSxyi8oo

---

The Benefits of Autogenics

The state of deep relaxation induced by autogenics has a powerful impact on the body. Its beneficial effects include:

Reduced heart and respiration rate

Lower blood pressure

Less muscle tension

Lower risk of cardiovascular disease

Relief of tension and migraine headaches

Relief of asthma symptoms

Improved sleep

Less anxiety

Improved mood

hypnotic suggestions
Statements that the mind believes to be true.

Relief of symptoms of post-traumatic stress disorder (PTSD)[1]

Relief of symptoms of digestive disorders and thyroid problems

Autogenics, often combined with visualization, is used by athletes to improve their performance and by pilots and first responders to remain calm during intensely stressful situations.

What You Need to Know

Unlike meditation techniques in which you consciously focus your mind, autogenics requires a passive state sometimes described as "effortless effort" or "allowing rather than doing." You do not consciously attempt to induce feelings of warmth and heaviness. Instead you allow these sensations to occur. If nothing happens, you accept this without judgment. If you do feel physical sensations, you observe them. Whatever happens happens.

To try autogenics, lie down on a bed, exercise mat, or carpet. Rest your arms on the surface, with the palms of your hands up and your fingers loosely extended. Your feet should form a "V" with the toes pointing outward and the heels close to each other but not touching. Support your head and neck with a pillow.

If you prefer to sit, choose a comfortable chair with a high back and armrests so your head and arms are supported. Keep your feet flat on the floor with your legs apart. Press your buttocks against the back of the chair. Your arms, hands, and fingers can rest on the arms of the chair, or you can put them in your lap.

Eliminate any possible distractions. Shut off your phone, laptop, or other devices. If possible, close and lock your door, or inform your roommates that you need some private time. Record the suggestions below and play the audio, or ask a friend or classmate to read them to you.

The Stages of Autogenics

A session of autogenic relaxation typically follows this sequence:

Stage 1: Heaviness
Give yourself commands such as:

My right arm is heavy.

My left arm is heavy.

Both arms are heavy.

My right leg is heavy.

My left leg is heavy.

Both of my legs are very heavy.

My arms and legs are very heavy.

Stage 2: Warmth

Follow the same sequence of instructions:

My right arm is warm.

My left arm is warm.

Both arms are warm.

Stage 3: Heart

Focus on sensations of heaviness and warmth in the area of the heart. Repeat the following command several times:

My heartbeat is strong and regular.

Stage 4: Respiration

Focus on breathing, giving yourself the following command several times:

My breathing is calm and relaxed.

Stage 5: Abdomen

Focus on sensations of warmth as you repeat to yourself:

My abdomen is warm.

Stage 6: Forehead

Focus on sensations of coolness as you repeat:

My forehead is cool.

It usually takes several months of practice of at least ten minutes daily to reach the point where you can induce feelings of warmth, heaviness, and calm throughout your body. Once you have reached this point, you can add relaxing images. This is sometimes called autogenic meditation. (See page 281 at the end of this chapter for an introductory autogenics exercise.)

Biofeedback

Biofeedback is a technique of becoming aware, with the aid of external monitoring devices, of internal physiological activities in order to develop the capability of altering them. The goal of biofeedback for stress reduction is a state of tranquility, usually associated with the brain's production of alpha waves (which are slower and more regular than normal waking brain activity).

Understanding Biofeedback

Biofeedback provides feedback, or information, about some physiological activity occurring in the body. A monitoring device attached to the body detects a change in an internal function and communicates it to an individual through a tone, light, or meter. By paying attention to this feedback, most people can gain some control over

functions once thought to be beyond conscious influence, such as body temperature, breathing, heart rate, muscle tension, and brain waves.

Biofeedback equipment is not meant to be used during a stressful experience, but as a means of training people to gain greater control of their physiological processes when they do encounter stress. The monitors described below teach individuals to recognize the sensations of relaxation and its physiological correlates: decreased muscle tension, heart rate, respiration, and blood pressure.

Clinical biofeedback employs various monitors to observe different bodily functions. The most widely used include:

- **Electromyelogram (EMG):** Electrodes or other sensors, usually attached to the forehead, jaw, or shoulder muscles, produce a signal, such as a sound or colored light, to indicate increased tension. Once alerted, a person immediately senses how this tension feels and can take steps to release this tightness. EMG is most often used to relax the muscles involved in back pain, neck pain, headaches, asthma, hypertension, ulcers, tinnitus, colitis, and bruxism (teeth grinding).

- **Temperature:** Sensors attached to the fingers indicate skin temperature, which typically decreases in the hands and feet during the stress response. A drop in temperature signals that it's time to relax. Thermal biofeedback is used to treat hypertension, migraine headaches, and **Raynaud's disease** (a condition that causes too little blood to flow into the fingers).

- **Galvanic Skin Response (GSR):** Specialized sensors measure the activity of the sweat glands by detecting perspiration on the skin, which typically increases during stress.

- **Electroencephalogram (EEG):** Sensors attached to the scalp are linked to a computer that monitors the activity of different brainwaves—beta, alpha, theta, and delta—associated with different states, such as normal wakefulness, various stages of sleep, and relaxation. With training, individuals can produce more of the alpha waves characteristic of relaxation and sleep.

Once individuals recognize their automatic responses to stress, they can employ techniques such as meditation, progressive muscle relaxation, or autogenics as interventions to return the body to homeostasis.

The Benefits of Biofeedback

With biofeedback, people can learn to control usually involuntary functions, such as circulation

biofeedback
A technique of becoming aware, with the aid of external monitoring devices, of internal physiological activities in order to develop the capability of consciously altering them.

Raynaud's disease A condition in which the fingers become painful and white when exposed to cold.

to the hands and feet, tension in the jaws, and heart rates. Biofeedback has been used to treat dozens of ailments, including asthma, Raynaud's disease, headaches, chronic pain, asthma, hypertension, irritable bowel syndrome, fibromyalgia, hot flashes, cardiac arrhythmia (irregular heartbeat), side effects of cancer chemotherapy, and epilepsy. Biofeedback, particularly of breathing, also helps individuals with PTSD.[2]

What You Need to Know

Biofeedback itself provides information about the body, but it is not a substitute for relaxation techniques. Once alerted to the physiological changes associated with stress, you can use breathing, relaxation, and other approaches to intercept the stress response and relax. With practice, you can recognize stress signals without monitors and machines and take steps to return your body to homeostasis.

If you are interested in biofeedback to help with a health problem, turn to a certified biofeedback specialist. Your primary care physician or your school's health service should be able to refer you. Biofeedback training may be available through psychology or health education departments on some campuses.

You can buy apps, software, wrist monitors, and products that offer biofeedback for stress management. Various tracking devices measure skin temperature, breathing patterns, heart rate variability, and skin conductance (a measure of electrical charge that reflects changes in arousal) to increase awareness of stress level. Software programs and apps for mobile devices guide you through activities that help you relax and focus your mind through games or entertaining challenges.

Do they work? No one really knows. Stress-monitoring products for consumers have not been scientifically tested. Read reviews online, or download free or inexpensive apps to see if they appeal to you.

yoga Traditionally associated with religion, yoga consists of various breathing and stretching exercises that unite all aspects of a person.

Wrist monitors and apps for mobile devices provide immediate feedback on heart rate, breathing patterns, and other stress indicators.

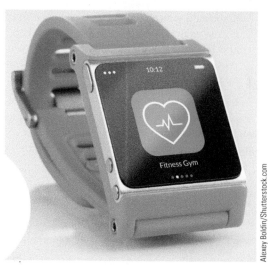

Alexey Boldin/Shutterstock.com

Yoga

One of the most ancient of mind-body practices, **yoga** comes from a Sanskrit word meaning "to yoke or join" and has been defined as a union of mental, physical, social, and spiritual components. Yoga consists of various breathing and stretching exercises and postures that unite all aspects of a person and that, according to traditional belief, unite your ordinary self (the one who thinks "I am reading these words") and your spiritual or true self (much bigger and a part of everything in the universe).[3]

About 31 million U.S. adults have tried yoga. Regular yoga practitioners are more likely to be:

- Female
- Younger
- Generally healthier than the general populations
- White
- College educated
- Higher earners
- Residents of western states

The most common reasons that people practice yoga are general wellness, disease prevention, more energy, improved immune function, relief of back pain, and relief of stress.[4]

> 🌀 **Stress Reliever:** Yoga Videos and Websites
>
> Check out instructional videos, such as the following:
>
> Yoga Camp Day 1: https://www.youtube.com/watch?v=AUJW1Kd4zik
>
> Yoga for Anxiety and Stress: https://www.youtube.com/watch?v=hJbRpHZr_d0
>
> Beginners' Yoga: https://www.youtube.com/watch?v=9jU6ASkhdsQ
>
> Also check out the websites listed below.
>
> http://www.yogasite.com
>
> http://www.yogabasics.com
>
> http://yoga.about.com
>
> http://www.yogajournal.com
>
> Did you gain any new ideas from exploring these sites?

Understanding Yoga

Yoga has been traced back nearly 5,000 years to ancient India. Traditional yoga instruction involved a master teacher who passed his teachings on to disciples through an integrated eightfold process called **ashtanga yoga**, which consists of:

- *Yama*—rules for productive living in society, such as honesty

- *Niyama*—self-rules that govern personal contentment and cleanliness

- *Asana*—physical exercises called postures

- *Pranayama*—deep-breathing exercises

- *Pratyhara*—freeing the mind from the senses

- *Dharana*—focused concentration on an object

- *Dhyana*—meditation

- *Samadhi*—cosmic meditation.

As students progressed through the eight stages of training, they liberated and mastered their life force, which was believed to be located in the spinal cord and vital organs.

The type of yoga used most often for fitness, flexibility and stress management is **hatha yoga**, which consists of breathing exercises *(pranayamas)* and stretching exercises called postures or *asanas*, which lengthen muscles, loosen connective tissue, and release the tension in tight or braced muscles. The poses flow from one to the other at a comfortable pace that allows time to focus on breathing and meditation.

The goal during yoga is to give complete mental attention to each movement to the exclusion of everything else. This awakens inner energy, increases blood flow to targeted areas, increases flexibility in the spine and joints, and stretches and relaxes muscles, ligaments, and tendons. Some postures develop balance more than flexibility, while others develop strength and power. Working on a wide variety of postures enhances each of these aspects of fitness throughout the entire body (see Figure 14.1 and Figure 14.2).

Yoga postures work on all dimensions of health and well-being. Physically, the body experiences healing, muscle strengthening, stretching, and relaxation. Mentally, the mind cultivates peacefulness, alertness, and a heightened ability to focus and concentrate. Emotionally, yoga frees the mind from anxiety, worry, and tension and transforms negative emotions and behaviors into positive higher states. Spiritually, yoga develops inner strength. Behaviorally, yoga redirects wasted energy away from activities and habits that could be detrimental to well-being.

ashtanga yoga
A training process in which a master teacher leads students through eight stages of training through which they liberate and master their life force.

hatha yoga A type of yoga used for fitness, flexibility, and stress management, which consists of various stretching exercises called postures, designed to reduce muscle tension and facilitate at relaxed state of being.

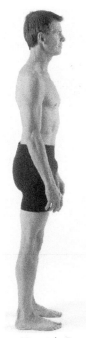
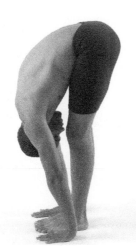
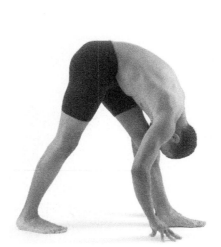
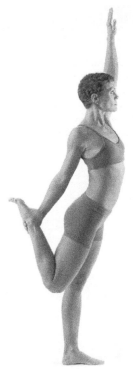

Mountain Pose · Standing Forward Bend · Side Angle Pose · Dancing Pose

FIGURE 14.1 Common yoga poses.

Source: Cengage Learning

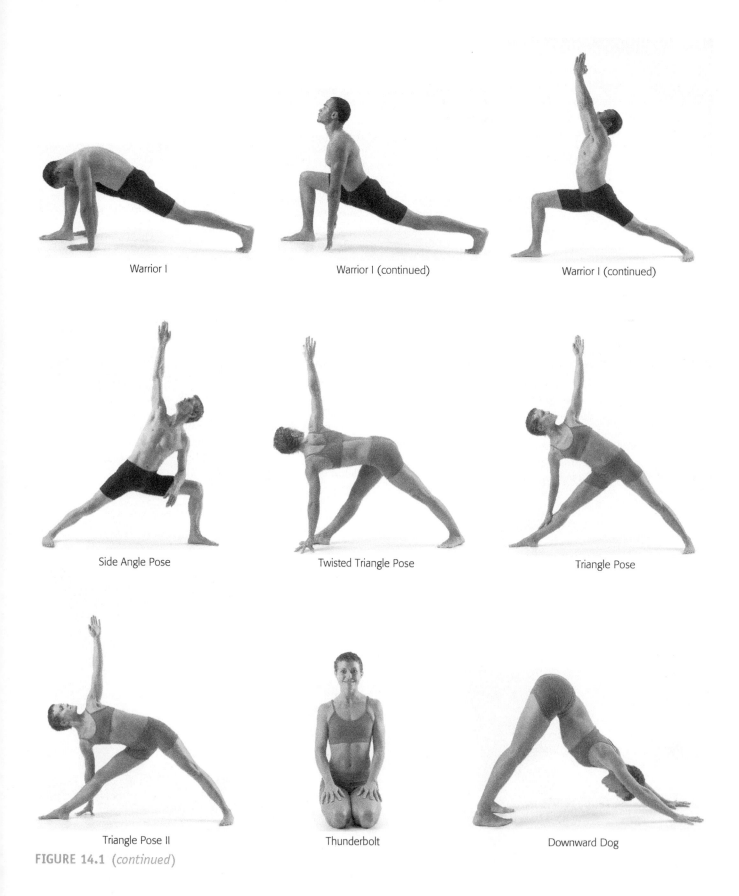

Warrior I

Warrior I (continued)

Warrior I (continued)

Side Angle Pose

Twisted Triangle Pose

Triangle Pose

Triangle Pose II

Thunderbolt

Downward Dog

FIGURE 14.1 (*continued*)

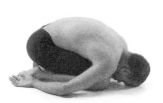

Child's Pose

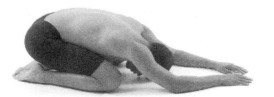

Stretched Child's Pose

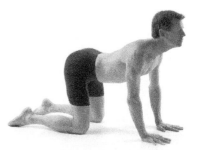

Tiger Breathing (inhale)

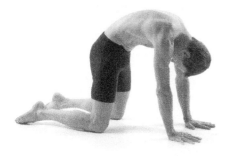

Tiger Breathing (exhale)

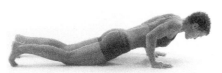

Half Boat

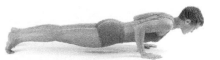

Half Boat (continued)

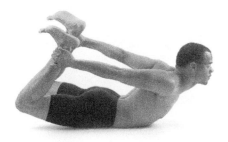

Bow

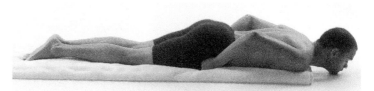

Full Locust

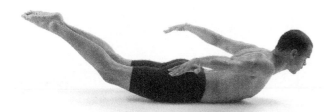

Full Locust (continued)

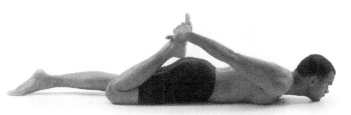

Half Bow

FIGURE 14.1 *(continued)*

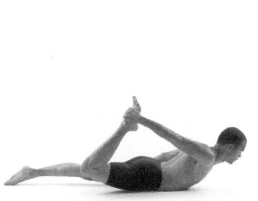

Half Bow (continued)

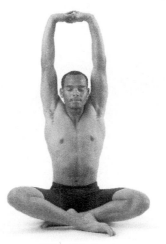

Sitting Side Bend

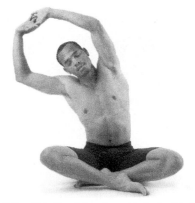

Sitting Side Bend (continued to both sides)

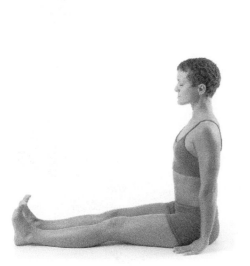

Staff Pose

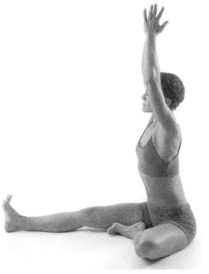

Head to the Knee

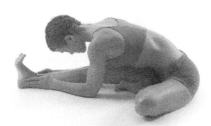

Head to the Knee (continued)

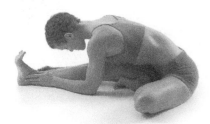

Head to the Knee (continued)

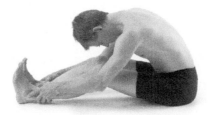

Back Stretch

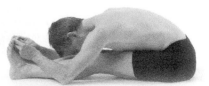

Back Stretch (continued)

FIGURE 14.1 *(continued)*

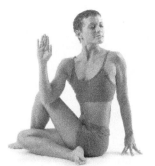

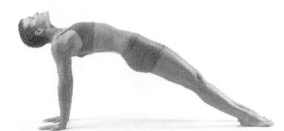

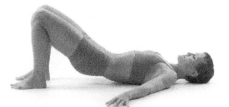

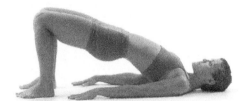

Spiral Twist (both sides)

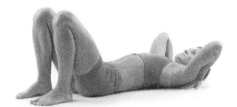

Front Body Stretch

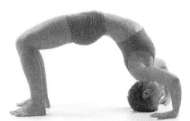

Bridge Pose

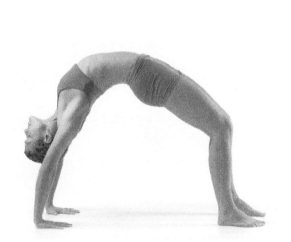

Bridge Pose (continued)

Upward Bow

Upward Bow (continued)

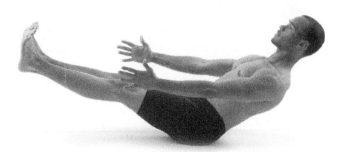

Boat Pose

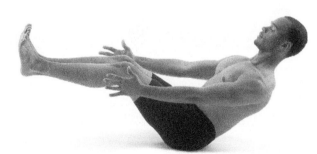

Upward Bow (continued)

Boat Pose (continued)

FIGURE 14.1 *(continued)*

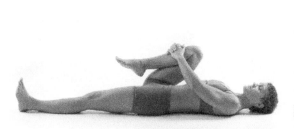

Single Knee to Chest (do each knee)

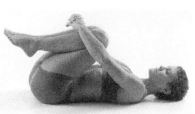

Knees to Chest

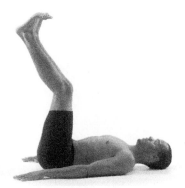

Upward Straight Legs

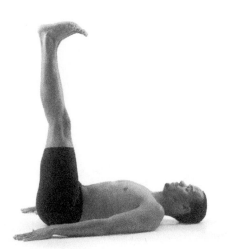

Upward Straight Legs (continued)

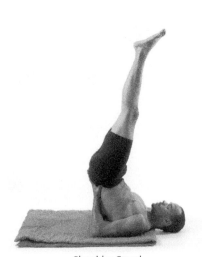

Shoulder Stand

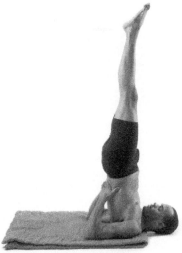

Shoulder Stand (continued)

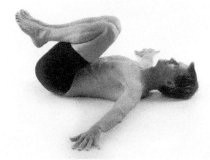

Belly Turning Pose

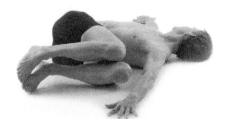

Belly Turning Pose (left side)

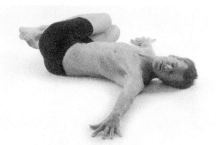

Belly Turning Pose (right side)

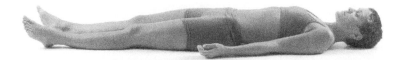

Corpse Pose

FIGURE 14.1 *(continued)*

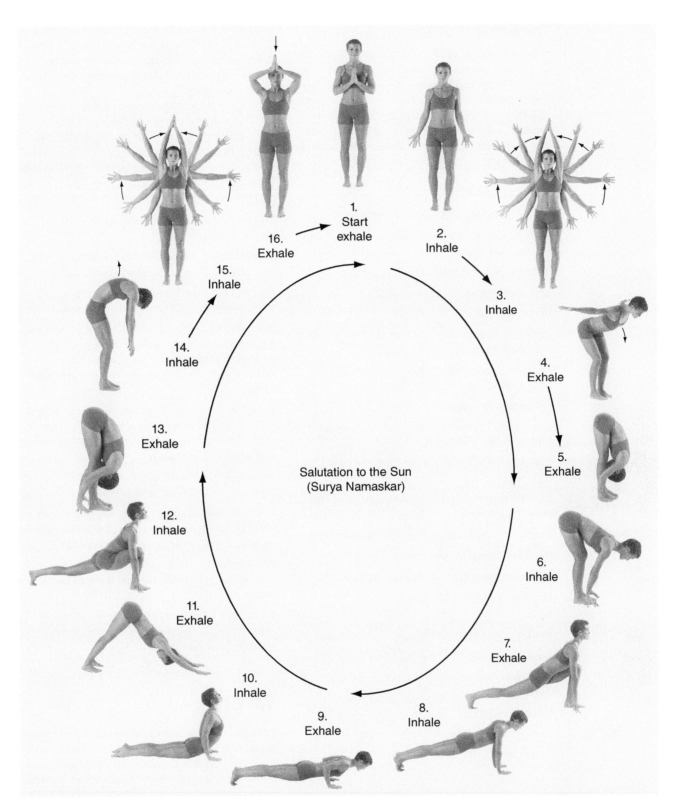

FIGURE 14.2 Salutations to the sun.

Source: Cengage Learning

The Benefits of Yoga

Although its biological mechanisms are not fully understood, studies to date suggest that yoga leads to better regulation of the sympathetic nervous system and hypothalamic-pituitary-adrenal system (described in Chapter 2), which help counter and control the stress response. Other ways in which yoga enhances well-being include the following:

Physical Benefits

Enhanced fitness and sense of well-being.[5]

Lower levels of the stress hormone cortisol[6] and of perceived stress.[7]

Reduced physical arousal during stress.[8]

Improved cardiovascular endurance.[9]

Better sleep.

Improved flexibility, which may offer protection from back pain and injuries.

Stronger, denser bones from yoga's weight-bearing postures.

Enhanced circulation.

Lower blood pressure and other risk factors for cardiovascular disease.[10]

Lower blood sugar in people with diabetes.

Reduced pain for those with backaches, arthritis, carpal tunnel syndrome, fibromyalgia, and other chronic problems.[11]

Improved lung function in people with asthma.

Improved mood for pregnant women.[12]

Less inflammation and enhanced immunity.[13]

Reversal of markers of aging.[14]

Psychological Benefits

Reduced anxiety.[15]

Positive impact on mood (similar to the effect of aerobic exercise).

Greater resilience.

Less perceived stress.[16]

Lessening of symptoms in PTSD.[17]

What You Need to Know

The best way to try yoga is to take an introductory class taught by a certified yoga instructor and learn a few yoga postures and breathing techniques. A typical yoga session consists of assuming a series of poses, being mindful of what is happening in the body, entering and ending each pose slowly, breathing fully and deeply in and out, and enjoying the process. You can practice yoga nearly anywhere: at home, at school, in a park, or anywhere you have some open space, peace, and quiet.

Yoga is generally considered safe, but check with your doctor if you have joint problems, back pain, or neck pain; balance problems; uncontrolled high blood pressure; certain eye conditions, including glaucoma; severe osteoporosis; pregnancy; or artificial joints.

Here are some other things to keep in mind:

To enhance your experience, do yoga on an empty stomach.

Yoga is usually done barefoot, wearing comfortable athletic attire or loose clothing.

Do not hold your breath, and never lock your joints when extending your arms or legs.

Yoga should help, not hurt. To prevent injuries to your knees, back, neck, shoulders, wrists, or ankles, avoid forcing your body into difficult postures. Proper technique is essential to safety.

Stretch to the point of tension (just short of any pain) and hold that position initially for a count of ten. In time you will be able to stretch farther and hold a pose longer.

Go at your own pace. Don't compare your progress or your flexibility with anyone else.

The more you do it, the more you will experience the positive effects of yoga. When possible, try to practice at the same time every day.

Enjoy the experience. Associate pleasure with stretching, breathing, and smooth body movement.

Be patient. After years of building up tension in your body, it takes time to loosen up and become more flexible.

Tai Chi

Tai chi is an exercise and relaxation technique developed in China that involves slow, focused, rhythmic moments combined with controlled breathing and meditation. Tai chi integrates mind and body through respiration and mental and visual concentration.

This ancient practice, originally a form of self-defense involving body, mind, and spirit, gently works muscles, focuses concentration, and improves the flow of *qi* or *chi*, the vital life energy that sustains health. Its blend of fluid physical activity and philosophical outlook stems from

tai chi An exercise and relaxation technique developed in China that involves slow, focused, smooth, rhythmic movements along with control of breathing and mental and visual concentration.

a belief in flowing and harmonizing with opponents rather than fighting them. This view is similar to that of Taoism, which emphasizes the balance of yin and yang, opposing forces in life that come together to form a whole. The concept of "going with the flow" sets tai chi apart from many other forms of self-defense.

Understanding Tai Chi

Tai chi rests on the belief that health involves the continual, unobstructed flow of *chi*. Disease is seen as a breakdown in the flow of this life-giving energy.

Sometimes described as "meditation in motion," tai chi teaches individuals to remain calm and centered against the forces of opposition. It emphasizes conserving energy, remaining balanced, and flowing into rather than fighting an opposing force. As an exercise in maintaining balance, tai chi teaches people how to maintain homeostasis in the face of stressors. Mental techniques (staying calm, not giving in to fear, harmonizing with the opposition) blend with physical ones (maintaining balance, keeping a low center of gravity, conserving energy) to maintain equilibrium.

The Benefits of Tai Chi

The basic concepts of tai chi all have stress-reducing qualities, including:

- Effortless deep breathing: Students get in touch with their breathing, making sure it comes from the abdomen rather than the chest.

- Relaxation and tension reduction: As they perform graceful moments, students look for signs of tension that may inhibit the flow of energy.

- Uniting yin and yang: Students bring together opposing forces such as speed and stillness, force and relaxation.

- Mind-body integration: Students concentrate on the body and visualize its movement. When their minds stray, they return to focusing on their movements.

Tai chi has been shown to improve sleep, reduce prenatal depression and anxiety,[18] lower levels of blood chemicals that may increase the risk of cardiovascular disease[19], and promote heart health.[20]

What You Need to Know

Tai chi incorporates strategies used in other stress management approaches, such as deep breathing, visualization, meditation, and muscle relaxation, with a philosophy of life that emphasizes the need to be flexible and adapt to change rather than fight it. Its fundamentals include:

- A perpendicular stance: keeping the spinal column straight during transitions from position to position.

- A low center of gravity: maintaining a stable base in order to remain centered.

- Moving the body as one rather than limb by limb to provide greater strength and balance.

- An even speed: Continuous, smooth movements to conserve energy compared with sudden, jerky ones.

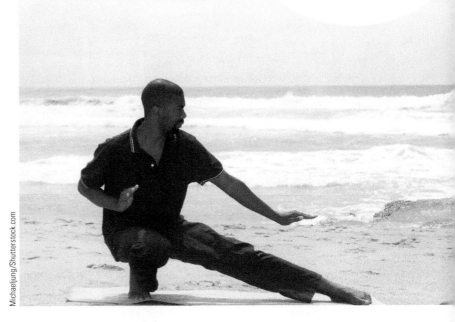

Michaeljung/Shutterstock.com

Tai chi combines mental techniques with physical ones, such as maintaining balance and a low center of gravity.

Classes are available on campuses and in fitness centers, community centers, and some martial arts schools. Full mastery of all the steps of tai chi can take years. Books and videos can supplement your practice but cannot substitute for formal instruction.

Pilates

Used by dancers for deep-body conditioning and injury rehabilitation, **Pilates** (pronounced Puh-lah-teez) is a mind-body approach that focuses on strength, core stability, flexibility, muscle control, posture, and breathing. Developed more than seven decades ago by German immigrant Joseph Pilates, it is increasingly used to complement aerobics and weight training.

Understanding Pilates

The basic principles of Pilates include centering, concentration, control, precision, flow, and breathing.[21] Pilates-trained instructors offer "mat" or "floor" classes that stress the stabilization and strengthening of the back and abdominal muscles. They also may provide training on Pilates equipment, primarily a device called the Reformer, a wooden contraption with various cables, pulleys, springs, and sliding boards that is used for a series of progressive range-of-motion exercises.

Pilates A technique for deep-body conditioning and injury rehabilitation, originally developed for dancers, that emphasizes flexibility and joint mobility and strengthening the core by developing pelvic stability and abdominal control.

Pilates "mat" or "floor" classes focus on stabilizing and strengthening back and abdominal muscles.

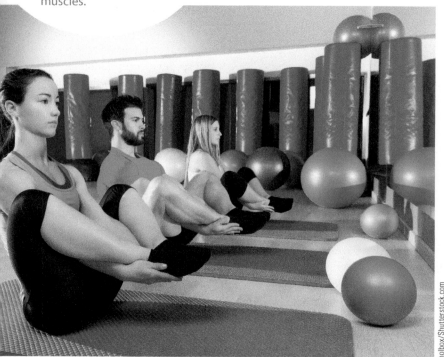

holbox/Shutterstock.com

Stress Reliever: Pilates Videos

Check out instructional videos, such as the following:

Pilates for Beginners: https://www.youtube.com/watch?v=gcgbXDPaFVw

Beginner Pilates Mat Exercises: https://www.youtube.com/watch?v=D3TC-tz3TeQ

Mat Pilates at Home: https://www.youtube.com/watch?v=3hhOObKIu8U

The Benefits of Pilates

Because it is a mind-body approach, Pilates yields both physical and psychological health dividends, including:

Improved flexibility and joint mobility.

Stronger abdominal "core" muscles.

Relief of lower back pain comparable with massage therapy and exercise.[22]

Improved balance and coordination.

Reduced risk of heart disease.

Stronger bones.

Increased cardiorespiratory capacity, but with less risk of injury than aerobic exercise because of low intensity.

Improved body image and self-esteem.

Improved concentration, mindfulness, and mood.

Greater energy and less fatigue.

Higher quality of life and life satisfaction.[23]

What You Need to Know

Pilates training is available on many campuses, gyms, and community centers. Group "mat" classes offer a less expensive alternative to more expensive private lessons on Pilates equipment.

Dance or Movement Therapy

Dance or movement therapy, as defined by the American Dance Therapy Association, is the psychotherapeutic use of movement to further the emotional, cognitive, physical, and social integration of the individual. Body movement serves as both a means of assessment and an intervention for individuals of all ages with developmental, medical, social, physical, and psychological impairments.[24]

Marian Chace, a pioneer in dance therapy, discovered in the 1940s that patients with what we now call post-traumatic stress disorder (PTSD) could express themselves through dance, thereby lessening tension in their bodies and minimizing isolation.[25] The core belief of dance therapy is that the mind and body are interconnected, so that what happens to the body influences the mind and vice versa. Compared with approaches such as exercise or music lessons, dance therapy has a greater impact on decreasing anxiety and boosting mood.[26]

> **Stress Reliever:** Dance it Out!
> ....
> You don't need training, rhythm, or special dance moves. Next time you're feeling stressed, choose music that moves you, get up on your feet, and dance—as if no one were looking.

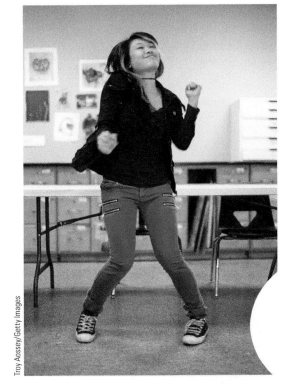

Troy Aossey/Getty Images

Dancing can decrease anxiety, brighten spirits, and fill you with joy.

Chapter Summary

- Autogenics is a self-directed relaxation technique based on suggestions to reduce muscle tension by means of controlled breathing and different physical sensations, such as relaxing different muscle groups.

- The beneficial effects of autogenics include slower heart rate, lower blood pressure, decreased respiration, less muscle tension, lower risk of cardiovascular disease, relief of tension and migraine headaches, improved sleep, less anxiety, better mood, and relief of symptoms of post-traumatic stress disorder.

- Biofeedback is a technique of becoming aware, with the aid of external monitoring devices, of internal physiological activities in order to develop the capability of consciously altering them. The goal of biofeedback for stress reduction is a state of tranquility, usually associated with the brain's production of alpha waves (slower and more regular than normal waking brain activity).

- Clinical biofeedback employs a range of technology to observe different bodily functions, including devices that measure bodily functions such as muscle tension, skin temperature, perspiration, and brainwaves.

- Various devices, software programs, and apps available on line and in stores offer biofeedback for stress management. They have not been scientifically tested.

- One of the most ancient of mind-body practices, yoga stems from an ancient Hindu tradition that includes mental, physical, social, and spiritual components. It consists of breathing and stretching exercises that unite all aspects of a person.

- The type of yoga most often used for fitness, flexibility, and stress management is hatha yoga, which consists of various stretching exercises called postures, designed to reduce muscle tension and facilitate relaxation.

- The benefits of yoga include reduced anxiety, lower levels of the stress hormone cortisol, improved mood and enhanced feelings of well-being, decreased resting heart rate, improved flexibility, stronger bones, enhanced circulation, lower blood pressure, reduced pain in people with back problems, arthritis, carpal tunnel syndrome, fibromyalgia, and other chronic problems; improved lung function in people with asthma, less inflammation, fatigue, and depression in breast cancer survivors.

- Used by dancers for deep-body conditioning and injury rehabilitation, Pilates exercises improve flexibility and joint mobility and strengthen the core by developing pelvic stability and abdominal control.

- Tai Chi is an exercise and relaxation technique that involves slow, focused, rhythmic movements that gently work muscles and improve the flow of *chi,* the vital life energy that sustains health.

- Dance/movement therapy is the psychotherapeutic use of movement to further the emotional, cognitive, physical and social integration of the individual.

STRESS RELIEVERS

Autogenic Videos

Check out instructional videos, such as the following:

- Autogenic Training I: https://www.youtube.com /watch?v=E_sdaDwa2Ek

- Autogenic Relaxation: https://www.youtube.com /watch?v=5Lzi4T6mu0U

- An autogenic exercise for sleep: https://www.youtube .com/watch?v=74aXSxyi8oo

Yoga Videos and Websites

Check out instructional videos, such as the following:

- Yoga Camp Day 1: https://www.youtube.com /watch?v=AUJW1Kd4zik

- Yoga for Anxiety and Stress: https://www.youtube.com /watch?v=hJbRpHZr_d0

- Beginners' Yoga: https://www.youtube.com /watch?v=9jU6ASkhdsQ

    Also check out the websites listed below.

- http://www.yogasite.com

- http://www.yogabasics.com

- http://yoga.about.com

- http://www.yogajournal.com

    Did you gain any new ideas from exploring these sites?

Tai Chi Videos

Check out instructional videos, such as the following:

- Top Tai Chi Moves for Beginners: https://www.youtube .com/watch?v=vHBR5MZmEsY

- Tai Chi for Beginners: https://www.youtube.com /watch?v=HpfWh1UXRBc

- Tai Chi Form 1: Beginning. https://www.youtube.com /watch?v=gyAN4MC0XBY

Pilates Videos

Check out instructional videos, such as the following:

- Pilates for Beginners: https://www.youtube.com /watch?v=gcgbXDPaFVw

- Beginner Pilates Mat Exercises: https://www.youtube .com/watch?v=D3TC-tz3TeQ

- Mat Pilates at Home; https://www.youtube.com /watch?v=3hh0ObKIu8U

Dance it Out!

You don't need training, rhythm, or special dance moves. Next time you're feeling stressed, choose music that moves you, get up on your feet, and dance—as if no one were looking.

YOUR PERSONAL STRESS MANAGEMENT TOOLKIT

REFLECTION: Why Try a Mind-Body Technique?

Answer the following questions:

_____ Do your muscles often feel tight or tense?
_____ Do you suffer from headaches?
_____ Do you have problems falling or staying asleep?
_____ Can you tune into sensations within your body?
_____ Would you like to feel more energized?
_____ Are you open to nontraditional ways of thinking?

The more "yeses" that you check, the more likely you are to enjoy and benefit from the approaches in this chapter because you will find new ways to move and connect body and mind. If physical activity hasn't been a major part of your life, these exercises can be an excellent introduction because they require no innate athletic ability or experience.

TECHNIQUE: Introductory Autogenics Exercise

- Make yourself as comfortable as possible on a floor, bed, or chair.

- Breathe in through your nose and exhale. Repeat several times.

- As you breathe, allow thoughts of past and future to drift away. Close your eyes. Bring yourself into the present moment and focus on inner sensations.

- Direct your attention to your right arm and hand. Note how they are supported by the surface below. As you breathe slowly and steadily, focus passively on your right arm and hand. Silently repeat to yourself: "My right hand and arm are heavy." Continue for several minutes.

- Shift your focus to your left hand and arm and sense how they are supported by the surface below. As you breathe slowly and evenly, repeatedly say to yourself: "My left hand and arm are heavy."

- After several minutes, focus on both hands and arms and how they feel. You may want to shift your attention back and forth from right to left. As you continue to breathe deeply and slowly, repeat silently to yourself: "My hands and arms are heavy." Continue to repeat this phrase for several minutes.

- Imagine the feelings of heaviness and warmth in your arms flowing to every other part of your body. Each time you breathe out, sink into deeper relaxation.

- With your eyes still closed, shift your focus to your right leg. Breathing evenly, say to yourself: "My right leg is heavy." Continue for a few minutes. Make note of the deepening feelings of relaxation in your right leg.

- Let your attention move to your left leg. As you breathe, repeat to yourself, "My left leg is heavy." Notice the deepening relaxation in your left leg.

- Focus on both legs. If this is difficult, shift from one leg to the other. With closed eyes and steady breaths, say to yourself, "My legs are heavy." Repeat several times.

- Let your attention travel to your arms, and say to yourself, "My arms are warm." Continue breathing steadily as the warmth spreads through your arms. Repeat several times.

- Once again focus on your legs, and say, "My legs are warm." Continue saying this to yourself as you breathe and let sensations of warmth travel through your legs.

- Take several minutes to notice how your arms and legs feel. Describe the sensations in your mind.

- Mentally scan your body and notice the feelings of warmth and heaviness spreading to your shoulders, chest, abdomen, hips, and feet. Breathing evenly, say to yourself, "My entire body is warm and heavy." Continue for several minutes.

- Pause and become aware of sensations of warmth and heaviness in every part of your body. Feel them spread as you pay more attention to them.

- As feelings of relaxation deepen, sense the regular beat of your heart. Become very quiet and aware of its rhythm. Inhale and exhale deeply, and repeat to yourself, "My heart is calm and regular."

- Shift attention to your breath, and say to yourself, "My breathing is slow and even." Continue for several minutes.

- Take note of your forehead, and say to yourself, "My forehead is cool and relaxed."

- For several minutes, observe how comfortable, quiet, and still your body feels. Notice your slow, regular breathing and the rhythm of your heart. Feel a sense of deep relaxation spread throughout your body. Enjoy these pleasant sensations.

- If you notice any areas of tension, imagine warmth flowing into them as you continue to breathe steadily.

- Passively accept the deep relaxation enveloping our body. Enjoy the feeling of being rested and at ease.

- To end the session after about 20 minutes, breathe deeply in and out. Completely fill your lungs, and then release the breath. Gently move your fingers, hands, arms, toes, feet, and legs to revive the muscles.

- With your eyes still closed, move your head from side to side.

- Gently stretch your entire body and extend your arms overhead. As you bring your arms down, turn to your side. Lift your knees toward your chest.

- Open your eyes, and slowly lift yourself to a sitting position.

- Remain seated for a few moments and enjoy the feeling of deep relaxation.

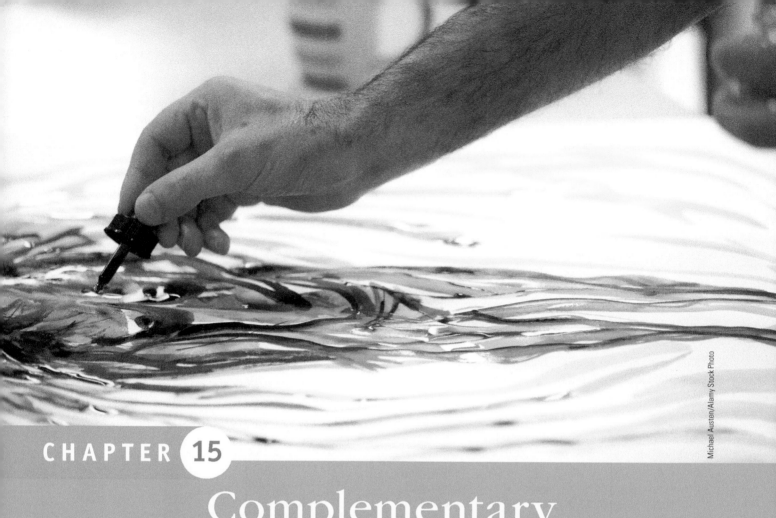

Michael Austen/Alamy Stock Photo

CHAPTER 15

Complementary, Alternative, and Creative Therapies

After reading this chapter, you should be able to:

15.1 Discuss the value of complementary and alternative medicine (CAM).

15.2 Identify the common premise for expressive and creative therapies.

Before you reply, answer the following questions:

_____ Have you ever had a massage?

_____ Do you ever drink chamomile or other soothing teas?

_____ Do you enjoy certain scents, such as eucalyptus or lavender?

_____ Do you doodle?

_____ Do you listen to songs that make you feel a certain way?

If you answered "yes" to any of these queries, you've used a nontraditional approach to stress management. This chapter explains how and why such techniques can help you relax and recover from excess stress.

Often people soothe themselves in ways they don't think of as stress remedies. Half of Americans, for instance, say they pray, yet many may not think of their conversation with a higher power as a stress-reducing technique. Others get a massage simply because it feels good or put a lavender sachet by their bedside because it smells nice, yet these too are alternative forms of stress management.

This chapter introduces an array of options, some imported from other cultures and traditions. Although we need more research on how they work and when to apply them most effectively, non-mainstream interventions have shown a positive impact on relieving stress and enhancing psychological well-being. As with any health-related program or product, you should ask questions and do research before trying these techniques. Weigh the potential risks and benefits, and make informed choices. (See "Reflection" in the Personal Stress Management Toolkit on page 294 at the end of this chapter.)

Complementary and Alternative Medicine (CAM)

CAM refers to various medical and health-care systems, practices, and products not considered part of conventional medicine because there is not yet sufficient proof of their safety and effectiveness. It encompasses:

- **Complementary medicine**, non-mainstream approaches used together with conventional medicine, and

- **Alternative medicine**, non-mainstream approaches used in place of conventional treatments.

According to recent surveys, about 30 percent of Americans have reported using CAM approaches such as relaxation, imagery, biofeedback, and hypnosis. A larger percentage have tried such techniques to prevent, treat, or recover from illness. In general, CAM users tend to be:

- female more often than male

- ages 18 to 44 rather than older

- white more often than Hispanic or black

- college graduates more often than those with less education.[1]

Understanding CAM

CAM's varied healing philosophies, approaches, and therapies include preventive techniques designed to delay or prevent serious health problems before they start and **holistic** methods that focus on the whole person and the physical, mental, emotional, and spiritual aspects of well-being. Some approaches are based on the same physiological principles as traditional Western

complementary and alternative medicine (CAM) A group of diverse medical and health care systems, practices, and products that are not presently considered to be part of conventional medicine.

complementary medicine Therapies that are used together with conventional medicine.

alternative medicine Therapies that are used in place of conventional medicine.

holistic medicine An approach that focuses on the whole person and the physical, mental, emotional, and spiritual aspects of well-being.

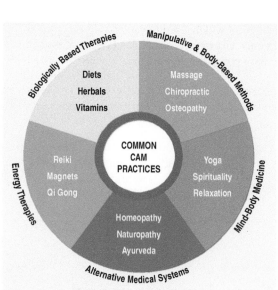

FIGURE 15.1 The five categories of CAM.

integrative or integrated medicine Therapies that combine mainstream medical therapies and CAM therapies.

alternative medical systems A type of CAM that refers to theories and practices based on non-Western medical systems.

mind–body interventions A type of CAM that uses techniques designed to enhance the mind's capacity to affect bodily function and symptoms.

manipulative and body-based methods A type of CAM that includes treatments based on manipulation and/or movement of the body.

Acupuncture uses needles to enhance the flow of energy through the body.

methods; others come from different healing systems. (See Figure 15.1.)

Some techniques once considered unconventional, such as hypnosis (see Chapter 13) and biofeedback (see Chapter 14), are now routinely used by health professionals in treating a broad range of problems and diseases. Many medical schools include training in CAM in their curricula. **Integrative or integrated medicine**, which combines selected elements of both conventional and alternative medicine in a comprehensive approach to diagnosis and treatment, has gained greater acceptance within the medical community.

The National Center for Complementary and Alternative Medicine (NCCAM) has classified CAM therapies into five categories or domains:

1. **Alternative Medical Systems:** Examples include homeopathic medicine, naturopathic medicine, traditional Chinese medicine, and ayurveda.

2. **Mind–Body Interventions:** Examples include meditation, prayer, biofeedback, and therapies that use creative outlets, such as art, music, or dance (discussed later in this chapter).

3. **Manipulative and Body-Based Methods:** Examples include chiropractic or osteopathic manipulation and massage (discussed later in this chapter).

4. **Biologically-based Therapies:** Examples include dietary supplements and herbal products.

5. **Energy Therapies:** Examples include Reiki and Qigong (discussed later in this chapter).

CAM for Stress Management

Each category of CAM techniques includes some therapies that are especially useful for reducing or relieving stress.

Alternative Medical Systems

Western medicine is often described as disease-oriented because of its focus on treating illness and injury. Others differ in both theory and practice.

Traditional Chinese medicine, which dates back some 3,000 years, includes techniques such as **acupuncture** and **acupressure** to enhance energy and reduce stress. These practices are based on the premise that a cycle of energy circulating through the body controls health.

Pain and disease are seen as the result of a disturbance in the energy flow, which can be corrected by inserting long, thin needles at specific points along longitudinal lines, or **meridians**, throughout the body. Each point controls a different corresponding part of the body. The meridian system consists of a network of interconnected points throughout the body that allow the passage of energy. If they are blocked or congested, they may not be able to supply adequate energy to particular organs. Acupuncture, acupressure, and shiatsu massage are healing practices that attempted to unblock congested meridians to allow the free flow of energy.

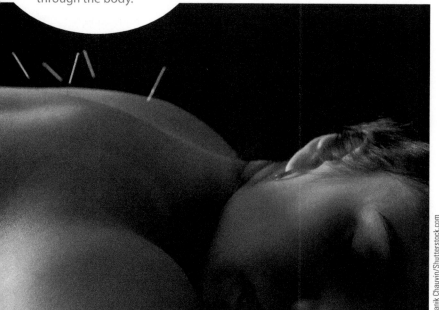

Yanik Chauvin/Shutterstock.com

In acupuncture, needles inserted along a meridian are rotated gently back and forth or charged with a small electric current for a short time. Western scientists aren't sure exactly how acupuncture works, but some believe that the needles alter the functioning of the nervous system. Recent studies have found that acupuncture and acupressure help stress-related conditions such as chronic lower back pain, irritable bowel syndrome, and some neurologic disorders. However, acupuncture can produce adverse effects, including infection and trauma.

Considered alternative in this country, **ayurveda** is a traditional form of medical treatment in India, where it has evolved over thousands of years. Its basic premise is that illness stems from incorrect mental attitudes, diet, and posture. Practitioners use a discipline of exercise, meditation, herbal medication, and proper nutrition to cope with such stress-induced conditions as hypertension, the desire to smoke, and obesity.

Homeopathy is based on three fundamental principles: like cures like; treatment must always be individualized; and less is more, based on the premise that increasing dilution (and lowering the dosage) can increase efficacy. By administering doses of animal, vegetable, or mineral substances to a large number of healthy people to see if they all develop the same symptoms, homeopaths determine which substances may be given, in small quantities, to alleviate the symptoms. Some of these substances are the same as those used in conventional medicine: nitroglycerin for certain heart conditions, for example, although the dose is minuscule.

Naturopathy emphasizes natural remedies, such as sunlight, water, heat, and air, as the best treatments for disease. Therapies might include dietary changes (such as more vegetables and no salt or stimulants), steam baths, and exercise. Some naturopathic physicians (who are not MDs) work closely with medical doctors in helping patients.

Mind–Body Medicine

Mind–body medicine uses techniques designed to enhance the mind's capacity to affect bodily function and symptoms. Stress-relieving approaches include guided imagery (see Chapter 12); meditation (see Chapter 13); yoga, tai chi, and biofeedback (see Chapter 14); and therapies that use creative outlets such as art and music. (discussed later in this chapter).

Manipulative and Body-based Methods

✔ **Check-in:** Have you ever had a massage?

The most widely used therapy based on manipulation and/or movement of the body is **massage**, which enhances the therapeutic effects of touch by stretching and loosening tight muscles and stimulating circulation. Usually it involves application of lotion and techniques such as caressing, gliding, and kneading to relax the muscles directly.

 Stress Reliever: Massage Videos

Check out instructional videos, such as the following:

How to Massage for Beginners: https://www.youtube.com/watch?v=aliKjIcDMQO

How to Give a Relaxing Back Massage: https://www.youtube.com/watch?v=bwB8ajhteKc

Best Relaxation Back Massage: https://www.youtube.com/watch?v=wunsbyF1XPA

Types of Massage

The most common forms of massage are Swedish, shiatsu, deep tissue, and medical/sports massage.

Swedish

Swedish or total body massage combines a variety of strokes that gradually increase in pressure. It starts with light, flowing strokes called effleurage, followed by a serious of shorter, more pressurized squeezes and roles (petrissage). These

biologically-based therapies CAM treatments that include herbal medicine (botanical medicine or phytotherapy), the use of individual herbs or combinations; and special diet therapies.

energy therapies CAM approaches that focus on energy fields believed to exist in and around the body.

traditional Chinese medicine Therapies that include a variety of carefully formulated techniques, such as acupuncture, herbal medicine, massage, qigong, and nutrition.

acupuncture A therapy that involves inserting hair-thin, sterile needles into the body at specific points (acupoints) to manipulate the body's flow of energy to balance the endocrine system.

Chair massage focuses on relieving tension in the back, shoulders, neck, and arms.

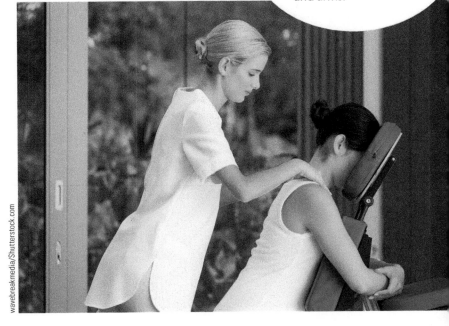

wavebreakmedia/Shutterstock.com

acupressure Therapy that uses direct finger pressure applied to points thought to be areas of chi concentration; described as acupuncture without the needles.

meridians Invisible channels of energy that flow in the body, or energy fields outside the body.

ayurveda India's traditional system of natural medicine that believes that all aspects of life contribute to health, including nutrition, hygiene, sleep, weather, and lifestyle, as well as physical, mental, and sexual activities.

homeopathy A system of medical practice that treats a disease by administering dosages of substances that would in healthy persons produce symptoms similar to those of the disease.

Various types of massage can release chronic patterns of tension in the body.

are followed by deeper, penetrating strokes that include vigorous pressure by circular motion of the thumb or fingertips (friction), kneading (a squeezing action across the width of a muscle), hacking (light slaps or karate chops), and deep vibrating movements. Usually done with lotions or oils, it affects nerves, muscles, glands, and circulation.

A Swedish massage usually progresses up and down the spine, working the neck, shoulders, buttocks, hamstrings, and calves, the areas most susceptible to the buildup of tension and associated aches, pains, strain, and fatigue.

Shiatsu

Shiatsu or acupressure massage, like acupuncture, is based on the theory that stress and disease are due in part to blocks in the flow of the body's vital energy. While acupuncture relieves such blockages by inserting needles, shiatsu applies pressure, usually with the thumbs in a series of circular movements, on points of the body where muscle tension usually builds. Shiatsu massage is shorter and simpler than a Swedish massage and does not require nudity.

Deep Tissue Massage

Deep tissue massage uses deep muscle compression to release the chronic patterns of tension in the body with the heel of the hand, the pads of the thumb, or the elbow pressing along the grain of the muscle. With continuous pressure, deeply held patterns of tension, as well as toxins, can be released.

Medical or Sports Massage

Medical or sports massage is performed to heal muscle tissue damaged by injury or

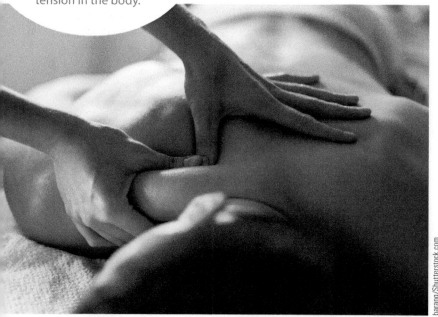

overexertion; this technique may employ a variety of strokes and touches combined with pressure. Often used to help athletes recover from strenuous workouts, it increases the circulation of blood to specific muscles. This increased circulation helps carry nutrients to the tissue, and facilitates the removal of waste products like lactic acid, which can contribute to fatigue and discomfort. This process can reduce stress, relieve pain, and restore a sense of emotional well-being.

Chair Massage

For chair massage, you remain clothed and sit in a special chair with your face resting in a cradle, your arms and legs resting on supports, and your gaze directed toward the floor. For about 10 to 15 minutes, the massage therapist focuses on relieving tension in your back, shoulders, neck, and arms with moves such as kneading and compression. Often offered at airports and shopping malls, chair massage is a good way to release muscle tension and prevent spasms.

The Benefits of Massage

Massage is regularly used in hospitals and clinics to help patients relax and to increase circulation to injured parts of the body. By stimulating blood flow to an injured area, massage reduces swelling, promotes healing, and speeds the healing process. Athletes, trainers, sports medicine, and dance specialists also use massage to prevent and treat soft-tissue injuries.

Other benefits for mind, body, and spirit include:

Reduced stress and anxiety

Improved range of motion

Relief of muscle cramps and spasms

Improved circulation

More efficient removal of the metabolic by-products of exercise

Increased flow of oxygen and nutrients through the blood vessels

Enhanced alertness

Improved sleep

Enhanced feelings of well-being

Relief of headache, muscle stiffness, pain, asthma, arthritis, temporo-mandibular disorder (TMD), carpal tunnel syndrome, and athletic injuries.

What You Need to Know

For most professional massages, you begin by lying on your stomach, with your face in a cradle so you don't have to strain your neck. Generally clients are naked or wearing only underwear beneath a towel or sheet. The massage therapist uncovers only the part of the body that is being worked on.

The therapist's hands should be warm; massage oil ensures that they glide smoothly over your skin. You can request a certain type of massage or a combination of styles. In addition to the strokes described on page 286, therapists may target a particularly "hot" or troublesome spot with their thumbs, fingers, or elbows to separate the tissues, restore circulation, and make the muscle softer and more pliable.

Be sure to let the therapist know if the pressure feels too intense. If possible, try different therapists and types of massage to determine which ones you like best.

Keep in mind that a massage is an intimate experience. Intention is particularly important. Giving a massage to relieve muscle tension—an act of healing—is quite different from giving a massage with the intent to arouse a partner sexually.

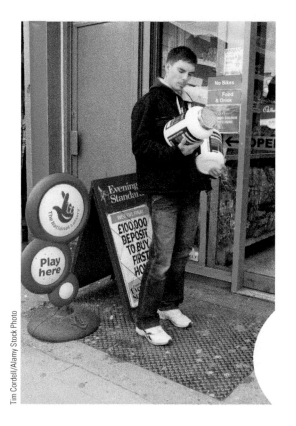
Tim Cordell/Alamy Stock Photo

Herbal and dietary supplements may contain potentially unsafe ingredients. Read labels carefully before you try them.

 Stress Reliever: How to Give a Massage

Most of us know how to give a back or shoulder rub, but the following steps may help you refine your technique:

Have the person lie down on a massage table or high bed. Place a pillow under his or her head.

Use some form of lubricating oil—although some people prefer powder.

Make sure the oil is warm or at room temperature. Warm the container in hot water in the sink if it seems cold.

Pour the oil onto your hands and rub it around before applying it to the other person's body.

You can start at the feet, work up to the head, and finish with the hands, or at the abdomen, the center of the body, and work outwards. Just remember to work the entire body in a systematic way.

Allow yourself enough room to move around the person without having to lean. You need to be able to position yourself so you can apply firm pressure.

Take your time, moving slowly and rhythmically.

Biologically-based Therapies

✔ **Check-in:** Have you ever used dietary supplements or herbs?

Biologically-based CAM therapies use substances such as herbs, foods, and vitamins. They include **herbal medicine** (botanical medicine or phytotherapy), the use of individual herbs or combinations; special diet therapies, such as macrobiotics, Ornish, Atkins, and high fiber; orthomolecular medicine (use of nutritional and food supplements for preventive or therapeutic purposes); and use of other products (such as shark cartilage) and procedures applied in an unconventional manner.

Although many natural substances are marketed as effective stress relievers, there have not been rigorous scientific studies to prove efficacy and safety. Unlike drugs, dietary supplements (vitamins, minerals, herbs, botanicals, amino acids, and enzymes sold as tablets, capsules, softgels, or gelcaps) are not regulated. Many contain active ingredients with strong and potentially unsafe biological effects in the body. This makes them particularly dangerous when used with medications (whether prescription or over-the-counter) or taken in high doses.

Liver injury related to herbal and dietary supplements has more than doubled in the past 10 years.[2] Several widely used herbs, including

naturopathy An alternative system of treatment of disease that emphasizes the use of natural remedies such as sun, water, heat, and air. Therapies may include dietary changes, steam baths, and exercise.

Swedish massage The most common type of basic relaxation massage usually performed with lotions or oils that includes long gliding strokes, kneading, friction, tapping, and shaking motions on the upper or more superficial layers of the muscles.

shiatsu Oriental-based therapy system, using finger pressure applied to specific points along acupuncture meridians.

deep tissue massage
Deep muscle compression with the heel of the hand, the pads of the thumb, and even the elbow pressing deliberately along the grain of the muscle to release the chronic patterns of tension in the body.

medical or sports massage A special type of massage, focusing on muscle systems specific to athletic and sporting events.

Herbal medicine The use of herbs, special diet therapies, nutritional and food supplements, and other products or procedures to prevent or treat disease.

Reiki A healing technique that channels the universal life energy to recipients by the laying on of hands.

Some alternative techniques employ energy fields believed to exist in and around the body.

ginger, garlic, and ginkgo biloba, are dangerous if taken prior to surgery. Consumer groups and state attorneys have accused major retailers of selling contaminated herbal supplements and called on Congress to provide the FDA with more power to regulate supplements.

Energy Therapies

Various approaches focus on energy fields believed to exist in and around the body. Some use external energy sources, such as electromagnetic fields or magnets, but there is little scientific evidence of their efficacy. In Chinese medicine, the vital energy called *chi* or *qi* flows through the body by way of the invisible channels called meridians, which can be blocked by stress. Several techniques, such as acupressure, acupuncture, and shiatsu, combine energy balance with massage to restore a healthy energy flow.

Reiki

Reiki, a Japanese technique for stress reduction and relaxation, involves the laying on of hands to promote the flow of an unseen "life force energy." When this force is low, people are more likely to feel stressed or sick. Higher levels boost health and happiness.

Reiki comes from two Japanese words—*Rei*, which means "God's Wisdom or the Higher Power," and *Ki*, for "life force energy." It involves the transfer of life force energy from a Reiki master to a student. Among the benefits attributed to it are relaxation and feelings of peace, security, and well-being.

Reiki is not a substitute for medical treatment, but can complement conventional therapies to relieve symptoms and promote recovery from illness. Although its roots are spiritual, Reiki is not a religion, and it is not necessary to hold certain beliefs in order for it to be effective.

Reiki is not taught in the usual sense. Through a process called "attainment," a Reiki master allows a student to tap into an unlimited supply of life force energy in order to improve health and quality of life. Some of its enthusiasts report that using Reiki puts them more in touch with their spirituality.

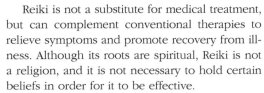

Stress Reliever: Reiki Videos

You can learn more about Reiki techniques and theory from videos, such as the following:

Reiki healing: https://www.youtube.com/watch?v=-iNPSlEFik4

Reiki meditation techniques: https://www.youtube.com/watch?v=NzmPvXgyqMA

Reiki treatment session: https://www.youtube.com/watch?v=eaCCjE1xuOA

Qigong

This ancient Chinese practice integrates physical postures, breathing techniques and focused intention. The word **Qigong** (also called Chi Kung) is made up of two Chinese words: *Qi* (pronounced chee) refers to the life force; *gong* (pronounced gung) describes a skill cultivated through steady practice. Together, Qigong means cultivating energy to maintain health, heal, and increase energy.

Its various styles all involve a posture (moving or stationary), breathing techniques, and mental focus. The gentle, rhythmic movements of Qigong are believed to reduce stress, build stamina, increase vitality, and enhance the immune, cardiovascular, respiratory, circulatory, lymphatic and digestive systems. You can see a demonstration of basic Qigong moves on the web at https://www.youtube.com/watch?v=3HMLtN7BOlY.

Other Complementary and Alternative Techniques

Some complementary and alternative therapies do not fit precisely into any one category. They include **hydrotherapy**, in which warm water draws blood from the body's core to relax the

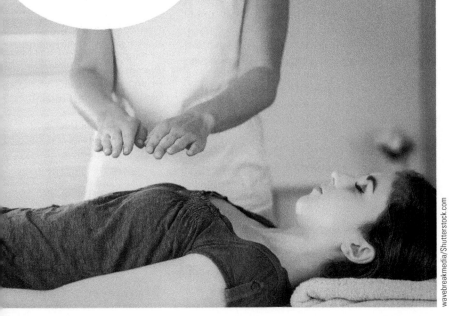

wavebreakmedia/Shutterstock.com

muscles, and **pet or animal-assisted therapy**, which has demonstrated that owning a pet or even petting an animal can lower heart rate, blood pressure, and muscle tension. (See Chapter 6 for more on support animals.)

Aromatherapy is the practice of using the natural or essential oils extracted from flowers, bark, stems, leaves, roots or other parts of a plant to enhance psychological and physical wellbeing. Essential oils are extracted by steaming or pressing the plant matter until it breaks down into a fragrant oil, which is cooled and filtered.

✔ **Check-in:** Do you have a favorite scent?

Aromatherapy is based on the principle that natural fragrances, or essential oils, from certain plants or flowers can affect brain function and how we think or feel at any given time. Breathing in aromas or absorbing them through the skin may produce benefits such as better circulation and digestion, improved sleep, enhanced immunity, and faster healing of cuts or other wounds.

Aromatherapy may date back to ancient Egypt, where oils from plants such as clove and cinnamon were used to bury the dead. The Chinese may have been the first to use infused aromatic oils as a mood enhancer. The Greeks, including Hippocrates, considered the father of medicine, used plant oils for healing purposes. The term "aromatherapy" originated in 1937 when a French chemist began studying the healing powers of essential oils.

Although "natural" oils may seem harmless, you need to be careful when using them. Keep in mind the following precautions:

- Read all warnings and precautions on the label. Dilute oils with water or massage oil as instructed. Be sure to check if certain oils should not be used with specific medications or medical conditions, such as low blood pressure or epilepsy.

- Use only the suggested amount; misuse can lead to headaches and/or nausea.

- Because they are so concentrated, do not rub essential oils directly onto the skin. This can cause redness, burning, itching, and irritation. If the oil comes into contact with your skin, coat the area in a cream or vegetable oil and then wash with warm, soapy water.

- Keep essential oils away from your eyes. If an oil comes into contact with your eye, flush it out with large quantities of warm water and immediately seek medical advice. Store essential oils out of the reach of children, who might attempt to touch or taste them.

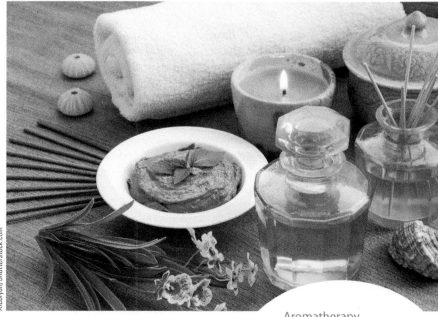

Xiebiyun/Shutterstock.com

Stress Reliever: Soothing Scents

The scents recommended for stress relief include Bergamot, Chamomile, Lavender, Lemon, Orange, Patchouli, Vanilla, and Ylang Ylang. Try several to identify those which you find most soothing.

Creative or Expressive Therapies

We humans have an innate urge to express ourselves in creative ways. Our early ancestors painted on the walls of their caves and made music with simple instruments. For centuries professional artists, musicians, and dancers have delighted and dazzled the world with their gifts. But you don't need talent or formal training to benefit from the process of transforming your ideas, feelings, and experiences into artistic statements.

Creative or expressive therapy focuses not on the final product, but on the process of creating. It encompasses drawing, painting, carving, sculpting, dance, drama, horticulture, music, photography, and film/video. All share the common premise that by tapping into the imagination, individuals can get in touch with emotions and thoughts that words alone cannot capture. By enhancing self-awareness and self-expression, the creative arts foster inner healing, growth, and development.

Aromatherapy uses essential oils extracted from flowers, roots, and other parts of plants to enhance wellbeing.

Qigong An ancient Chinese practice that involves postures, breathing techniques, and mental focus.

hydrotherapy The use of warm water to draw blood from the body's core to relax the muscles.

pet or animal-assisted therapy The inclusion of animals as a form of treatment to relieve stress or improve social, emotional, or cognitive functioning. Animals include domesticated pets, farm animals, and marine mammals (such as dolphins).

aromatherapy The practice of using the natural or essential oils extracted from flowers, bark, stems, leaves, roots, or other parts of a plant to enhance psychological and physical well-being.

Art Therapy

The American Art Therapy Association defines **art therapy** as "the therapeutic use of art making, within a professional relationship, by people who experience illness, trauma, or challenges in living, and by people who seek personal development." By creating art and reflecting on art, people can increase awareness of self and others; cope with symptoms, stress and traumatic experiences; enhance cognitive abilities; and enjoy the life-affirming pleasures of making art.

The creative and expressive arts tap into the unconscious, the source of the thoughts and feelings that set the stress response in motion. Because nonverbal images, symbols, colors, forms, and movements stem from the same source, they can provide insights that enable us to become aware of and cope better with the stressors we confront in life.

Understanding Art Therapy

Art therapy, which emerged as a mental health discipline in the mid-twentieth century, integrates art and creativity into counseling and psychotherapy for the purpose of healing. It has been used to help individuals of all ages with physical, mental, or emotional problems. As an alternative healing opportunity for those who may not respond fully to conventional treatments such as psychotherapy, art therapy can, as the AATA states, help individuals "explore their feelings, reconcile emotional conflicts, foster self-awareness, manage behavior and addictions, develop social skills, improve reality orientation, reduce anxiety, and increase self-esteem."

Art therapy is offered in hospitals, psychiatric and rehabilitation facilities, wellness centers, schools, crisis centers, senior communities, and private practice. By tapping into an individual's inherent creativity, art therapy can benefit a wide range of people, including survivors of trauma and abuse and patients with physical and psychological disabilities and disorders. Art therapy also helps people reduce stress, resolve conflicts, improve interpersonal skills, achieve personal insight, and deepen their enjoyment of life.

A career in art therapy usually requires a master's degree, professional certification, and knowledge of the visual arts (drawing, painting, sculpture, and other art forms) and the creative process, as well as of human development, psychology, and counseling theories and techniques.

Yet art ultimately is more than a therapeutic tool. It is an expression of your deepest thoughts and feelings. Trying your hand at a creative project can lead to a journey of personal self-discovery that releases pent-up emotions from your unconscious and yields deeper understanding of where you are in life.

The Benefits of Art Therapy

Finding an artistic outlet for self-expression has proven beneficial in:

reducing stress

aiding recovery after trauma

increasing self-esteem

achieving insight

managing problematic behaviors such as smoking

developing interpersonal skills

resolving conflicts and problems

improving memory

easing depression

soothing symptoms of chronic diseases and age-related disorders.[3]

What You Need to Know

Don't worry about your artistic skills or lack thereof. Even doodling has been recognized as a nonverbal message from the unconscious. You can draw stick figures, paint abstract forms, mold clay animals, or paste together words and images from magazines. Art therapy is not a competition; you won't be graded or criticized for your creation.

Art Therapy Exercises

Although you can choose any medium that appeals to you, art therapists suggest starting with a blank sheet of white paper of any size and as wide a range of colors as possible—in crayons, colored

creative or expressive therapy Therapeutic approaches that encompass art, dance, drama, horticulture, music, photography, and film/video as ways of tapping into the imagination so individuals can get in touch with emotions and thoughts that words alone cannot capture.

art therapy The therapeutic use of art making for people who experience illness, trauma, or challenges in living, and those who seek personal development.

Art therapy helps people reduce stress, express emotions, and deepen appreciation of life and beauty.

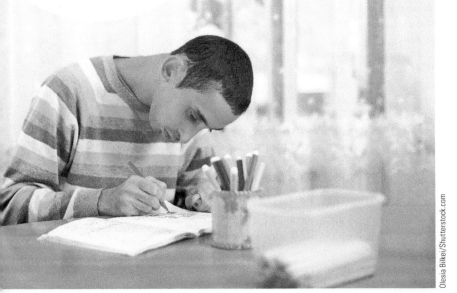

Olesia Bilkei/Shutterstock.com

pencils, watercolors, or oil paints. Once you've assembled your materials, you can start drawing anything until you come up with an inspiration. Or you try these suggestions from art therapists:

- Create something that represents you. It doesn't have to be a self-portrait, but it should reflect something that matters to you.

- Close your eyes and draw a line on the paper. It can be any shape you choose. Keep your eyes closed until you've finished. Once you open them, you can rotate the paper in any direction and then complete the drawing, creating something meaningful out of the random line you drew without looking.

- Draw a dream. Can you recall an image from a recent dream? You might not be able to describe it in words, so try showing what it looks like.

- If you have a medical problem, draw the part of your body that hurts, such as your aching head or sore arm. Then draw another image of this same region of your body, this time showing it fully healed.

- You also may enjoy the adult coloring books that have been growing in popularity as a simple way of focusing and soothing the mind.

 Stress Reliever: Capture Moments

If you have a camera on your cell phone, keep your eye open for images that strike you. Take photos, not for the sake of showing a scene, but to tell a story of how you felt in that moment in time.

Music Therapy

Music can reach our deepest thoughts and feelings in a way that verbal language cannot. Even before birth a fetus responds to sounds.[4] Children as young as age five are able to express emotions in their singing by using pitch, intensity, and tempo; even younger children can pick out emotional cues in music.[5]

As humans we appear to be wired to listen for musical patterns—melodies, rhythms, and lyrics. Anticipating these patterns activates reward centers in the brain.[6] Auditory sensations stimulate neurons in the limbic system, particularly the hypothalamus, known as the "seat of emotions." While we recognize at a conscious level that music can influence mood, auditory stimuli can also penetrate the unconscious mind and promote their own changes in our perceptions.

Music breaks down strong emotional defenses and allows for freer expression of feelings.[7] It heightens positive emotions by stimulating hits of dopamine that can make us feel good, comforted, excited, or elated. Some musicologists believe that listening to certain types of music accesses the creative right brain and enhances the mind's receptivity to new ideas. In one study, volunteers listening to Mozart's *Eine Kleine Nachtmusik* (*A Little Night Music*) reported less stress and more relaxation than those who listened to New Age music.[8] Other studies have confirmed the power of the "Mozart effect" in relieving pain and tension.[9]

Loud, rapid-tempo music may release latent anger; uplifting, slow, rhythmic music can sedate and rejuvenate. Athletes use the subliminal power of music to motivate themselves with "power anthems." "Soft" music—classical, solo piano, instrumental—played as background in dental offices significantly reduces levels of stress, anxiety, and depression.[10] In one study, volunteers were asked to identify happy and sad "smiley icons" while listening to happy or sad music. When a happy song was playing, the participants often "saw" a smiley face even when a neutral face was shown, but a sad one when sad music was playing.[11]

 Stress Reliever: Mood Music

Experiment with songs to identify those that resonate most with your moods. Find and name three songs that infuse a sense of hope and optimism when you're dealing with hardships; three that soothe when you want to calm down; and three that energize you for an upbeat workout. For an even greater impact, watch music videos of your selected songs.

Understanding Music Therapy

Music therapy, as defined by American Music Therapy Association, is "the clinical and evidence-based use of music interventions to accomplish individualized goals within a therapeutic relationship."[12] According to a broader, less formal definition, "music therapy" refers to active music-making or passive listening to music for the sake of relaxation and stress reduction.

Music therapists employ music within a therapeutic relationship to address a client's physical, emotional, cognitive, and social needs. Depending on abilities, individuals may listen, sing, or create music. Music therapy provides an alternative form of communication for those who find it difficult to express themselves in words. It has

music therapy The use of music interventions to accomplish individualized goals within a therapeutic relationship.

proven effective in improving motivation, facilitating movement, providing emotional support, and engaging patients in their treatment.

Credentialed music therapists, who may have bachelor's or master's degrees, work in medical facilities, nursing homes, schools, and other clinical settings to provide music-based treatments for patients with disabilities, chronic pain, brain injuries, dementia, and other mental health needs.

The Benefits of Music Therapy

Music has long played a role in healing rituals, and modern researchers have confirmed its benefits for a wide range of clinical applications. As one researcher put it, "The promise of music as medicine is that it's natural and it's cheap and it doesn't have the unwanted side effects that many pharmaceutical products do."[13] As recent studies have shown, music therapy:

Prevents stress-induced increases in cortisol, heart rate, and blood pressure.[14]

Aids in post-surgery recovery.[15]

Improves mood, memory, and cognitive function in people with Alzheimer's, and their caregivers.[16]

Reduces anxiety and stress in hospitalized children.[17]

Relieves pain in patients with fibromyalgia.[18]

Bolsters immune functioning.[19]

Enhances memory and learning.[20]

Boosts exercise/sports motivation and performance.[21]

Hastens the recovery and return to their jobs of workers on disability.[22]

Listening to music can re-energize you during a study break and boost your concentration and memory.

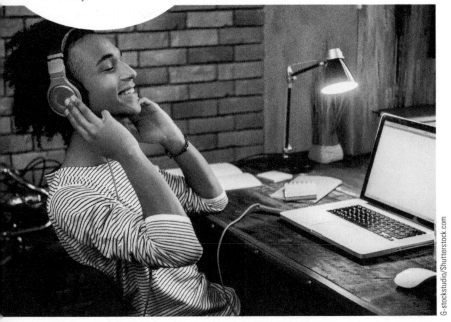

G-stockstudio/Shutterstock.com

 Stress Reliever: Music Meditation

As explained in Chapter 13, you can focus on your breath, a mantra, or a visual image during meditation. Music provides another option; if you are feeling frazzled, melodic music with a slower rhythm can help slow down your breathing, heart rate, and muscular activity. Experiment with listening to Indian and other Eastern musical compositions specifically designed for meditation.

What You Need to Know

Thanks to modern technology, you can take music everywhere you go—as you walk, drive, do your laundry, wait for a friend—to create a more tranquil setting. As background sound, soothing music can promote physiological calmness while you go about other tasks.

In order to make the most of music as a relaxation technique, keep in mind the following suggestions:

- Create stress-soothing playlists for times when you want to unwind from a long day or end it on a relaxing note. Music that is grating to your ear will promote stress rather than reduce it.

- Music therapists recommend instrumental or acoustic music with a slow tempo. This can include classical, improvisational jazz, or New Age music—although not all types are slow or relaxing. Find something you like and build on this style.

- Set aside some time solely for music. During your listening session, minimize or eliminate interruptions. Choose a comfortable, peaceful environment. Sit or recline in a comfortable position with eyes closed to minimize distractions. Breathe deeply and evenly.

 Stress Reliever: Make Music

Don't worry about carrying a tune. Sing to yourself in the shower or car. Hum; whistle; play an instrument. For an even greater benefit, join a choir. Making music together tends to synch breathing and heart rates, producing a group-wide calming effect.

Chapter Summary

- Complementary and Alternative Medicine (CAM) refers to various medical and health-care systems, practices, and products not considered part of conventional medicine because there is not yet sufficient proof of their safety and effectiveness.

- Complementary medicine consists of non-mainstream approaches used together with conventional medicine. Alternative medicine includes non-mainstream approaches used in place of conventional treatments.

- CAM emphasizes holistic methods that focus on the whole person and all aspects of well-being. Integrative or integrated medicine combines selected elements of both conventional and alternative medicine in a comprehensive approach to diagnosis and treatment.

- The National Center for Complementary and Alternative Medicine (NCCAM) has classified CAM therapies into five categories or domains: Alternative Medical Systems, Mind-Body Interventions, Manipulative and Body-based Methods, Biologically-based Therapies, and Energy Therapies.

- Ayurveda is a traditional form of medical treatment in India, where it has evolved over thousands of years. Its basic premise is that illness stems from incorrect mental attitudes, diet, and posture.

- Traditional Chinese medicine, which dates back some 3,000 years, includes techniques such as acupuncture and acupressure to enhance energy and reduce stress. These practices are based on the premise that a cycle of energy circulating through the body controls health.

- The most widely used therapy based on manipulation and/or movement of the body is massage, which enhances the therapeutic effects of touch by stretching and loosening tight muscles and stimulating circulation.

- Massage is a direct way of relaxing tense muscles and stimulating circulation to the tissues and muscles. Its benefits include reduced stress and anxiety, improved range of motion, relief of muscle cramps and spasms, more efficient removal of the metabolic by-products of exercise, improved sleep, and enhanced feelings of well-being.

- The most common forms of massage are Swedish or total body, shiatsu or acupressure, deep tissue massage, and medical or sports massage.

- Biologically based CAM therapies include herbal medicine (botanical medicine or phytotherapy), the use of individual herbs or combinations; and special diet therapies. There have not been rigorous scientific studies to prove their efficacy and safety.

- Reiki, a Japanese technique for stress reduction and relaxation, involves the laying on of hands to promote the flow of an unseen "life force energy." When this force is low, people are more likely to feel stressed or sick.

- Creative or expressive therapy encompasses several forms, including art, dance, drama, horticulture, music, photography, and film/video. By tapping into the imagination, individuals can get in touch with emotions and thoughts that words alone cannot capture.

- The American Art Therapy Association defines art therapy as " . . . the therapeutic use of art making, within a professional relationship, by people who experience illness, trauma or challenges in living, and by people who seek personal development."

- Finding an artistic outlet for self-expression has proven beneficial in reducing stress, increasing self-esteem, achieving insight, managing problematic behaviors such as smoking, developing interpersonal skills, and resolving conflicts and problems.

- Music therapy, as defined by American Music Therapy Association, is "the clinical and evidence-based use of music interventions to accomplish individualized goals within a therapeutic relationship." According to a broader, less formal definition, "music therapy" refers to active music-making or passive listening to music for the sake of relaxation and stress reduction.

- To reduce stress, music therapists recommend instrumental or acoustic music with a slow tempo. This can include classical, improvisational jazz, or New Age music.

 STRESS RELIEVERS

Massage Videos
Check out instructional videos, such as the following:

- How to Massage for Beginners: https://www.youtube.com/watch?v=aliKjIcDMQ0

- How to Give a Relaxing Back Massage: https://www.youtube.com/watch?v=bwB8ajhteKc

- Best Relaxation Back Massage: https://www.youtube.com/watch?v=wunsbyF1XPA

How to Give a Massage

Most of us know how to give a back or shoulder rub, but the following steps may help you refine your technique:

- Have the person lie down on a massage table or high bed. Place a pillow under his or her head.

- Use some form of lubricating oil—although some people prefer powder.

- Make sure the oil is warm or at room temperature. Warm the container in hot water in the sink if it seems cold.

- Pour the oil onto your hands and rub it around before applying it to the other person's body.

- You can start at the feet, work up to the head, and finish with the hands, or at the abdomen, the center of the body, and work outwards. Just remember to work the entire body in a systematic way.

- Allow yourself enough room to move around the person without having to lean. You need to be able to position yourself so you can apply firm pressure.

- Take your time, moving slowly and rhythmically.

Reiki Videos

You can learn more about Reiki techniques and theory from videos, such as the following:

- Reiki healing: https://www.youtube.com/watch?v=-iNPSlEFik4

- Reiki meditation techniques: https://www.youtube.com/watch?v=NzmPvXgyqMA

- Reiki treatment session: https://www.youtube.com/watch?v=eaCCjE1xuOA

Soothing Scents

The scents recommended for stress relief include Bergamot, Chamomile, Lavender, Lemon, Orange, Patchouli, Vanilla, and Ylang Ylang. Try several to identify those which you find most soothing.

Capture Moments

If you have a camera on your cell phone, keep your eye open for images that strike you. Take photos, not for the sake of showing a scene, but to tell a story of how you felt in that moment in time.

Mood Music

Experiment with songs to identify those that resonate most with your moods. Find and name three songs that infuse a sense of hope and optimism when you're dealing with hardships; three that soothe when you want to calm down; and three that energize you for an upbeat workout. For an even greater impact, watch music videos of your selected songs.

Music Meditation

As explained in Chapter 13, you can focus on your breath, a mantra, or a visual image during meditation. Music provides another option; if you are feeling frazzled, melodic music with a slower rhythm can help slow down your breathing, heart rate, and muscular activity. Experiment with listening to Indian and other Eastern musical compositions specifically designed for meditation.

Make Music

Don't worry about carrying a tune. Sing to yourself in the shower or car. Hum; whistle; play an instrument. For an even greater benefit, join a choir. Making music together tends to synch breathing and heart rates, producing a group-wide calming effect.

⊜ YOUR PERSONAL STRESS MANAGEMENT TOOLKIT

REFLECTION: Should You Try a Complementary, Alternative, or Creative Therapy?

Here are some key questions to ask:

- **Is it safe?** Be particularly wary of unregulated products like stress tablets or supplements.

- **Is it effective?** You can find the latest research on the website of the National Center for CAM: http://nccam.nih.gov.

- **Will it interact with other medicines or conventional treatments?** Check with your physician if you have a chronic health problem or are taking prescription medications.

- **Is the practitioner/therapist/trainer qualified?** Check out the credentials and training of anyone to whom you entrust your health and well-being.

- **What do others say?** Talk to or go online to find comments from people who have used these therapies for a similar problem, both recently and in the past.

- **Can you talk openly and easily with the person offering treatment?** You should feel comfortable asking questions and confident in the answers you receive. And the practitioner's office, studio, or workout space should put you at ease.

- **What are the costs?** Many CAM services are not covered by HMOs or health insurers, so you will probably be paying out of pocket. Make sure you are getting your money's worth.

TECHNIQUE: Express Your Stress

- Choose any medium: paper and pen, paints, clay, photography, collage, digital imaging, music, film, and so on.

- Think back to the last time you were feeling stressed, and focus on the feelings you had: anxiety, fear, dread, panic, frustration, anger. Imagine ways you can express these emotons—in a song, dance, bold colors, abstract shapes, photographs, or video.

- Don't worry about artistic technique. You're not creating a work of art; you're releasing inner feelings. Draw, sing, dance, paint it out!

Glossary

A

ABC relaxation The theory that relaxation or "centering" consists of three stages: Attention (sustained focus on a single thing); Behavior (minimal purposeful activity); and Cognition (passive observation rather than analysis, planning, and other thoughts).

academic entitlement Students' belief that they are owed more—more attention from instructors, easier assignments, higher grades on papers and tests, etc.— than is merited by their effort.

academic procrastination An intentional delay in beginning or completing important and time-sensitive academic activities.

acculturation A complex psychosocial process in which an ethnic minority changes, both as individuals and as a group, as a consequence of contact with the ethnic majority.

acetylcholine A neurotransmitter that decreases metabolic activity and returns the body to homeostasis.

action The stage of change in which you actively modify your behavior according to your plan.

active or reflective listening Hearing what's being said non-verbally as well as verbally, processing the information, reflecting back the content, and utilizing appropriate verbal and non-verbal responses.

active meditation The use of repetitive motion, such as dancing, swimming, or walking, as the focus of meditation.

acupressure Therapy that uses direct finger pressure applied to points thought to be areas of chi concentration; described as acupuncture without the needles.

acupuncture A therapy that involves inserting hair-thin, sterile needles into the body at specific points (acupoints) to manipulate the body's flow of energy to balance the endocrine system.

acute academic stressor A short-term intellectual challenge, such as a zoology test or a presentation in an urban studies class.

acute stress disorder Development of disabling symptoms, such as recurrent and intrusive distressing memories or dreams related to the trauma, within three days to a month after exposure to a traumatic event.

acute stressor A short-term event or situation that an individual perceives as a threat.

adjustment disorder Development of mild to moderate emotional or behavioral symptoms within three months of an identifiable stressor, whether a single event (such as being robbed) or multiple or recurrent stressors (such as conflict with a roommate or partner).

adrenal cortex Outer portion of adrenal glands.

adrenal glands Two triangle-shaped glands, one positioned on top of each kidney, that secrete the stress hormones epinephrine and norepinephrine during the stress response.

adrenal medulla Inner portion of adrenal glands, where epinephrine and norepinephrine are secreted.

affirmation A positive statement repeated to oneself for emotional encouragement and support.

allostatic load The cumulative biological burden caused by daily adaptation to physical and emotional stress.

alpha waves Slow, low-amplitude brain waves associated with a low-stress, resting state.

alternative medical systems A type of CAM that refers to theories and practices based on non-Western medical systems.

alternative medicine Therapies that are used in place of conventional medicine.

altruism Helping or giving to others without thought of self-benefit in order to promote their welfare.

altruistic egotism Offering support to others in ways that satisfy the needs of both giver and recipient.

alveoli Elastic air sacs in the lungs that expand when air is inhaled and contract when it is exhaled.

AmED (Alcohol mixed with energy drinks) Any combination of alcohol with caffeine and other stimulants.

amygdala An almond-shaped structure within the brain that plays a critical role in processing emotions, including anxiety and fear.

anorexia nervosa A psychological disorder in which refusal to eat and/or an extreme loss of appetite leads to malnutrition, severe weight loss, and possibly death.

anticipatory academic stressor A long-term intellectual challenge, such as a qualifying exam, that has the potential to influence a major goal in the future.

APR (annual percentage rate) The amount of interest a credit card company charges each year on the unpaid balance.

aromatherapy The practice of using the natural or essential oils extracted from flowers, bark, stems, leaves, roots, or other parts of a plant to enhance psychological and physical well-being.

art therapy The therapeutic process of creating art by people who experience illness, trauma, or challenges in living or who seek personal development.

ashtanga yoga A system of yoga that involves synchronizing the breath with a progressive series of postures to calm the mind and enhance well-being.

attention Focused observation of thoughts, feelings, and physical sensations as they occur.

autogenics or autogenic relaxation A technique that uses both visual imagery and body awareness to control blood pressure, breathing, and heart rate in order to achieve deep relaxation and reduce stress.

autonomic nervous system The branch of the nervous system responsible for essential involuntary body functions that occur without our thinking about them, such as breathing, blood pressure, heartbeat, temperature, appetite, and sleep cycles.

autonomy Ability to draw on internal resources; independence from familial and societal influences.

ayurveda India's traditional system of natural medicine that believes that all aspects of life contribute to health, including nutrition, hygiene, sleep, weather, and lifestyle, as well as physical, mental, and sexual activities.

B

binge Pattern of drinking alcohol that brings blood-alcohol concentration (BAC) to 0.08 gram-percent or above—typically by consuming five or more drinks in about two hours for a man and four or more drinks for a woman.

binge eating The rapid consumption of an abnormally large amount of food in a relatively short time.

binge-eating disorder A psychiatric disorder characterized by bingeing once a week or more for at least a three-month period.

biofeedback A technique of becoming aware, with the aid of external monitoring devices, of internal physiological activities in order to develop the capability of consciously altering them.

biologically-based therapies CAM treatments that include herbal medicine (botanical medicine or phytotherapy), the use of individual herbs or combinations; and special diet therapies.

biracial Term used to describe individuals who genetically belong to more than one race.

blended families Families formed when one or both of the partners bring children from a previous union to the new marriage.

bracing Chronic tensing of muscles.

bruxism Clenching or grinding of teeth as a result of stress.

bulimia nervosa A psychological disorder characterized by episodic binge eating, often followed by forced vomiting or laxative abuse, and a persistent preoccupation with body shape and weight.

burnout A state of physical, emotional, and mental exhaustion that occurs when workers or caregivers feel overwhelmed and unable to meet constant demands.

C

capillaries Small blood vessels surrounding the alveoli that receive oxygen and carry it to the heart.

challenge response A physiological response that strengthens connections between the parts of the brain that suppress fear and enhance learning and positive motivation so as to prepare and enable a person to face a stressor directly.

chest or thoracic breathing A shallow breathing pattern, in which the chest expands and the shoulders rise with every inhalation, that delivers less oxygen to the heart and lungs.

chronic procrastination Regular delaying of work or other activities to the extent that it interferes with your functioning and performance.

chronic stressor Unrelenting demands and pressures that go on for an extended time.

codependency An emotional and psychological behavioral pattern in which the spouses, partners, parents, children, and friends of individuals with addictive behaviors allow or enable their loved ones to continue their self-destructive habits.

cognition The mental process that consists of thinking and reasoning.

cognitive behavioral therapy (CBT) A form of psychotherapy that targets irrational or inaccurate thoughts or beliefs to help individuals break out of a distorted way of thinking.

cognitive restructuring or reframing An approach to changing the meaning or interpretation of stressors.

cohabitation Two people living together as a couple, without official ties such as marriage.

compassion Desire to help another on the basis of feelings of empathy.

complementary and alternative medicine (CAM) A group of diverse medical and health care systems, practices, and products that are not presently considered to be part of conventional medicine.

complementary medicine Therapies that are used together with conventional medicine.

computer-mediated communication The conveying of written text via ever-evolving new networks, sites, and apps.

concentration The learned control of keeping one's awareness on a particular object or thought.

conscientiousness Striving for competence and achievement, self-discipline, orderliness, reliability, deliberativeness.

contemplation The stage of change in which, although you might prefer not to change, you start to realize that you must.

cortisol A stress hormone produced by the adrenal cortex that spurs the metabolism of nutrients to provide energy and fuel for your body and brain.

creative or expressive therapy Therapeutic approaches that encompass art, dance, drama, horticulture, music, photography, and film/video as ways of tapping into the imagination so individuals can get in touch with emotions and thoughts that words alone cannot capture.

credit score A rating based on your history of paying credit card, utilities, loans, rent, and other debts.

culture The shared attitudes, values, goals, and practices of a group that are internalized by an individual within the group.

cyberbullying Deliberate, repeated, and hostile actions that use information and communication technologies, including social media and text messages, with the intent of harming others by means of intimidation, control, manipulation, false accusations, or humiliation.

cyberstalking A form of cyberbullying that uses websites, Twitter, e-mail messages, and social media to harass victims and try to damage their reputation or turn others against them.

D

decibels (dB) Units for measuring the intensity of sounds.

deep tissue massage Deep muscle compression with the heel of the hand, the pads of the thumb, and even the elbow pressing deliberately along the grain of the muscle to release the chronic patterns of tension in the body.

diaphragm The muscle separating the lungs and the abdomen that contracts and relaxes as you breathe in and out.

diaphragmatic or abdominal breathing Inhaling in a way that causes the diaphragm to contract and move down, drawing air deep into the lungs.

diaphragmatic or abdominal breathing A breathing pattern that draws air deep into the lungs as the abdominal cavity expands and the diaphragm contracts downward. Deeper and slower than chest breathing, it enhances the flow of energizing oxygen.

diathesis stress model The theory that a predisposition stemming from genetic, developmental, psychological, biological, or situational factors makes people more or less susceptible to stress.

distress A negative stress that may result in illness.

dopamine A neurotransmitter involved in reward and pleasure.

downward spiral A progression of negative thoughts and feelings that can lead to depression or self-destructive behaviors.

dysfunctional Characterized by negative and destructive patterns of behavior between partners or between parents and children.

E

ecosystem A community of organisms sharing a physical and chemical environment and interacting with each other.

emotional health The ability to express and acknowledge one's feelings and moods and exhibit adaptability and compassion for others.

emotional intelligence A set of skills that contribute to the accurate appraisal, expression, and regulation of emotion in oneself and in others and the use of feelings to motivate, plan, and achieve in one's life.

empathy Ability to take the perspective of and feel the emotions of another person.

enabling Unwittingly contributing to a person's addictive or abusive behavior. Components of enabling include shielding or covering up for an abuser/addict, controlling him or her, taking over responsibilities, rationalizing addictive behavior, and cooperating with him or her.

energy therapies CAM approaches that focus on energy fields believed to exist in and around the body.

environmental health The impact the world around you has on well-being and the impact you can have by protecting and preserving the environment.

epinephrine A powerful chemical, also called adrenalin, produced during the stress response that increases blood pressure, stimulates heart muscle, and accelerates the heart rate so the heart pumps more blood.

episodic acute stressor Frequent and repeated experience of an acute stressor.

EQ (emotional quotient) The ability to monitor and use emotions to guide thinking and actions.

ethnicity The common heritage—the customs, language, history, and characteristics—of a certain group.

eudaemonic Happiness based on a sense of higher purpose and service to others.

eustress Beneficial or positive stress.

exclusive, concentration, or focused meditation Focused meditation.

exercise A type of physical activity that requires planned, structured, and repetitive bodily movement with the intent of improving one or more components of physical fitness.

expressive writing Disclosing one's deepest thoughts and feelings about a stressful life event.

extraversion A personality trait correlated with being active, talkative, assertive, social, stimulation- seeking.

F

families Persons united by marriage, blood, or adoption—each residing in the same household; maintaining a common culture; and interacting with one another on the basis of their roles within the group.

family stress A crisis that occurs in the response to an event; its impact depends on its magnitude and the meaning attached to the event by family members.

fight or flight response The body's automatic physiological response that prepares the individual to take action upon facing a perceived threat or danger.

fixed interest rate An interest rate that stays the same over time.

freezing A survival mechanism that stems from some of the oldest circuits within the brain; freezing gives a person time to stop, look, listen, and assess what is happening in the face of a stressor.

G

GERD (gastroesophageal reflux disease) A digestive disorder characterized by the return (reflux) of the contents of the stomach to the esophagus.

guided imagery A program of directed suggestions that involve all the senses—sounds, tastes, smells, textures, sights—to relax the body, promote healing, or improve performance.

H

hardiness A personality trait characterized by being committed to something that is meaningful, believing it is possible to take control, and viewing change, whether positive or negative, as an opportunity to learn.

hatha yoga A type of yoga used for fitness, flexibility, and stress management that consists of various stretching exercises called postures, designed to reduce muscle tension and facilitate at relaxed state of being.

health A state of complete well-being, including physical, psychological, spiritual, social, intellectual, and environmental dimensions.

hedonic Happiness derived from accumulating material things and enjoying pleasurable activities.

herbal medicine The use of herbs, special diet therapies, nutritional and food supplements, and other products or procedures to prevent or treat disease.

holistic A view of health and the individual as a whole rather than part by part.

holistic medicine An approach that focuses on the whole person and the physical, mental, emotional, and spiritual aspects of well-being.

homeostasis The body's natural state of balance or stability.

homophobia A fear of and aversion to homosexuals that can result in discrimination and gay and "trans" bashing (attacking homosexuals and transgender individuals).

hookup Refers to a range of physically intimate behaviors—from kissing to intercourse—with no expectation of emotional intimacy or a romantic relationship.

humor or laughter therapy The use of humor and laughter to promote overall health and relieve stress.

hydrotherapy The use of warm water to draw blood from the body's core to relax the muscles.

hyperventilation Extremely rapid and shallow breathing.

hypnosis A state of concentration characterized by focused attention, deep relaxation, greater responsiveness to suggestions, more openness, and a suspension of belief and criticism.

hypnotic suggestion A statement used to narrow awareness and deepen relaxation that the mind believes is accurate or true.

hypothalamus Chief region of the brain that acts as the command center for higher-order thinking.

I

insomnia A lack of sleep so severe that it interferes with functioning during the day.

integrative or integrated medicine Therapies that combine mainstream medical and CAM approaches.

intellectual health ability to learn from life experience, accept new ideas, and question and evaluate information.

intimacy A state of closeness between two people, characterized by the desire and ability to share one's innermost thoughts and feelings with each other.

introductory interest rate A rate that starts low but increases after a certain period of time.

J

journaling Translating thoughts and feelings into words, photos, or video.

K

koans Unsolvable, illogical riddles that force the mind to focus on a concept that has no answer.

L

locus of control The sense of whether external or internal influences determine what happens in life.

loneliness Feelings of distress resulting from a discrepancy between a person's desired and actual social relations.

lovingkindness meditation A form of concentration meditation in which you focus on a sacred object or being, weaving feelings of love and gratitude into your thoughts.

M

maintenance The ongoing stage of change that involves locking in and consolidating gains to make a change permanent.

mandala A figure with intricate designs and intense colors that serves as the focus of concentration during meditation.

manipulative and body-based m ethods A type of CAM that includes treatments based on manipulation and/or movement of the body.

mantra A word or phrase repeated during a meditative state.

mantra meditation A type of meditation that focuses on a repeated word, sound, or phrase.

medical or sports massage A special type of massage, focusing on muscle systems specific to athletic and sporting events.

meditation The intentional process of deepening attention and focus.

mental health The ability to perceive reality as it is, respond to its challenges, and develop rational strategies for living.

meridians Invisible channels of energy that flow in the body.

microaggressions Subtle pressures or expressions of hostility based on bias toward individuals or members of any minority.

microassaults Conscious and intentional actions or slurs, such as racial or sexual epithets.

microinsults Verbal and nonverbal communications that subtly convey rudeness and insensitivity and demean a person's racial heritage or identity.

microinvalidations Communications that subtly exclude, negate, or nullify the thoughts, feelings or experiential reality of an individual.

mind–body interventions A type of CAM that uses techniques designed to enhance the mind's capacity to affect bodily function and symptoms.

mindfulness A form of concentration that involves fully experiencing the physical and mental sensations of the present moment without being judgmental or reactive.

mindfulness-based stress reduction A program based on mindfulness meditation that uses awareness techniques to reduce stress and promote wellness.

mindset The mental frame or lens that selectively organizes information, thereby orienting individuals toward a unique way of understanding experiences that shapes their choices and behaviors.

minority stress The unique pressures experienced by students in any racial, ethnic, or gender.

mood Sustained emotional state that colors one's view of the world for hours or days.

multiracial Term used to describe individuals who genetically belong to more than one race.

muscle dysmorphia A dangerous obsession, primarily among men, characterized by the belief that one's own body is too small, too skinny, and not muscular or lean enough. Also known as reverse anorexia, this obsession puts men at risk for depression, anxiety, and abuse of substances such as anabolic steroids.

music therapy The use of music interventions to accomplish individualized goals within a therapeutic relationship.

N

nadam A repeated sound that meditators listen to or imagine.

neuroplasticity Ability of the brain to produce new neurons and synapses throughout life.

neustress Neutral stressors that do not affect an individual immediately or directly but that may trigger anxiety, sadness, fear, and other stressful feelings.

norepinephrine A hormone, also known as noradrenalin, that, together with epinephrine, brings about the stress response.

O

occupational health The ability to work productively, to meet job requirements, and to gain satisfaction from workplace roles and responsibilities.

occupational stress The distress related to any aspect of a job that can take a physical or psychological toll.

open or inclusive meditation A form of meditation that allows the mind to wander and to observe any and all thoughts with "detached observation"—that is, without emotion, judgment, consideration, or contemplation.

optimism The tendency to seek out, remember, and expect pleasurable experiences.

oxytocin A hormone (sometimes called the "cuddle chemical") produced by the pituitary gland that fine-tunes the brain's social network, increases empathy, fosters willingness to help and support others, and helps protect the cardiovascular system.

P

parasympathetic nervous system The branch of the autonomic nervous system that returns the body to a state of homeostasis, or balance, after a possible threat has passed.

passive progressive relaxation A focused observation technique, such as a body scan, that monitors tension in various parts of the body.

perception The process of becoming aware of something through the senses; a way of understanding and interpreting something.

persistence Continuing to work and to keep moving forward.

pet or animal-assisted therapy The inclusion of animals as a form of treatment to relieve stress or improve social, emotional, or cognitive functioning.

physical activity Any movement produced by the muscles that results in expenditure of energy.

physical fitness The ability to respond to routine physical demands with enough reserve energy to cope with a sudden challenge.

physical health The functioning of the cells, tissues, organs, and systems that make up the body.

Pilates A technique for deep-body conditioning and injury rehabilitation, originally developed for dancers, that emphasizes flexibility, joint mobility, and strengthening the core by developing pelvic stability and abdominal control.

pituitary gland The key regulator of all hormonal functions in the body.

pollution Any change in the air, water, or soil that could reduce its ability to support life.

positive spiral A progression of positive thoughts and feelings that leads to fulfilling events and experiences.

post-traumatic stress disorder (PTSD) A psychological response to a trauma such as a life-threatening accident, a natural disaster, or sexual assault that causes symptoms that interfere with normal functioning.

pranayama The Sanskrit term for yogic breathing practices.

precontemplation The period prior to behavioral change when a person has no intention of making a change.

prefrontal cortex The part of the frontal lobe in the brain that regulates cognitive processes such as planning and problem solving and functions as the center for postponing gratification, self-discipline, and emotional regulation.

preparation The stage of change in which individuals begin to think, plan, and act with change specifically in mind.

progressive muscle relaxation (PMR) Alternate tensing and relaxing of various muscle groups in the body.

psychological health Psychological health encompasses both our emotional and mental states—that is, our feelings and our thoughts—and involves the ability to recognize and express emotions, to function independently, and to cope with the challenges of stress.

psychoneuroimmunology A multidisciplinary field that studies the interaction between psychological processes and the nervous and immune systems.

Q

Qigong An ancient Chinese practice that involves postures, breathing techniques, and mental focus.

R

race Genetic patterns, inherited characteristics, and physical traits, such as skin, hair, and eyes, shared by a unique population.

rational emotive behavior therapy (REBT) Treatment based on the theory that irrational, self-defeating thoughts and behaviors that cause stress can be challenged and changed.

Raynaud's disease A condition in which the fingers become painful and white when exposed to cold.

Reiki A healing technique that channels the universal life energy to recipients by the laying on of hands.

relapse Reverting to old behaviors.

relaxation A process of letting go of the residual stress that builds up in the mind and body.

resilience The process of adapting well to adversity and significant sources of stress.

rumination The continuous processing of negative thoughts and feelings.

S

same-sex marriage A marriage in which two people of the same sex commit to each other and live together as a family.

self-actualization A state of wellness and fulfillment that can be achieved once certain human needs are satisfied; living to one's full potential.

self-compassion A healthy form of self-acceptance and self-care.

self-disclosure Sharing personal information and experiences.

self-efficacy Belief in one's ability to accomplish a goal or change a behavior.

self-esteem Confidence and satisfaction in oneself.

sexting Sending sexually explicit text messages or digital photos.

Shiatsu Oriental-based therapy system, using finger pressure applied to specific points along acupuncture meridians.

social anxiety disorder A fear and avoidance of social situations.

social health The ability to interact effectively with other people and with the social environment, develop satisfying interpersonal relationships, and fulfill social roles.

social intelligence The skills that foster harmony and create satisfying relationships.

social isolation A lack of social contacts or activities.

social physique anxiety A type of distress that occurs most often in women who feel they do not measure up in terms of weight or appearance to what they or others consider most desirable.

social support An individual's knowledge or belief that he or she is cared for and loved and belongs to a network or community; the ways in which individuals provide comfort, information, or assistance to others.

Soto Zen meditation A form of concentration meditation that involves concentration on and memorization of a visual mantra.

spiritual health The ability to identify one's basic purpose in life, to engage in meaningful pursuits, and to achieve one's full potential.

spiritual intelligence The capacity to sense, understand, and tap into ourselves, others, and the world around us.

spirituality A belief in someone or something that transcends the boundaries of self.

static stretching Exercises, derived from hatha yoga, that utilize the elastic properties of muscles and connective tissue.

stress The nonspecific response of the body to any demands or perceived threat.

stress paradox The observation that the most stressful aspects of life also bring the greatest satisfaction and joy.

stressor An event or situation that an individual perceives as a threat.

submission If unable to flee from or "fight off" a stressor, a person may give up or give in, agree with others, or surrender their aspirations.

Swedish massage The most common type of basic relaxation massage that includes long gliding strokes, kneading, friction, tapping, and shaking motions on the upper or more superficial layers of the muscles.

sympathetic nervous system The branch of the autonomic nervous system responsible for initiating the fight-or-flight response.

synapses The connections by which neurons transmit electrical impulses.

T

Tai Chi An exercise and relaxation technique that involves slow, focused, smooth, rhythmic movements along with control of breathing and mental and visual concentration.

technostress Tension and anxiety associated with technology and the nonstop barrage of digital media.

telomeres Protective strips of DNA at the ends of chromosomes that prevent the chromosomes from shredding.

temporomandibular disorder (TMD) A malfunctioning of the joint that connects the upper and lower jaw.

tend and befriend A behavioral response to stress characterized by increased feelings of trust and compassion and a desire to forge social connections.

tension myositis syndrome (TMS) A term coined by Dr. John Sarno for the unconscious tensing of muscles caused by repressed emotions that constricts blood vessels, reduces the supply of oxygen, and causes pain in the back or neck.

test anxiety A negative emotional state that can cause physiological and cognitive changes before, during, and after an exam.

therapeutic humor Any intervention that uses the power of smiles, laughter, and playfulness to help heal physical or mental illness.

thriving Enhanced psychological and physical functioning after successful adaptation to stressors and change; also referred to as hardiness, grit, resilience, or post-traumatic growth.

traditional Chinese medicine Therapies that include a variety of carefully formulated techniques, such as acupuncture, herbal medicine, massage, qigong, and nutrition.

transactional or cognitive reappraisal model A framework for evaluating the process of coping with a stressful event in four stages (primary appraisal, secondary appraisal, coping, and reevaluation); based on the theory that the level of stress that people experience depends on their assessment of a stressor and on the resources available to deal with it.

transcendental meditation (TM) A type of meditation that involves inducing a meditative state by repeating a special, individualized mantra.

trauma An intensely upsetting, frightening, or disturbing event.

trichotillomania A mental disorder characterized by pulling out chunks of hair from the scalp or elsewhere on the body.

V

values The criteria by which one makes choices about one's thoughts, actions, goals, and ideals.

variable interest rate A rate that changes over time and can be raised at any time, or in response to your credit behavior.

visualization Use of the imagination to "see" a place, person, or object in your mind.

Y

Yerkes-Dodson Principle The theory that increased stress or arousal can help improve performance, but only up to a certain point when excess stress diminishes performance and may undermine health.

yoga An approach that consists of various breathing and stretching exercises that unite all aspects of a person.

yogic breathing Breathing practices such as slowing down breathing, making inhalations and exhalations even, then holding the breath briefly during each cycle; used along with yoga postures. Also called **pranayama**.

Z

Zazen meditation A form of open meditation that focuses on subjective states of consciousness and detachment from emotional thoughts.

References

Chapter 1

1. American College Health Association. (2016). *American College Health Association-National College Health Assessment II: Reference Group Executive Summary Fall 2015.* Hanover, MD: American College Health Association: 2016.
2. Hurst, C.S. et al. (2013), "College Student Stressors: A Review of the Qualitative Research." *Stress and Health* 29(4): 275-285. doi: 10.1002/smi.2465. Epub 2012 Oct 1. Review. PMID: 23023893
3. Park, C. I., and Helgeson, V. S. (2006). "Growth Following Highly Stressful Life Events—Current Status and Future Directions." *Journal of Consulting and Clinical Psychology* 74: 791–796.
4. American Institute of Stress. http://www.stress.org/daily-life/
5. American Psychological Association. (2016). *Stress in America,* March 2016. www.stressinamerica.org
6. *Ibid.*
7. Gouin, J. P. et al. (2012). "Chronic Stress, Daily Stressors and Circulating Inflammatory Markers." *Health Psychology* 31(2): 264-8. doi: 10.1037/a0025536. Epub 2011 Sep 19.
8. Charles, S. T. et al. (2013). "The Wear and Tear of Mental Stressors on Mental Health," *Psychological Science* 24(5): 733–741. doi: 10.1177/0956797612462222. Epub 2013 Mar 26.
9. Miller, G. et al. (2009). "Chronic Interpersonal Stress Predict Activation of Pro- and Anti-Inflammatory Signaling Pathways Six Months Later." *Psychosomatic Medicine* 71(1): 57–62. doi: 10.1097/PSY.0b013e318190d7de. Epub 2008 Dec 10.
10. Uchino, B. N. et al. (2012). "Social Support and Immunity," in Segerstrom, S. S. (edit) *The Oxford Handbook of Psychoneuroimmunology.* New York: Oxford University Press.
11. Cohen, S. et al. (2006). "Socioeconomic Status is Associated with Stress Hormones." *Psychosomatic Medicine* 68(3): 414–420.
12. Kaplan, S. A. (2013). "The Perception of Stress and Its Impact on Health in Poor Communities." *Journal of Community Health* 38(1): 142–149. doi: 10.1007/s10900-012-9593-5.
13. Derry, H. M. et al. (2013). "Lower Subjective Social Status Exaggerates Interleukin-6 Responses to a Laboratory Stressor." *Psychoneuroendocrinology* 38(11): 2676–2685. doi: 10.1016/j.psyneuen.2013.06.026. Epub 2013 Jul 9.
14. Schauer, M., and Elbert, T. (2010). "Dissociation Following Traumatic Stress," *Journal of Psychology* 218(2): 109–127.
15. McGonigal, Kelly. (2015). *The Upside of Stress.* New York: Avery Press.
16. *Ibid.*, p. 113.
17. Taylor, S. E. et al. (2000). "Biobehavioral Responses to Stress in Females: Tend-and-Befriend, not Fight-or-Flight." *Psychological Review*, 107(3): 411–429.
18. Eisenberger, M. D. (2007). "Neural Pathways Link Social Support to Attenuated Neuroendocrine Stress Responses." *Neuroimage* 35(4): 1601–1612
19. McGonigal, p. 136
20. McGonigal, p. 139
21. Poulin, M. J., Brown, S. L., Dillard, A. J., & Smith, D. M. 2013. "Giving to Others and The Association Between Stress and Mortality." *American Journal of Public Health* 103(9): 1649–1655. doi: 10.2105/AJPH.2012.300876. Epub 2013 Jan 17.
22. Lazarus, R, and Launier, R. (1978). "Stress-Related Transactions between Person and Environment." *Perspectives in Interactional Psychology.* New York: Plenum.
23. Berjot S and Gillet N. "Stress and Coping with Discrimination and Stigmatization." *Frontiers in Psychology* 2011 Mar 1;2:33. doi: 10.3389/fpsyg.2011.00033. eCollection 2011.
24. McGonigal, K. xxi
25. Park, C. I., and Helgeson, V. S. (2006). "Growth Following Highly Stressful Life Events—Current Status and Future Directions." *Journal of Consulting and Clinical Psychology* 74: 791–796.
26. Keller, A., Litzelman, K., Wisk, L. E., Maddox, T., Cheng, E. R., Creswell, P. D., & Witt, W. P. (2012). "Does The Perception That Stress Affects Health Matter? The Association with Health and Mortality." *Health Psychology* 31(5): 677–684. doi: 10.1037/a0026743. Epub 2011 Dec 26
27. *Ibid.*
28. Crum, A. J. et al. (2013). "Rethinking Stress: The Role of Mindsets in Determining the Stress Response." *Journal of Personality and Social Psychology* 104(4): 716–733. doi: 10.1037/a0031201. Epub 2013 Feb 25.
29. Brooks, A. W. 2014. "Get Excited: Reappraising Pre-Performance Anxiety as Excitement," *Journal of Experimental Psychology: General* 143(3): 1144–1158. doi: 10.1037/a0035325. Epub 2013 Dec 23.
30. Park, C. I., and Helgeson, V. S. (2006). "Growth Following Highly Stressful Life Events—Current Status and Future Directions." *Journal of Consulting and Clinical Psychology* 74(5): 791–796.
31. Epel, E. S. et al. (1998). "Embodying Psychological Thriving: Physical Thriving in Response to Stress." *Journal of Social Issues* 53(2): 301–322.
32. Garland, E. L. et al. (2010). "Upward Spirals of Positive Emotions Counter Downward Spirals of Negativity: Insights from the Broaden-and-Build Theory and Affective Neuroscience on The Treatment of Emotion Dysfunctions and Deficits in Psychopathology." *Clinical Psychology Review* 30(7): 849–864.

Chapter 2

1. Cohen, S. et al. (1993). "Negative Life Events, Perceived Stress, Negative Affect and Susceptibility to the Common Cold." *Journal of Personality and Social Psychology* 64: 131–140.
2. McGonigal, Kelly. (2015). *The Upside of Stress.* New York: Avery Press.
3. Poulin, M. J., Brown, S. L., Dillard, A. J., & Smith, D. M. 2013. "Giving to Others and The Association Between Stress and Mortality." *American Journal of Public Health* 103(9): 1649–1655. DOI: 10.2105/AJPH.2012.300876. Epub 2013 Jan 17
4. Cardoso, D. et al. (2013). "Stress-Induced Negative Mood Moderates The Relation Between Oxytocin Administration and Trust: Evidence For The Tend-and-Befriend Response to Stress?" *Psychoneuroendocrinology* 38(11): 2800–2804. DOI: 10.1016/j.psyneuen.2013.05.006. Epub 2013 Jun 12.
5. van den Bos, R. et al. (2015). "Sex matters, as do individual differences..." *Trends in Neuroscience* 38(7): 401–402. DOI: 10.1016/j.tins.2015.05.001. Epub 2015 May 25.
6. Darnall, B. D., and Suarez, E. C. (2009). "Sex and Gender in Psychoneuroimmunology Research: Past, Present, and Future." *Brain, Behavior, and Immunity* 23(3): 595–604. DOI: 10.1016/j.bbi.2009.02.019. Epub 2009 Mar 9.
7. Rao, K. (2009). "Recent Research in Stress, Coping, and Women's Health." *Current Opinion in Psychiatry* 22(2): 188–193. DOI: 10.1097/YCO.0b013e328320794a.
8. Youssef, F. F. et al. (2012). "Stress Alters Personal Moral Decision-Making." *Psychoneuroendocrinology* 37: 491–498. DOI: 10.1016/j.psyneuen.2011.07.017. Epub 2011 Sep 6.
9. Nauert, R. (2008). "Genetic Disposition for Anxiety." *Psych Central*.; Levinson & Nichols, Stanford 2014
10. Gouin, J. P. et al. (2012). "Childhood Abuse and Inflammatory Responses to Daily Stressors." *Annals of Behavioral Medicine* 44(2): 287–292. DOI: 10.1007/s12160-012-9386-1.
11. Solomon, G. F., and Moos, R. H. (1964). "Emotions, Immunity, and Disease: A Speculative Theoretical Integration." *Archives of General Psychiatry* 11: 657–674.
12. Chen, E. et al. (2011). "Maternal Warmth Buffers the Effects of Low Early-Life Socioeconomic Status on Pro-Inflammatory Signaling in Adulthood." *Molecular Psychiatry* 16(7): 729–737. DOI: 10.1038/mp.2010.53. Epub 2010 May 18.
13. McEwen, B. S., and Gianaro, P. I. (2010). "Central Role of the Brain in Stress and Adaptation: Links to Socioeconomic Stress, Health, and Disease." *Annals of the New York Academy of Sciences* 1186: 190–222. DOI: 10.1111/j.1749-6632.2009.05331.x.
14. Kelly, S. J., and Ismial, M. (2015). "Stress and Type 2 Diabetes: A Review of How Stress Contributes to the Development of Type 2 Diabetes," *Annual Review of Public Health* 36: 441–462. DOI: 10.1146/annurev-publhealth-031914-122921. Epub 2015 Jan 12.
15. Cohen, S. et al. (2012). "Chronic Stress, Glucocorticoid Receptor Resistance, Inflammation, and Disease Risk." *Proceedings of the National Academy of Sciences* 109(16): 5995–5999. DOI: 10.1073/pnas.1118355109. Epub 2012 Apr 2.
16. Trueba, A. F., and Ritz, T. (2013). "Stress, Asthma, and Respiratory Infections." *Brain, Behavior, and Immunity* 29: 11–27. DOI: 10.1016/j.bbi.2012.09.012. Epub 2012 Oct 2.
17. Gayman, M. D. et al. (2011). "Depressive symptoms and bodily pain: The role of physical disability and social stress." *Stress and Health* 27(1): 52–63.
18. Wood, W., and Drolet, A. (2013). "How Do People Adhere to Goals When Willpower is Low? The Profits (and Pitfalls) of Strong Habits." *Journal of Personality and Social Psychology* 104(6): 959–975. DOI: 10.1037/a0032626.
19. Karatsoreos, I. N., and McEwen, B. S. (2013). "Resilience and Vulnerability: A Neurobiological Perspective." *F1000Prime Reports* 2013 5(13): (May 1, 2013). DOI: 10.12703/P5-13. Print 2013
20. Chrousos, G. P. (2010). "Stress and Sex versus Immunity and Inflammation." *Science Signaling* 3(143): 36. DOI: 10.1126/scisignal.3143pe36.
21. Gouin, J. P., and Kiecolt-Glaser, J. K. (2011). "The Impact of Psychological Stress on Wound Healing: Methods and Mechanisms." *Critical Care Nursing Clinics of North America* 24(2): 201–213. DOI: 10.1016/j.ccell.2012.03.006.
22. Chrousos, G. P. (2010). "Stress and Sex versus Immunity and Inflammation." *Science Signaling* 3(143): 36. DOI: 10.1126/scisignal.3143pe36.
23. Leiker, C., Roper, V. et al. (2014). "Cross-Sectional and Longitudinal Relationships between Perceived Stress and C-Reactive Protein in Men and Women." *Stress and Health* 30(2): 158–165. DOI: 10.1002/smi.2507. Epub 2013 Jul 1.
24. Trudel, X. et al. (2015). Adverse Psychosocial Work Factors, Blood Pressure and Hypertension Incidence: Repeated Exposure in a 5-year Prospective Cohort Study. *Journal of Epidemiology & Community Health* 2015 Nov 3. pii: jech-2014-204914. DOI: 10.1136/jech-2014-204914.

25. Hoekstra, T. et al. (2013). "Vital Exhaustion and Markers of Low-Grade Inflammation in Healthy Adults: The Amsterdam Growth and Health Longitudinal Study." *Stress and Health* 29(5): 392–400. DOI: 10.1002/smi.2485. Epub 2013 Mar 8.

26. Bergh, C. et al. (2015). "Stress Resilience and Physical Fitness in Adolescence and Risk of Coronary Heart Disease in Middle Age." *Heart* 101(8): 623–629. DOI: 10.1136/heartjnl-2014-306703. Epub 2015 Mar 4.

27. Cohen, B. E. et al. (2015). State of the Art Review: "Depression, Stress, Anxiety, and Cardiovascular Disease." *American Journal of Hypertension* 28(11): 1295–1302. DOI: 10.1093/ajh/hpv047. Epub 2015 Apr 24.

28. Gouin, J. P. et al. (2012). "Chronic Stress, Daily Stressors, and Circulating Inflammatory Markers." *Health Psychology* 31(2): 264–268. DOI: 10.1037/a0025536. Epub 2011 Sep 19. PMID: 21928900

29. Barbosa-Leiker, C. et al. (2014). "Cross-Sectional and Longitudinal Relationships Between Perceived Stress and C-Reactive Protein in Men and Women." *Stress and Health* 30(2): 158–165. DOI: 10.1002/smi.2507. Epub 2013 Jul 1.

30. Bonaz, B. L., and Bernstein, C. N. (2013). "Brain-Gut Interactions in Inflammatory Bowel Disease." *Gastroenterology* 144(1): 36–49. DOI: 10.1053/j.gastro.2012.10.003. Epub 2012 Oct 12.

31. Chung, C. S. et al. (2015). "A Systematic Approach for the Diagnosis and Treatment of Idiopathic Peptic Ulcers." *Korean Journal of Internal Medicine* 30(5): 559–570. DOI: 10.3904/kjim.2015.30.5.559.

32. Groesz, L. M. et al. (2012). "What is Eating You? Stress and The Drive to Eat." *Appetite* 58(2): 717–721. DOI: 10.1016/j.appet.2011.11.028. Epub 2011 Dec 4.

33. Sarno, John. (2010). *Healing Back Pain: The Mind-Body Connection*. New York: Grand Central.

34. DeWeerdt, Sarah. (2012). "Psychodermatology: An Emotional Response." *Nature* 492(7429): S62–S63. DOI: 10.1038/492S62a.

35. Hall, J. M. et al. (2012). "Psychological Stress and Cutaneous Immune Response: Roles of the HPA Axis and the Sympathetic Nervous System in Atopic Dermatitis and Psoriasis." *Dermatology Research and Practice* 2012: p. 1155. DOI: 10.1155/2012/403908.

36. Traish, A. M. et al. (2002). "Biochemical and Physiological Mechanisms of Female Genital Sexual Arousal." *Archives of Sexual Behavior* 31(5): 393–400.

37. Vellani, E. et al. (2013). "Association of State and Trait Anxiety to Semen Quality of in vitro Fertilization Patients: A Controlled Study." *Fertility and Sterility* 99(6): 1565–1572. DOI: 10.1016/j.fertnstert.2013.01.098. Epub 2013 Feb 13.

38. Keenan, K. et al. (2014). "Stress During Pregnancy: Impact and Potential Treatment." *Obstetrics & Gynecology*. December 2014. p. 1080.

39. Dvivedi, J. et al. (2008). "The Effects of a 61-Points Relaxation Technique on Stress Parameters in Premenstrual Syndrome." *Indian Journal of Physiology and Pharmacology* 52(1): 69–76.

40. McDonald, P. G. et al. (2013). "Psychoneuroimmunology and Cancer: A Decade of Discovery, Paradigm Shifts, and Methodological Innovations." *Brain, Behavior, and Immunity* 30: S1–S9. DOI: 10.1016/j.bbi.2013.01.003. Epub 2013 Jan 16.

41. Spiegel, David. (2014). "Minding the Body: Psychotherapy and Cancer." *British Journal of Health Psychology* 19(3): 465–485. DOI: 10.1111/bjhp.12061. Epub 2013 Aug 26.

42. Spiegel, David. (2012). "Mind Matters in Cancer Survival." *Psycho-Oncology* 21(6): 588–593. DOI: 10.1002/pon.3067. Epub 2012 Mar 21.

43. Zalli, A. et al. (2014). "Shorter Telomeres with High Telomerase Activity are Associated with Raised Allostatic Load and Impoverished Psychosocial Resources." *Proceedings of the National Academy of Sciences of the United States of America* 111(12): 4519–4524. DOI: 10.1073/pnas.1322145111. Epub 2014 Mar 10.

44. Ornish, D. et al. (2013). "Effect of Comprehensive Lifestyle Changes on Telomerase Activity and Telomere Length in Men with Biopsy-Proven Low-Risk Prostate Cancer: 5-Year Follow-Up of a Descriptive Pilot Study." *The Lancet Oncology* 14(11): 1112–1120. DOI: 10.1016/S1470-2045(13)70366-8. Epub 2013 Sep 17.

45. Hoge, E. A. (2013). "Loving-Kindness Meditation Practice Associated with Longer Telomeres in Women." *Brain, Behavior, and Immunity* 32: 159–163. DOI: 10.1016/j.bbi.2013.04.005. Epub 2013 Apr 19.

Chapter 3

1. Teh Hui Chian et al. (2015). "Mental Well-Being Mediates the Relationship between Perceived Stress and Perceived Health." *Stress and Health* 31(1): 71–77. DOI: 10.1002/smi.2510.

2. Crum, A. J. et al. (2013). "Rethinking Stress: The Role of Mindsets in Determining the Stress Response." *Journal of Personality and Social Psychology* 104(4): 716–733.

3. Starcke, K., and Brand, M. (2012). "Decision Making under Stress: A Selective Review." *Neuroscience and Biobehavioral Reviews* 36(4): 1228–1248.

4. Mason, J. W. (1975). "A Historical View of the Stress Field." *Journal of Human Stress* 1(2): 22–36. DOI: 10.1080/0097840X.1975.9940405.

5. Ellis, A., and Grieger, R. (1977). *RET Handbook of Rational Emotive Therapy*. New York: Springer Publishing Company.

6. *Ibid*.

7. Jamieson, J. P. et al. (2012). "Mind over Matter: Reappraising Arousal Improves Cardiovascular and Cognitive Responses to Stress." *Journal of Experimental Psychology* 141(3): 417–422. DOI: http://dx.doi.org/10.1037/a0025719.

8. American College Health Association. (2016). *American College Health Association-National College Health Assessment II: Reference Group Executive Summary Fall 2015*. Hanover, MD: American College Health Association: 2016.

9. Harkness, K. L. et al. (2010). "Gender Differences in Life Events Prior to Onset of Major Depressive Disorder: The Moderating Effect of Age." *Journal of Abnormal Psychology* 119(4): 791–803.

10. Hales, R. E. et al. (eds.). (2014). *American Psychiatric Press Textbook of Psychiatry*. Arlington, VA: American Psychiatric Press.

11. Greenberg, N. et al. (2015). "Latest Developments in Post-Traumatic Stress Disorder: Diagnosis and Treatment," British Medical Bulletin 114(1): 147–155. DOI: 10.1093/bmb/ldv014.

12. Sullivan, E. M. et al. (2015). "Suicide Trends Among Persons Aged 10-24 Years—United States, 1994–2012." *Morbidity and Mortality Weekly Report (MMWR)* 64(08): 201–205. Atlanta: Centers for Disease Control and Prevention. (http://www.cdc.gov/mmwr/preview/mmwrhtml/mm6408a1.htm)

13. American College Health Association. (2016). *American College Health Association-National College Health Assessment II: Reference Group Executive Summary Fall 2015*. Hanover, MD: American College Health Association: 2016.

14. Siqueira L et al. (2015). "Binge Drinking." *Pediatrics* 136(3): e718–e726. DOI: 10.1542/peds.2015-2337.

15. Shapiro, S. L., and Carlson, L. (2009). *The Art and Science of Mindfulness: Integrating Mindfulness into Psychology and the Helping Professions*. Washington, D.C.: American Psychological Association.

16. Kabat-Zinn J. (1990). *Full Catastrophic Living: Using the Wisdom of Your Body and Mind to Overcome Pain*. New York: Delacourt.

17. Braden, B. B. et al. "Brain and Behavior Changes Associated with an Abbreviated 4-week Mindfulness-Based Stress Reduction Course in Back Pain Patients." *Brain and Behavior* 2016 Feb 16:e00443 [Epub ahead of print].

18. McEwen, B. S. "In Pursuit of Resilience: Stress, Epigenetics, and Brain Plasticity".: *Annals of the New York Academy of Sciences* 2016 Feb 25. DOI: 10.1111/nyas.13020. [Epub ahead of print]. American Psychiatric Association. (2013).

Chapter 4

1. National Center of Education Statistics.http://nces.ed.gov/programs/digest/d14/tables/dt14_105.20.asp?current=yes

2. American College Health Association. (2016). *American College Health Association-National College Health Assessment II: Reference Group Executive Summary Fall 2015*. Hanover, MD: American College Health Association: 2016.

3. American College Health Association. (2016).

4. Hintz, S., et al. (2015). "Evaluating an Online Stress Management Intervention for College Students." *Journal of Counseling Psychology* 62(2): 137–147. DOI: 10.1037/cou0000014. Epub 2014 Mar 17.

5. Schut, Christina, et al. (2015). "Psychological Stress and Skin Symptoms in College Students: Results of a Cross-sectional Web-based Questionnaire Study."*Acta dermato-venereologica*. DOI: 10.2340/00015555-2291. [Epub ahead of print.]

6. Sribanditmongkol, V. et al. (2015). "Effect of Perceived Stress on Cytokine Production in Healthy College Students." *Western Journal of Nursing Research* 37(4): 481–493. DOI: 10.1177/0193945914545658. Epub 2014 Aug 13. PMID: 25125502.

7. Wagner, M., and Rhee, Y. (2013). "Stress, Sleep, Grief: Are College Students Receiving Information That Interests Them?" *College Student Journal* 47(1): 24–33.

8. Zascavage, V. et al. (2012). "Student-life Stress in Education and Health Service Majors." *Higher Education Research and Development* 31(4): 599–610.

9. Gilbert, Meghan. (2015). "The Relationship Between Gender and Perceived Stress Levels in College Students." (May 21, 2015). Symposium of University Research and Creative Expression. Paper 151. http://digitalcommons.cwu.edu/source/2015/posters/151/. (2016)

10. American College Health Association. (2016).

11. Lewis, T. et al. (2015). "Gender Differences of Coping Strategies in Dealing with College Stress." (October 4, 2015). 18th Annual Georgia College Student Research Conference. http://kb.gcsu.edu/src/2015/friday/12/

12. Deatherage, S. et al. (2014). "Stress, Coping, and Internet Use of College Students." *Journal of American College Health* 62(1): 40–46. DOI: 10.1080/07448481.2013.843536.

13. Dill, P. L., and Henley, T. B. (1998). "Stressors of College: A Comparison of Traditional and Nontraditional Students." *The Journal of Psychology* 132(1): 25–32.

14. Whitman, D. K. et al. (2013). "The Development and Implications of Peer Emotional Support for Student Service Members/Veterans and Civilian College Students." *Journal of Counseling Psychiatry* 60(2): 265–278. DOI: 10.1037/a0031650. Epub 2013 Feb 18.

15. Kayla, J. et al. (2016). "The Effects of Sex and Gender Role Identity on Perceived Stress and Coping among Traditional and Non-Traditional Students." *Journal of American College Health*, DOI: 10.1080/07448481.2015.1117462

16. Dill, P. L., and Henley, T. B. (1998). "Stressors of College: A Comparison of Traditional and Nontraditional Students." *The Journal of Psychology* 132(1): 25–32.

17. Bryant, Scott E., and Malone, Timothy I. (2015). "An Empirical Study of Emotional Intelligence

and Stress in College Students." *Business Education & Accreditation* 7(1): 1–11.

18. Conley, C. et al. "Promoting Psychosocial and Stress Management in First-Year College Students." *Journal of American College Health* 61(2): 75–86. DOI: 10.1080/07448481.2012.754757.

19. Pepperoni, L. "First Generation Students Unite." *The New York Times* (April 8, 2015).

20. Hurst, C. S. et al. (2013). "College Student Stressors: A Review of the Qualitative Research." *Stress and Health* 29(4): 275–285. 10.1002/smi.2465. Epub 2012 Oct 1. Review. PMID: 23023893.

21. Besser, A. et al. (2014). "Positive Personality Features and Stress among First-Year University Students: Implications for Psychological Distress, Functional Impairment, and Self-esteem." *Self and Identity* 13(1): 24–44.

22. Jackson, L. M., Pancer, S. M., Pratt, M. W., & Hunsberger, B. E. (2000). "Great Expectations: The Relation Between Expectancies and Adjustment During the Transition to University." *Journal of Applied Social Psychology* 30(10): 2100–2125.

23. Wei, M. et al. (2011). "Minority Stress and College Persistence Attitudes Among African American, Asian American, and Latino Students: Perception of University Environment as a Mediator." *Cultural Diversity and Ethnic Minority Psychology* 17(2): 195–203. DOI: http://dx.doi.org/10.1037/a0023359.

24. Kaholokula, J. et al. (2010). "Effects of Perceived Racism and Acculturation on Hypertension in Native Hawaiians." *Hawaii Medical Journal* 69(5 suppl 2): 11–15

25. Peek, M. et al.(2011). "Self-reported Racial Discrimination in Health Care and Diabetes Outcomes." *Medical Care* 49(7): 618–625. DOI: 10.1097/MLR.0b013e318215d925.

26. Wagner, J. A. et al. "Self-reported Racial Discrimination and Endothelial Reactivity to Acute Stress in Women." Stress and Health (2013) 29(3): 214–221. DOI: 10.1002/smi.2449. Epub 2012 Sep 7.PMID: 22962001.

27. Nuru-Jetter, A. et al. (2009) "It's The Skin You're In": African American Women Talk about Their Experiences of Racism. An Exploratory Study to Develop Measures of Racism for Birth Outcome Studies. *Maternal and Child Health Journal* 13(1): 29–39. DOI: 10.1007/s10995-008-0357-x.

28. Sirin, Selcuk R., et al. (2015). "Discrimination-Related Stress Effects on the Development of Internalizing Symptoms Among Latino Adolescents." *Child Development* 86(3): 709–725. DOI: 10.1111/cdev.12343. Epub 2015 Feb 11. PMID: 25676605.

29. deCastro, A. et al. (2008). "Workplace and Discrimination and Health Among Filipinos in the United States." *American Journal of Public Health* 98(3): 520–526. DOI: 10.2105/AJPH.2007.110163. Epub 2008 Jan 30.

30. Ehlers, C. et al (2009). "Acculturation Stress, Anxiety Disorders, and Alcohol Dependence in a Select Population of Young Adult Mexican Americans." *Journal of Addiction Medicine* 3(4): 227–233. DOI: 10.1097/ADM.0b013e3181ab6db7. PMID: 20161543.

31. Bai, Jieru. (2016). "Perceived Support as a Predictor of Acculturative Stress among International Students in the United States," *Journal of International Students* 6(1): 93–106.

32. O'hara, Ross E. et al. (2015). "Perceived Racial Discrimination and Negative-Mood–Related Drinking Among African American College Students." *Journal of Studies on Alcohol and Drugs* 76(2): 229–236. PMID: 25785798.

33. Turner, D. T. (2015). "The Relationship between Race-related Stress and the Career Planning and Confidence for African-American College Students." Dissertation, University of Iowa. http://ir.uiowa.edu/etd/1920/

34. Hurst, C. S. et al. (2013). "College Student Stressors: A Review of the Qualitative Research." *Stress and Health* 29(4):275–285.

35. Smith, W. A., Allen, W. R., & Danley, L. L. (2007). "'Assume the Position…You Fit the Description':

Psychosocial Experiences and Racial Battle Fatigue among African American Male College Students." *American Behavioral Scientist*, 51(4): 551–578.

36. Sue, D. W. (2007). "Microaggressions in Everyday Life: Implications for Clinical Practice." *American Psychologist* 62(4): 271–286. Review. PMID: 17516773.

37. Pozos-Radillo, Blanca Elizabeth et al. (2014). "Academic Stress as a Predictor of Chronic Stress in University Students." *Psicología Educativa* 20(1): 47–52.

38. Conley, K. M., and Lehman, B. J. (2012). "Test Anxiety and Cardiovascular Responses to Daily Academic Stressors." *Stress and Health* 28(1): 41–50. DOI: 10.1002/smi.1399. Epub 2011 May 24

39. Feldman, D. B. et al. (2014). "Personal Resources, Hope, and Achievement Among College Students." *Journal of Happiness Studies* 16(3): 543–560.

40. Komarraju, M., and Nadler, D. (2013). "Self-efficacy and Academic Achievement: Why do Implicit Beliefs, Goals, and Effort Regulation Matter?" *Learning and Individual Differences* 25: 67–72.

41. Barton, Alison L., and Hirsch, Jameson K. (2016) "Permissive Parenting and Mental Health in College Students: Mediating Effects of Academic Entitlement." *Journal of American College Health* 64(1): 1–8. DOI: 10.1080/07448481.2015.1060597.

42. Turner, J. et al. (2015). "Students' Perceived Stress and Perception of Barriers to Effective Study: Impact on Academic Performance in Examinations." *British Dental Journal* 219(9): 453–458. DOI: 10.1038/sj.bdj.2015.850.

43. Hurst, C. S. et al.

44. Panek, E. (2014). "Left to Their Own Devices: College Students' 'Guilty Pleasure' Media Use and Time Management." *Communication Research* 41(4): 561–577.

45. Wang, J. L. et al. (2015). "The Role of Stress and Motivation in Problematic Smartphone Use Among College Students." *Computers in Human Behavior* 53: 181–188.

46. Mikdiff, Madison et al. (2015). "The Relationship Between Social Media Use and Stress in College Students." Georgia College Research Conference. October 4, 2015. http://kb.gcsu.edu/src/2015/friday/28/

47. Lepp, A. et al. (2014). "The Relationship between Cell Phone Use, Academic Performance, Anxiety, and Satisfaction with Life in College Students." *Computers in Human Behavior.* (2016) 31: 343–350.

48. American College Health Association. (2016).

49. Gayman, M. D. et al. (2011). "Depressive Symptoms and Bodily Pain: The Role of Physical Disability and Social Stress." *Stress and Health* 27(1): 52–53. Published online: 11 May 2010. DOI: 10.1002/smi.1319.

50. American College Health Association. (2016).

51. Hintz, Samuel Mathew. (2013). *Evaluating an online intervention to increase present control over stress.* Dissertation, University of Minnesota. http://conservancy.umn.edu/handle/11299/158336

52. Pignata, Silvia, and Winefield, Anthony H. (2015). "Stress-reduction Interventions in an Australian University: A Case Study." *Stress and Health* 31(1): 24–34. DOI: 10.1002/smi.2517. Epub 2013 Jul 23. PMID: 23878071

53. Ramler, T. R. et al. (2016). "Mindfulness and the College Transition: The Efficacy of an Adapted Mindfulness-based Stress Reduction Intervention in Fostering Adjustment among First-Year Students." *Mindfulness* 7(1): 179–188.

54. Conley, C. S. et al. (2015). "A Meta-analysis of Universal Mental Health Prevention Programs for Higher Education Students." *Prevention Science* 16(4): 487–507. DOI: 10.1007/s11121-015-0543-1.

55. Ramler, T. R.

56. Rogers, H. B. (2013)."Mindfulness Meditation for Increasing Resilience in College Students." *Psychiatric Annals* 43(12): 545–548. DOI: 10.3928/00485713-20131206-06.

Chapter 5

1. Rabin, L.A. et al. (2011). "Academic Procrastination in College Students: The Role of Self-Reported Executive Function." *Journal of Clinical and Experimental Neuropsychology* 33(3): 344–357.

2. Rothbart, Mary K., and Michael I. Posner. (2015). "The developing brain in a multitasking world." *Developmental Review* 35: 42–63. PMID: 25821335.

3. Vine, C. L. "College Students Think They Manage Money Well, But They Don't, Survey Finds." *Journal of Accountancy.* www.journalofaccountancy.com

4. American College Health Association. (2016). *American College Health Association-National College Health Assessment II: Reference Group Executive Summary Fall 2015.* Hanover, MD: American College Health Association: 2016.

5. National Student Financial Wellness Study. http://cssl.osu.edu/national-student-financial-wellness-study/

6. Xu, Yilan, et al. (2015). "Personality and Young Adult Financial Distress." *Journal of Economic Psychology* 51: 90–100.

7. Beiter, R., et al. (2015). "The Prevalence and Correlates of Depression, Anxiety, and Stress in a Sample of College Students." *Journal of Affective Disorders* 173: 90–96. DOI: 10.1016/j.jad.2014.10.054. Epub 2014 Nov 8. PMID: 25462401.

8. McCarthy, Patricia Curran. *Today's College Student: Measuring the Effectiveness of Financial Literacy Education and Effect on Subsequent Student Debt.* Diss. 2015. https://dspace.iup.edu/handle/2069/2339.

9. National Student Financial Wellness Study.

Chapter 6

1. American College Health Association. (2016). *American College Health Association-National College Health Assessment II: Reference Group Executive Summary Fall 2015.* Hanover, MD: American College Health Association: 2016.

2. Ploskonka, Rachel A., and Servaty-Seib, Heather L. (2015). "Belongingness and Suicidal Ideation in College Students." *Journal of American College Health* 63(2): 81–87. DOI: 10.1080/07448481.2014.983928. Epub 2015 Jan 20.

3. Cohen, Sheldon et al. (2015). "Does Hugging Provide Stress-Buffering Social Support? A Study of Susceptibility to Upper Respiratory Infection and Illness." *Psychological Science* 26(2): 135–147. *PMC.* Web. 9 Feb. 2016. Published online before print December 19, 2015, DOI: 10.1177/0956797614559284.

4. Picard, Mariah J. (2015). "Study of the Effect of Dogs on College Students' Mood and Anxiety" *Honors College.* Paper 233. http://digitalcommons.library.umaine.edu/honors/233/

5. Valdez, C. R. et al. (2013). "Emerging Adults' Lived Experience of Formative Family Stress: The Family's Lasting Influence." *Qualitative Health Research* 23(8): 1089–1102. DOI: 10.1177/1049732313494271. Epub 2013 Jun 14.

6. *Ibid.*

7. Hawkley, L. C. (2010). "Loneliness Matters: A Theoretical and Empirical Review of Consequences and Mechanisms." The Society of Behavioral Medicine *Annals of Behavioral Medicine* 40(2): 218–227. DOI: 10.1007/s12160-010-9210-8.

8. Jaremka, L. M., et al. (2013). "Loneliness Predicts Pain, Depression, and Fatigue: Understanding the Role of Immune Dysregulation." *Psychoneuroendocrinology* 38(8): 1310–1317. DOI: 10.1016/j.psyneuen.2012.11.016. Epub 2012 Dec 27.

9. VanderWeele, T. J. et al. (2012). "On the Reciprocal Association between Loneliness and Subjective Well-being." *American Journal of*

Epidemiology 176 (9): 777–784. DOI: 10.1093/aje/kws173. Epub 2012 Oct 16.

10. Holt-Lunstad, J. et al. (2015). "Loneliness and Social Isolation as Risk Factors for Mortality: A Meta-Analytic Review." *Perspectives on Psychological Science* 10(2): 227–237. DOI: 10.1177/1745691614568352.

11. American Psychiatric Association. (2013). *Diagnostic and Statistical Manual of Mental Disorders* (5th ed.). Arlington, VA: American Psychiatric Association.

12. Derbyshire, K. L. et al. (2013). "Problematic Internet Use and Associated Risks in a College Sample." *Comprehensive Psychiatry* 54(5): 415–422.

13. Yang, C. C., and Brown, B. B. (2013). "Motives for Using Facebook, Patterns of Facebook Activities, and Late Adolescents' Social Adjustment to College." *Journal of Youth and Adolescence* 42(3): 403–416. DOI: 10.1007/s10964-012-9836-x.

14. Hampton, K. et al. "Social Media and the Cost of Caring," Pew Research Internet Project. www.pewresearch.org

15. Aston-Lebold, Me. (2013). Online Socializing vs. In-Person Socializing: Psychological Sense of Community Is Equivalent. Ann Arbor, MI: ProQuest Information and Learning (2013). adworks.umi.com/35/01/3501757.htm

16. Egan, K. G. et al. (2013). "College Students' Responses to Mental Health Status Updates on Facebook." *Issues in Mental Health Nursing* 34(1): 46–51.

17. Toma, C., and Hancock, J. (2013). "Self-Affirmation Underlies Facebook Use." *Personality and Social Psychology Bulletin* 39(3): 321–331. DOI: 10.1177/0146167212474694. Epub 2013 Jan 28.

18. Hampton, K. et al.

19. Tandoc, Edson C., Ferruci, Patrick, and Duffy, Margaret. (2015). "Facebook Use, Envy, and Depression Among College Students: Is Facebooking Depressing?" *Computers in Human Behavior* 43: 139–146.

20. Martin, Ryan C., Kelsey Ryan Coyier, VanSistine, Leah M. VanSistine, and Schroeder, Kelly L.. (2013). *Cyberpsychology, Behavior, and Social Networking* 16(2): 119–122.

21. Crosslin, K., & Golman, M. (2014). "Maybe you don't want to face it"—College Students' Perspectives on Cyberbullying." *Computers in Human Behavior* 41: 14–20.

22. Selkie, E. M., Kota, R., Chan, Y., & Moreno, M. (2015). "Cyberbullying, Depression, and Problem Alcohol Use in Female College Students: A Multisite Study." *Cyberpsychology, Behavior, and Social Networking* 18(2): 79–86.

23. Dressing, H., et al. (2014). "Cyberstalking in a Large Sample of Social Network Users: Prevalence, Characteristics, and Impact Upon Victims." *Cyberpsychology, Behavior, and Social Networking* 17(2): 61–67.

24. Liu, G. et al. (2015). "Trends and Patterns of Sexual Behavior among Adolescents and Adults Aged 14 to 59 Years, United States." *Sexually Transmitted Diseases* 42(1): 20–27. DOI: 10.1097/OLQ.0000000000000231.

25. Galinsky, Adena M., and Freya Lund Sonenstein. (2013). "Relationship Commitment, Perceived Equity, and Sexual Enjoyment among Young Adults in the United States." *Archives of Sexual Behavior* 42(1): 93–104. DOI: 10.1007/s10508-012-0003-y. Epub 2012 Sep 22.

26. Juster, R. P. et al. (2013). "Sexual Orientation and Disclosure in Relation to Psychiatric Symptoms, Diurnal Cortisol, and Allostatic Load." *Psychosomatic Medicine* 75(2): 103–116. DOI: 10.1097/PSY.0b013e3182826881. Epub 2013 Jan 29.

27. Schrimshaw, E. W. et al. (2013). "Disclosure and Concealment of Sexual Orientation and the Mental Health of Non-Gay-Identified, Behaviorally Bisexual Men." *Journal of Consulting and Clinical Psychology* 81(1): 141–153. DOI: 10.1037/a0031272. Epub 2012 Dec 31.

28. American Academy of Pediatrics. (2015). "Four Stages of Coming Out." www.healthychildren.org

/English/ages-stages/teen/dating-sex/Pages/Four-Stages-of-Coming-Out.aspx

29. Bachtel, M. K. (2013). "Do Hookups Hurt? Exploring College Students' Experiences and Perceptions." *Journal of Midwifery and Women's Health* 58(1): 41–48. DOI: 10.1111/j.1542-2011.2012.00256.x.

30. Monto, M. A., Carey, A. G. (2014). "A New Standard of Sexual Behavior? Are Claims Associated With the "Hookup Culture" Supported by General Social Survey Data?" *Journal of Sex Research* 51(6): 605–615. DOI: 10.1080/00224499.2014.906031. Epub 2014 Apr 21.

31. Robertson, P. N. et al. (2015). "Hooking Up During the College Years: Is There a Pattern?" *Culture, Health & Sexuality* 17(5): 576–591. DOI: 10.1080/13691058.2014.972458. Epub 2014 Nov 17.

32. Braithwaite, Scott R. et al. (2015). "The Influence of Pornography on Sexual Scripts and Hooking Up among Emerging Adults in College." *Archives of Sexual Behavior* 44(1): 111–123. DOI: 10.1007/s10508-014-0351-x. Epub 2014 Sep 20. PMID: 25239659.

33. Fielder, R. L., et al. (2014). "Sexual Hookups and Adverse Health Outcomes: A Longitudinal Study of First-Year College Women." *Journal of Sex Research* 51(2): 131–144. DOI: 10.1080/00224499.2013.848255. Epub 2013 Dec 18.

34. Kenney, Shannon R. et al. (2014). "Development and Validation of the Hookup Motives Questionnaire (HMQ)." *Psychological Assessment* 26(4): p. 1127–1137. DOI: 10.1037/a0037131. Epub 2014 Jun 16.

35. Bersamin, M. M. et al. (2014). "Risky Business: Is There an Association between Casual Sex and Mental Health in Emerging Adults?" *Journal of Sex Research* 51(1): 43–51. DOI: 10.1080/00224499.2013.772088. Epub 2013 Jun 7.

36. Fielder, R. L. et al. (2014). "Sexual Hookups and Adverse Health Outcomes: A Longitudinal Study of First-Year College Women." *Journal of Sex Research* 51(2): 131–144. DOI: 10.1080/00224499.2013.848255. Epub 2013 Dec 18.

37. Vrangalova, Z. (2015). "Does Casual Sex Harm College Students' Well-Being? A Longitudinal Investigation of the Role of Motivation." *Archives of Sexual Behavior* 44(4): 945–959. DOI: 10.1007/s10508-013-0255-1. Epub 2014 Feb 5.

38. French, M. T. et al. (2014). "Personal Traits, Cohabitation, and Marriage." *Social Science Research* 45: 184–199. DOI: 10.1016/j.ssresearch.2014.01.002. Epub 2014 Jan 16.

39. Haas, S. M., and Whitton, S. W. (2015). "The Significance of Living Together and Importance of Marriage in Same-Sex Couples." *Journal of Homosexuality*. (April 7, 2015). DOI: 10.1080/00918369.2015.1037137. Epub 2015 Apr 7.

40. Uchino, B. N. et al. (2014). "Spousal Relationship Quality and Cardiovascular Risk: Dyadic Perceptions of Relationship Ambivalence Are Associated with Coronary-Artery Calcification." *Psychological Science* 25(4): 1037–1042.

41. Wight, R. G., et al. (2013). "Same-Sex Legal Marriage and Psychological Well-Being: Findings from the California Health Interview Survey." *American Journal of Public Health* 103(2): 339–346. DOI: 10.2105/AJPH.2012.301113. Epub 2012 Dec 13.

42. Campion, E. W. et al. (2015). "In Support of Same-Sex Marriage." *New England Journal of Medicine* 372: 1852–1853. DOI: 10.1056/NEJMe1505179. Epub 2015 Apr 22.

43. Jaremka, Lisa M. et al. "Marital Distress Prospectively Predicts Poorer Cellular Immune Function." *Psychoneuroendocrinology* 38(11): 2713–2719.

44. Doss, D. B., et al. (2009). "Marital Therapy, Retreats, and Books: The Who, What, When, and Why of Relationship Help-Seeking." *Journal of Marital and Family Therapy* 35(1): 18–29. DOI: 10.1111/j.1752-0606.2008.00093.x.

45. Heller, S. "Resolution, Not Conflict." *Psychology Today.* May 30, 2013. psychologytoday.com

46. Jaremka, L. M. et al. (2013). "Synergistic Relationships among Stress, Depression,

and Troubled Relationships: Insights from Psychoneuroimmunology." *Depression and Anxiety* 30(4): 288–296. DOI: 10.1002/da.22078. Epub 2013 Feb 14.

47. American College Health Association. (2016).

48. Johnson, W. I. et al. (2014). "Intimate Partner Violence and Depressive Symptoms during Adolescence and Young Adulthood." *Journal of Health and Social Behavior* 55: 39–55. DOI: 10.1177/0022146513520430.

49. Dardis, C. M. et al. (2015). "An Examination of the Factors Related to Dating Violence Perpetration Among Young Men and Women and Associated Theoretical Explanations: A Review of the Literature." *Trauma, Violence, & Abuse* 16(2): 136–152. (Epub Jan 10, 2014). DOI: 10.1177/1524838013517559. Epub 2014 Jan 10. Review. PMID: 24415138.

50. Littleton H. (2014). "Interpersonal Violence on College Campuses: Understanding Risk Factors and Working to Find Solutions." *Trauma, Violence, & Abuse* 15(4): 297–303. (Epub Jan 30, 2014). DOI: 10.1177/1524838013517559. Epub 2014 Jan 10.

51. Tsui, E. K., Santamaria, E. K. (2015). "Intimate Partner Violence Risk among Undergraduate Women from an Urban Commuter College: The Role of Navigating Off- and On-Campus Social Environments." *Journal of Urban Health.* (February 3, 2015). DOI: 10.1007/s11524-014-9933-0.

52. Sylaska, K. M., Edwards, K. M. "Disclosure Experiences of Sexual Minority College Student Victims of Intimate Partner Violence." *American Journal of Community Psychology* 55(3–4): 326–335. DOI: 10.1007/s10464-015-9717-z.

53. Sorenson, S. B. et al. (2012). "Knowing a Sexual Assault Victim or Perpetrator: A Stratified Random Sample of Undergraduates at One University." *Social Work in Health Care* 51(9): 798–814. DOI: 10.1080/00981389.2012.692352. PMID: 23078012.

54. Kohler, Rachel. "Campus sexual assault: Effects of trauma on student survivors and how campuses intervene." *7th Biennial National Conference on Health and Domestic Violence.* nchdv, 2015. www.futureswithoutviolence.org/

55. Slavich, G. M. et al. (2010). "Neural Sensitivity to Social Rejection is Associated with Inflammatory Response to Social Stress." *Proceedings of the National Academy of Sciences* 107(33): 14817–14822. DOI: 10.1073/pnas.1009164107. Epub 2010 Aug 2.

56. Slavich, G. M. et al. (2010). "Black Sheep Get The Blues: A Psychobiological Model of Social Rejection and Depression." *Neuroscience and Biobehavioral Reviews* 35(1): 39–45. DOI: 10.1016/j.neubiorev.2010.01.003. Epub 2010 Jan 18.

57. Tach, Laura M., and Eads, Alicia. (2015). "Trends in the Economic Consequences of Marital and Cohabitation Dissolution in the United States." *Demography* 52(2): 401–432.

58. Sbarra, D. A. et al. (2015). "Divorce and Health: Beyond Individual Differences." *Current Directions in Psychological Science* 24(2): 109–113. PMID: 25892857.

59. *Ibid.*

60. Dupree, M. E. et al. "Association Between Divorce and Risks for Acute Myocardial Infarction." *Circulation: Cardiovascular Quality and Outcomes* 8(3) 244–251. DOI: 10.1161/CIRCOUTCOMES.114.001291. Epub 2015 Apr 14.

61. Dardis, C. M. et al (2015). "An Examination of the Factors Related to Dating Violence Perpetration Among Young Men and Women and Associated Theoretical Explanations: A Review of the Literature." *Trauma, Violence, & Abuse* 16(2): 136–152. DOI: 10.1177/1524838013517559. Epub 2014 Jan 10. Review. PMID: 24415138.

62. Littleton, H. (2014). "Interpersonal Violence on College Campuses: Understanding Risk Factors and Working to Find Solutions." *Trauma, Violence, & Abuse* 15(4): 297–303. DOI: 10.1177/1524838014521030. Epub 2014 Jan 30.

Chapter 7

1. Lipschitz, Jessica M. et al. (2015) "Co-occurrence and Coaction of Stress Management with Other Health Risk Behaviors." *Journal of Health Psychology* 20(7): 1002–1012. DOI: 10.1177/1359105313506026. Epub 2013 Oct 28. PMID: 24165862.
2. Hales, D., and Christian, K. (2009). *An Invitation to Personal Change.* Belmont, CA: Wadsworth Cengage Learning.
3. Neal, D. T. et al. (2013). ""How Do People Adhere to Goals When Willpower Is Low? The Profits (and Pitfalls) of Strong Habits." *Journal of Personality and Social Psychology* 104(6): 959–975. DOI: 10.1037/a0032626. PMID: 23730907
4. Prochaska, James, Norcross, John, and DiClemente, Carlo. (1992). *Changing for Good.* New York: William Morrow.
5. Prochaska, J. O., and DiClemente, C. C. (2005). "The Transtheoretical Approach." In: Norcross, J. C., and Goldfried, M. R. (eds.) *Handbook of Psychotherapy Integration* (2nd ed) New York: Oxford University Press, 147–171.
6. Fadiman, James. (1990). *Unlimit Your Life: Setting and Getting Goals.* Berkeley: Celestial Arts.
7. Ent, Michael R., Baumeister, Roy F., and Tice, Dianne M. (2015). "Trait Self-Control and The Avoidance of Temptation." *Personality and Individual Differences* 74: 12–15.
8. Achtziger, A et al. (2008). "Implementation Intentions and Shielding Goal Striving from Unwanted Thoughts and Feelings." *Personality and Social Psychology Bulletin* 34(3): 381–393. DOI: 10.1177/0146167207311201. PMID: 18272806.

Chapter 8

1. Bryant, S. E. et al. (2015). "An Empirical Study of Emotional Intelligence and Stress in College Students." *Business Education & Accreditation* 7(1): 1–11. http://www.theibfr.com/ARCHIVE/BEA-V7N1-2015.pdf
2. Barbey, A. K. et al. (2014). "Distributed Neural System for Emotional Intelligence Revealed by Lesion Mapping." *Social Cognitive and Affective Neuroscience* 9(3): 265–272, Epub 19 November 2012. DOI: 10.1093/scan/nss124.
3. Jeste, D. V., and Palmer, B. W. (2015). "What Is Positive Psychiatry?" In *Positive Psychiatry,* edited by Dilip V. Jeste and Barton W. Palmer. Washington, D.C.: American Psychiatric Publishing. pp. 1–18.
4. Seligman, M. E. (2015). "Foreword." In *Positive Psychiatry,* edited by Dilip V. Jeste and Barton W. Palmer. Washington, D.C.: American Psychiatric Publishing. p. xvii.
5. Garland, E. L. et al. (2010). "Upward Spirals of Positive Emotions Counter Downward Spirals of Negativity: Insights from the Broaden-and-Build Theory and Affective Neuroscience on The Treatment of Emotion Dysfunctions and Deficits in Psychopathology." *Clinical Psychology Review* 30(7): 849–864.
6. Parks, A. C. et al. "Positive Psychotherapeutic and Behavioral Intervention." In *Positive Psychiatry,* edited by Dilip V. Jeste and Barton W. Palmer. Washington, D.C.: American Psychiatric Publishing. pp. 261–284.
7. Moore, R. C., et al. (2015). "Biology of Positive Psychiatry." In *Positive Psychiatry,* edited by Dilip V. Jeste and Barton W. Palmer. Washington, D.C.: American Psychiatric Publishing. pp. 261–284.
8. Winch, Guy. (2013). *Emotional First Aid: Practical Strategies for Treating Failure, Rejection, Guilt, and other Everyday Psychological Injuries.* Wollombi, New South Wales, Australia: Exisle Publishing.
9. Gartland, Nicola, et al. (2014). "Investigating the Effects of Conscientiousness on Daily Stress, Affect and Physical Symptom Processes: A Daily Diary Study." *British Journal of Health Psychology* 19(2): 311–328. DOI: 10.1111/bjhp.12077. Epub 2013 Nov 15. PMID: 24237707
10. Jazaieri, Hooria, et al. (2014). "A Randomized Controlled Trial of Compassion Cultivation Training: Effects on Mindfulness, Affect, and Emotion Regulation." *Motivation and Emotion* 38(1): 23–35. DOI: 10.1007/s11031-013-9368-z#/page-1
11. Zeller, M. et al. "Self-Compassion in Recovery Following Potentially Traumatic Stress: Longitudinal Study of At-Risk Youth." *Journal of Abnormal Child Psychology* 43(4): 645–653. DOI: 10.1007/s10802-014-9937-y.
12. Breines, Juliana G., and Serena Chen. (2012). "Self-Compassion Increases Self-Improvement Motivation." *Personality and Social Psychology Bulletin* 38(9): 1133–1143. DOI: 10.1177/0146167212445599.
13. Lyubominsky, S. (2013). *The Myths of Happiness.* New York: Penguin.
14. *Ibid.*
15. Nelson, S. K. et al. (2013). "In Defense of Parenthood: Children Are Associated with More Joy Than Misery." *Psychological Science* 24(1): 3–10. DOI: 10.1177/0956797612447798. Epub 2012 Nov 30.
16. Layous, K. et al. (2014). "Positive Activities as Protective Factors Against Mental Health Conditions." *Journal of Abnormal Psychology* 123(1): 3–12. DOI: 10.1037/a0034709. Review. PMID: 24661154.
17. Parks, Acacia C. et al. (2012). "Pursuing Happiness in Everyday Life: The Characteristics and Behaviors of Online Happiness Seekers." *Emotion* 12(6): 1222–1234. DOI: http://dx.doi.org/10.1037/a0028587.
18. Nittono, H. et al. (2012). "The Power of Kawai: Viewing Cute Images Promotes a Careful Behavior and Narrows Attentional Focus." *PLOS ONE* September 26, 2012. DOI: 10.1371/journal.pone.0046362.
19. Summers, R. F., and Lord, J. A. (2015). "Positivity in Supportive and Psychodynamic Therapy." In *Positive Psychiatry,* edited by Dilip V. Jeste and Barton W. Palmer. Washington, D.C.: American Psychiatric Publishing. pp. 167–192.
20. Martin, A. S. et al. (2015). "Positive Psychological Traits." Socioeconomic gradients and mental health: implications for public health. In *Positive Psychiatry,* edited by Dilip V. Jeste and Barton W. Palmer. Washington, D.C.: American Psychiatric Publishing. pp. 19–44.
21. Jobin, J. et al. (2014). "Associations between Dispositional Optimism and Diurnal Cortisol in a Community Sample: When Stress is Perceived as Higher Than Normal." *Health Psychology* 33(4): 382–391. DOI: 10.1037/a0032736. Epub 2013 May 13. PMID: 23668853.
22. Visser, Preston L. et al. (2013). "Hope as a Moderator of Negative Life Events and Depressive Symptoms in a Diverse Sample." *Stress and Health* 29(1): 82–88. DOI: 10.1002/smi.2433. Epub 2012 May 2.
23. American College Health Association. (2016). *American College Health Association-National College Health Assessment II: Reference Group Executive Summary Fall 2015.* Hanover, MD: American College Health Association: 2016.
24. Armeli, S. et al. (2016). "Episode-Specific Drinking-to-Cope Motivation and Next-Day Stress-Reactivity." *Anxiety, Stress & Coping.* 2016 Jan 29: 1–12. DOI: 10.1080/10615806.2015.1134787
25. Henslee, A. M. et al. "The Impact of Campus Traditions and Event-Specific Drinking." *Addictive Behaviors* 45: 180–183. DOI: 10.1016/j. addbeh.2015.01.033.
26. Coleman, J., and Trunzo, J. (2015). "Personality, Social Stress, and Drug Use Among College Students." *Psi Chi Journal of Psychological Research* 20(1): 52–56.
27. American College Health Association. (2016).
28. Gabert-Quillen. C. A. et al. (2015). "Post-Traumatic Stress Disorder Symptoms Mediate the Relationship Between Trauma Exposure and Smoking Status in College Students." *Stress and Health* 31(1): 78–82. DOI: 10.1002/smi.2543. Epub 2014 Jan 14. PMID: 24424717.

Chapter 9

1. Van Kim, N. A., and T. F. Nelson. (2013). "Vigorous Physical Activity, Mental Health, Perceived Stress, and Socializing among College Students." *American Journal of Health Promotion* 28(1): 7–15. DOI: 10.4278/ajhp.111101-QUAN-395.
2. Cooney, G. et al. (2014). "Exercise for Depression." *Journal of the American Medical Association* 311(23): 2432–2433. DOI: 10.1001/jama.2014.4930. PMID: 24938566.
3. American College Health Association. (2016). *American College Health Association-National College Health Assessment II: Reference Group Executive Summary Fall 2015.* Hanover, MD: American College Health Association: 2016.
4. Beddhu, S. et al. (2015). "Light-Intensity Physical Activities and Mortality in the United States General Population and CKD Subpopulation." *Clinical Journal of the American Society of Nephrology* 10(7): 1145–1153. DOI: 10.2215/CJN.08410814. Epub 2015 Apr 30.
5. Ratey, John. (2008). *Spark: The Revolutionary New Science of Exercise and the Brain.* New York: Little Brown.
6. Nokia, M. S. et al. (2016). "Physical Exercise Increases Adult Hippocampal Neurogenesis in Male Rats Provided it is Aerobic and Sustained." *The Journal of Physiology* 2016 Feb 4. DOI: 10.1113/JP271552.
7. Ratey, John
8. Richards, J. et al. (2015). "Don't Worry, Be Happy: Cross-sectional Associations between Physical Activity and Happiness in 15 European Countries." *BMC Public Health 2015* 15:53 DOI: 10.1186/s12889-015-1391-4.
9. Janssen, I. et al. (2013). "Years of Life Gained Due to Leisure-Time Physical Activity in the U.S." *American Journal of Preventive Medicine* 44(1): 23–29. DOI: 10.1016/j.amepre.2012.09.056. PMID: 23253646.
10. Gebel, K et al. (2015). "Physical Activity and Successful Aging-Reply: Even a Little Is Good." *JAMA Internal Medicine* 175(11):1862–1863. DOI: 10.1001/jamainternmed.2015.4747.
11. Watson, K., and Baar, K. (2014). "MTOR and the Health Benefits of Exercise." *Seminars in Cell & Developmental Biology* 36: 130–139. DOI: 10.1016/j.semcdb.2014.08.013. Epub 2014 Sep 16. Review. PMID: 25218794.
12. Weinberg L et al. (2014). "A Single Bout of Resistance Exercise Can Enhance Episodic Memory Performance." *Acta Psychologica* 153: 13–19. DOI: 10.1016/j.actpsy.2014.06.011. Epub 2014 Sep 28.
13. Physical Activity Guidelines for Americans. ODPHP. http://health.gov/paguidelines/guidelines/
14. Arem, H. et al. (2015). "Leisure Time Physical Activity and Mortality: A Detailed Pooled Analysis of the Dose-Response Relationship." *JAMA Internal Medicine* 175(6): 959–967. DOI: 10.1001/jamainternmed.2015.0533. PMID: 25844730.
15. American College Health Association. (2016).
16. Magsamen-Conrad, Kate. (2015). *Sleep Well, Be Well: Teaching students positive sleeping habits to create a less stressful environment.* http://works.bepress.com/kate_magsamen-conrad/9/
17. Mitchell, J. A. et al. (2013). "Sleep Duration and Adolescent Obesity." *Pediatrics* 131(5): e1428–e1434. DOI: 10.1542/peds.2012–2368. Epub 2013 Apr 8. PMID: 23569090.
18. Cedernaes, J. et al. (2015). "Short Sleep Makes Declarative Memories Vulnerable to Stress in Humans." *SLEEP* 38(12): 1861–1868. DOI: 10.5665/sleep.5228. PMID: 26158890.
19. American College Health Association. (2016).
20. Faraut, B. et al. (2015). "Napping Reverses the Salivary Interleukin-6 and Urinary Norepinephrine

Changes Induced by Sleep Restriction." *Journal of Clinical Endocrinology & Metabolism* 100(3): pp. E416–E426. DOI: http://dx.doi.org/10.1210/jc.2014-2566#sthash.asrYSJgO.dpuf

21. Ye, L. et al. (2015). "Napping in College Students and Its Relationship With Nighttime Sleep." *Journal of American College Health* 63(2): 88–97. DOI: 10.1080/07448481.2014.983926. Epub 2015 Jan 14.

22. *Dietary Guidelines For Americans, 2015–2020.* Washington, D.C.: ODPHP http://health.gov/DietaryGuidelines/

23. Han, E., and Powell, L. M. (2013). "Consumption Patterns of Sugar-Sweetened Beverages in the United States." *Journal of the Academy of Nutrition and Dietetics* 113(1): 43–53. doi:10.1016/j.jand.2012.09.016.

24. Lieberman, Harris, et al. (2015). "Intake of Caffeine from All Sources Including Energy Drinks and Reasons for Use in US College Students." *The FASEB Journal* 29(1) Supplement (2015): 392–401.

25. Doepker, Candace et al. (2016). "Caffeine: Friend or Foe?" *Annual Review of Food Science and Technology* 7: 113–137. DOI: 10.1146/annurev-food-041715-033243.

26. Mabe, A.G. et al. (2014). "Do you 'like' my photo? Facebook use maintains eating disorder risk," *International Journal of Eating Disorders* 47(5): 516–523. DOI:10.1002/eat.22254.

27. Nanney, M. S. et al. (2015). "Weight and Weight-Related Behaviors Among 2-Year College Students." *Journal of American College Health* 63(4): 221–229. DOI: 10.1080/07448481.2015.1015022. Epub 2015 Feb 18. PMID: 25692380.

28. Smith, S. S. et al. (2015). "Mediating Effects of Stress, Weight-Related Issues, and Depression on Suicidality in College Students." *Journal of American College Health* 63(1): 1–12. DOI: 10.1080/07448481.2014.960420. Epub 2014 Nov 24.

29. Tribole, E., and Resch, E. (2012). *Intuitive Eating.* New York: St. Martin's Griffin.

30. Bennett, J. et al. "Perceptions of emotional eating behavior. A qualitative study of college students." *Appetite* 60(1): 187–192. DOI: 10.1016/j.appet.2012.09.023. Epub 2012 Oct 6.

31. Groesz, Lisa M. et al. "What is eating you? Stress and the drive to eat." *Appetite* 58(2): 717–721. DOI: 10.1016/j.appet.2011.11.028. Epub 2011 Dec 4. PMID: 22166677.

Chapter 10

1. Egbert, Nichole. (2016). "Communication, Spirituality, and Health." In *The International Encyclopedia of Interpersonal Communication*, edited by Charles R. Berger, Michael E. Roloff, Steve R. Wilson, James Price Dillard, John Caughlin, and Denise Solomon. Wiley-Blackwell (2016). DOI:10.1002/9781118540190.wbeic230. Epub 2015 Dec 2.

2. Brechting, Emily H., and Charles R. Carlson. (2015). "Religiousness and Alcohol Use in College Students: Examining Descriptive Drinking Norms as Mediators." *Journal of Child & Adolescent Substance Abuse* 24(1): 1–11. DOI: 10.1080/1067828X.2014.958000.

3. Phillips, L., et al. (2015). "Eating Disorders and Spirituality in College Students." *Journal of Psychosocial Nursing and Mental Health Services* 53(1): 30–37. DOI: 10.3928/02793695-20141201-01. Epub 2014 Dec 10. PMID: 25490775.

4. Van Cappellen, Patty et al. (2016). "Religion and Well-Being: The Mediating Role of Positive Emotions." *Journal of Happiness Studies* 17(2): 485–505. DOI: 10.1007/s10902-014-9605-5. Epub 2014 Dec 18.

5. Yu, L. et al. (2015). "Purpose in Life and Cerebral Infarcts in Community-Dwelling Older People." *Stroke* 46(4): 1071–1076. DOI: 10.1161/STROKEAHA.114.008010. PMID: 25791714.

6. Goyal, M. et al. (2014). "Meditation Programs for Psychological Stress and Well-being: A Systematic Review and Meta-analysis." *JAMA Internal Medicine* 174(3):357–368. DOI: 10.1001/jamainternmed.2013.13018.

7. Olver, L. (2013). *Investigation Prayer: Impact on Health and Quality of Life.* New York: Springer.

8. Mills, Paul J.; Redwine, Laura; Chopra, Deepak. (2015). "A Grateful Heart May Be a Healthier Heart." *Spirituality in Clinical Practice* 2(1): 23–24. DOI: http://dx.doi.org/10.1037/scp0000063.

9. Fowler, James H. and Christakis, Nicholas A. (2009). "Dynamic Spread of Happiness in a Large Social Network: Longitudinal Analysis Over 20 Years in the Framingham Heart Study." *British Medical Journal* 3, January 2009. Available at SSRN: http://ssrn.com/abstract=1312605.

10. Lowe, Sarah R. et al. "Psychological Resilience after Hurricane Sandy: The Influence of Individual- and Community-Level Factors on Mental Health after a Large-Scale Natural Disaster." *PLOS ONE* 10.5 (2015): e0125761. DOI: 10.1371/journal.pone.0125761.

11. Southwick. S., and Charney, D. S. (2012). *Resilience: The Science of Mastering Life's Greatest Challenges.* London: Cambridge University Press.

12. Haase, Lori et al. (2016). "When the Brain does not Adequately Feel the Body: Links between Low Resilience and Interoception." *Biological Psychology* 113: 37–45. DOI: 10.1016/j.biopsycho.2015.11.004.

13. Knaevelsrud, C., and Böttche, M. (2013). "Writing Therapy after Traumatic Events: Therapeutic Approaches and Mechanisms of Change." Psychotherapie, Psychosomatik, Medizinische Psychologie 63(9–10): 391–397. DOI: 10.1055/s-0033-1349078. Epub 2013 Oct 11.

14. Andersson, M. A., and Conley, C. S. (2013). "Optimizing the Perceived Benefits and Health Outcomes of Writing about Traumatic Events." *Stress and Health* 29(1): 40–49. DOI: 10.1002/smi.2423. Epub 2012 Mar 9.

15. Leist, Anja K., and Müller, Daniela. (2013). "Humor Types Show Different Patterns of Self-Regulation, Self-Esteem, and Well-Being." *Journal of Happiness Studies* 14(2): 551–569. DOI: 10.1007/s10902-012-9342-6.

16. Scott, Ciera V., Hyer, Lee A., and McKenzie, Laura C. (2015). "The Healing Power of Laughter: The Applicability of Humor as a Psychotherapy Technique With Depressed and Anxious Older Adults." *Social Work in Mental Health* 13(1): 48–60. DOI: 10.1080/15332985.2014.972493.

17. Kim, S. H., Kim, Y. H., and Kim, H. J. (2015). "Laughter and Stress Relief in Cancer Patients: A Pilot Study." *Evidence-Based Complementary and Alternative Medicine* 2015;2015: Article 864739. DOI: 10.1155/2015/864739. Epub 2015 May 24.

18. Simons, J. (2015). "Hospital Clowns Boost Healing Through The Power of Laughter." *Nursing Children and Young People* 27(2): 15. DOI: 10.7748/ncyp.27.2.15.s17.

Chapter 11

1. Liu, S. et al. (2014). "Effectiveness of Job Search Interventions: A Meta-analytic Review." *Psychological Bulletin* 140(4): 1009–1041. DOI: http://dx.doi.org/10.1037/a0035923H.

2. Salanova, M. et al. (2013). "Engaged, Workaholic, Burned-Out or Just 9-to-5? Toward a Typology of Employee Well-being." *Stress and Health* 30(1): 71–81. DOI: 10.1002/smi.2499. Epub 2013 May 31. PMID: 23723156

3. deBloom, J. et al. (2013). "Vacation (After-) Effects on Employee Health and Well-Being, and the Role of Vacation Activities, Experiences and Sleep." *Journal of Happiness Studies* 14(2): 613–633. DOI: 10.1007/s10902-012-9345-3.

4. deBloom, J. et al. (2012). "Effects of Short Vacations, Vacation Activities and Experiences on Employee Health and Well-Being." *Stress and*

Health 28(4): 305–318. DOI: 10.1002/smi.1434. Epub 2011 Dec 28. PMID: 22213478.

5. Newton, C. and Teo, S. (2014). "Identification and Occupational Stress: A Stress-Buffering Perspective." *Human Resource Management* 53(1): 89–113. DOI: 10.1002/hrm.21598.

6. Manderson, Cameron. (2014). "Life Stress, Work Stress and Job Performance: Does Conscientiousness Make a Difference?" Dissertation, University of Iowa. December 2014. http://gradworks.umi.com/15/67/1567953.html

7. Goh, J et al. (2015). "Exposure To Harmful Workplace Practices Could Account For Inequality In Life Spans Across Different Demographic Groups." *Health Affairs* 34(10): 1761–1768. DOI: 10.1377/hlthaff.2015.0022.

8. *Ibid.*

9. American Psychological Association "Stress in the Workplace." www.apa.org

10. Hogh, A. et al. (2012). "Exposure to Negative Acts at Work, Psychological Stress Reactions and Physiological Stress Response." *Journal of Psychosomatic Research* 73(1): 47–52. DOI: 10.1016/j.jpsychores.2012.04.004. Epub 2012 May 7.

11. Matthews, R. A. et al. (2012). "Work hours and Work-Family Conflict." *Stress and Health* 28(3): 234–247. DOI: 10.1002/smi.1431. Epub 2011 Nov 3. PMID: 22282174.

12. Fodor. D. P. et al. (2014). "Healthy Eating at Different Risk Levels for Job Stress: Testing a Moderated Mediation." *Journal of Occupational Health Psychology* 19(2): 259–267. DOI: http://dx.doi.org/10.1037/a0036267.

13. Periera, D., and Elfering, A. (2014). "Social Stressors at Work, Sleep Quality and Psychosomatic Health Complaints." *Stress and Health* 30(1):43–52. DOI: 10.1002/smi.2494. Epub 2013 Jul 4.

14. Cieslak, Roman et al. (2014). "A Meta-Analysis of the Relationship between Job Burnout and Secondary Traumatic Stress among Workers with Indirect Exposure to Trauma." *Psychological Services* 11(1): 75–86. DOI: 10.1037/a0033798. Epub 2013 Aug 12. PMID: 23937082.

15. Naswali, K. et al. (2012). Job Insecurity as a Predictor of Physiological Indicators of Health in Healthy Working Women: An Extension of Previous Research. *Stress and Health* 28(3):255–263. DOI: 10.1002/smi.1430. Epub 2011 Dec 14.

16. Wenger, M et al. (2013). "Health and Quality of Life within the Context of Unemployment and Job Worries." *Psychotherapie, Psychosomatik, Medizinische Psychologie* 63(3–4): 129–137. DOI: 10.1055/s-0032-1332989.

17. Curtin P. (2016). "The Use of Emotional Intelligence and Positive Emotions in Coping with Chronic Unemployment." Dissertation, North Central University, 2016. http://gradworks.umi.com/10/01/10018937.html.

18. Gold, D. R., and Samet, J. M. (2013). "Air Pollution, Climate, and Heart Disease." *Circulation* 128(21): e411–e414. DOI: 10.1161/CIRCULATIONAHA.113.003988.

19. *Ibid.*

20. Moshammer, H. et al. (2015). "Early Prognosis of Noise-Induced Hearing Loss." *Occupational & Environmental Medicine* 72(2): 85–89. DOI: 10.1136/oemed-2014-102200. Epub 2014 Jul 25. PMID: 25063775.

21. Kim, Ki-Hyun, Kabir, Ehsanul, and Shamin Ara Jahan. "The Use of Cell Phone and Insight into its Potential Human Health Impacts." *Environmental Monitoring and Assessment* 188(4): 1–11. DOI: 10.1007/s10661-016-5227-1.

Chapter 12

1. Smith J, Jackson L. (2001). "Breathing Exercises and Relaxation States." Pp. 202–204 in *Advances in ABC Relaxation: Applications and Inventories*, edited by Jonathan C. Smith. New York: Springer.

2. El Malky, M. I., Atia, M. M., and El-Amrosy, S. H. (2015). "The Effectiveness of Stress Management Programme on Depression, Stress, and Anxiety of Depressed Patients." *Journal of Nursing Science* 1(2): 15–24.

3. Jerath, R. et al. (2015). "Self-Regulation of Breathing as a Primary Treatment for Anxiety." *Applied Psychophysiology and Biofeedback* 40(2): 107–115. DOI: 10.1007/s10484-015-9279-8. Review. PMID: 25869930

4. Dykema Ravi. (2006). *Yoga for Fitness and Wellness*. Belmont, CA: Wadsworth.

5. Chang, K. L. et al. (2015). "Chronic Pain Management: Nonpharmacological Therapies for Chronic Pain." *FP Essentials* 432: 21–6.

6. Beck, B. D. et al. (2015). "Coping with Work-Related Stress through Guided Imagery and Music (GIM): Randomized Controlled Trial." *Journal of Music Therapy* 52(3): 323–352. DOI: 10.1093/jmt/thv011. Epub 2015 Sep 30. PMID: 26424362.

7. Bhasin, M. K. et al. (2013). "Relaxation Response Induces Temporal Transcriptome Changes in Energy Metabolism, Insulin Secretion and Inflammatory Pathways." *PLOS ONE* 8(5): e62817. DOI: 10.1371/journal.pone.0062817. Print 2013. PMID: 23650531.

8. *Ibid.*

9. Jallo, N. et al. (2015). "Perceptions of Guided Imagery for Stress Management in Pregnant African American Women." *Archives of Psychiatric Nursing* 29(4): 249–254. DOI: 10.1016/j.apnu.2015.04.004. Epub 2015 Apr 24.

10. Stahl, J. E. et al. (2015). "Relaxation Response and Resiliency Training and Its Effect on Healthcare Resource Utilization." *PLOS ONE* 10(10): e0140212. DOI: 10.1371/journal.pone.0140212. eCollection 2015. PMID: 26461184.

11. *Ibid.*

12. Dolbeir, C. L. and Rush, T. E. (2012). "Efficacy of Abbreviated Progressive Muscle Relaxation in a High-Stress College Sample." *International Journal of Stress Management* 19(1): 48–68.

13. Benson, Herbert. (2009). *The Relaxation Response*. New York: HarperCollins.

14. Smith, Jonathan. (1999). *ABC Relaxation Theory*. New York: Springer.

15. Smith J, Jackson L. (2001). "Breathing Exercises and Relaxation States." Pp. 202–204 in Advances in ABC Relaxation: Application and Inventories, edited by Jonathan C. Smith. New York: Springer.

16. *Ibid.*

17. Smith, J. C. et al. (2000). "ABC Relaxation Theory and the Factor Structure of Relaxation States, Recalled Relaxation Activities, Dispositions, and Motivations." *Psychological Reports* 86(3c): 1201–1208. PMID: 10932580.

Chapter 13

1. Brown, K.W. and Ryan, R.M. (2003). "The benefits of being present: Mindfulness and its Role in Psychological Well-being." *Journal of Personality and Social Psychology* 84(4): 822–848. DOI: http://dx.doi.org/10.1037/0022-3514.84.4.822

2. Goroll, A. H. (2014). "Moving Toward Evidence-Based Complementary Care." *JAMA Internal Medicine* 174(3): 368–369. DOI: 10.1001/jamainternmed.2013.12995.

3. Goyal, M. et al. (2014). "Meditation Programs for Psychological Stress and Well-being: A Systematic Review and Meta-analysis." *JAMA Internal Medicine* 174(3): 357–368. DOI: 10.1001/jamainternmed.2013.13018.

4. Kabat-Zinn, J. (1994). *Wherever You Go, There You Are: Mindfulness Meditation in Everyday Life*. New York: Hyperion.

5. Robins, C. J. et al. (2012). "Effects of Mindfulness-Based Stress Reduction on Emotional Experience and Expression: A Randomized Controlled Trial." *Journal of Clinical Psychology* 68(1): 117–131. DOI: 10.1002/jclp.20857. Epub 2011 Dec 5.

6. Garland, Eric L. et al. (2015). "Mindfulness Training Promotes Upward Spirals of Positive Affect and Cognition: Multilevel and Autoregressive Latent Trajectory Modeling Analyses." *Frontiers in Psychology* 6: 15. Epub 2015 Feb 2. DOI: 10.3389/fpsyg.2015.00015. eCollection 2015. PMID: 25698988.

7. Garland, E. L. et al. (2010). "Upward Spirals of Positive Emotions Counter Downward Spirals of Negativity: Insights from the Broaden-and-Build Theory and Affective Neuroscience on The Treatment of Emotion Dysfunctions and Deficits in Psychopathology." *Clinical Psychology Review* 30(7): 849–864. DOI: 10.1016/j.cpr.2010.03.002.

8. Shapiro, S. L., and Carlson, L. E. (2009). *The Art and Science of Mindfulness*. Washington, DC: American Psychological Association.

9. Mikulas, W. L. (2015). "Cultivating Mindfulness: A Comprehensive Approach." *Mindfulness* 6(2): 398–401. DOI: 10.1007/s12671-014-0339-6.

10. Kuyken, W. et al. (2010). "How Does Mindfulness-based Cognitive Therapy Work?" *Behaviour Research and Therapy* 48(11): 1105–1112. DOI: 10.1016/j.brat.2010.08.003

11. Fjorback, L. O. et al. (2011). (2011). "Mindfulness-Based Stress Reduction and Mindfulness-Based Cognitive Therapy – A Systematic Review of Randomized Controlled Trials." *Acta Psychiatrica Scandinavica* 124(2): 102–119. DOI: 10.1111/j.1600-0447.2011.01704.x. Epub 2011 Apr 28. Review.

12. Bamber, M.D. and Schneider, J. K. (2015). "Mindfulness-Based Meditation to Decrease Stress and Anxiety in College Students: A Narrative Synthesis of the Research." *Educational Research Review* 18: 1–32. DOI: 10.1016/j.edurev.2015.12.004

13. Greeson, J. M. et al. (2015). "An Adapted, Four- Week Mind–Body Skills Group for Medical Students: Reducing Stress, Increasing Mindfulness, and Enhancing Self-Care." *Explore: The Journal of Science and Healing* 11(3): 186–192. DOI: 10.1186/s13063-014-0533-9. Epub 2015 Feb 16.

14. Kuhlmann, S. M. et al. (2015). "A Mindfulness-based Stress Prevention Training for Medical Students (MediMind): Study Protocol for a Randomized Controlled Trial." *Trials* 16: 40. DOI: 10.1186/s13063-014-0533-9.

15. Grossman, P. et al. (2004). "Mindfulness-based Stress Reduction and Health Benefits: A Meta-analysis." *Journal of Psychosomatic Research* 57(1): 35–43. DOI: 10.1016/S0022-3999(03)00573-7. PMID: 15256293.

16. Jacobs, Tonya. (2013). "Self-reported Mindfulness and Cortisol during a Shamatha Meditation Retreat." *Health Psychology* 32(10): 1104–1109. DOI: 10.1037/a0031362. Epub 2013 Mar 25. PMID: 23527522.

17. Rosenberg, E. L. et al. (2015). "Intensive Meditation Training Influences Emotional Responses to Suffering." *Emotion* 15(6): 775–790. DOI: 10.1037/emo0000080. Epub 2015 May 4.

18. Creswell, J. D. et al. (2009). "Mindfulness Meditation Training Effects on CD4+ T Lymphocytes in HIV-1 Infected Adults: A Small Randomized Controlled Trial." *Brain, Behavior, and Immunity* 23(2): 184–188. DOI: 10.1016/j.bbi.2008.07.004. Epub 2008 Jul 19.

19. Chiesa, A., and Serretti, A. (2011). "Mindfulness-based Interventions for Chronic Pain: A Systematic Review of the Evidence." *Journal of Alternative and Complementary Medicine* 17(1): 83–93. DOI: 10.1089/acm.2009.0546.

20. Davis, M. C. et al. (2015). "Mindfulness and Cognitive-Behavioral Interventions for Chronic Pain: Differential Effects on Daily Pain Reactivity and Stress Reactivity." *Journal of Consulting and Clinical Psychology* 83(1): 24–35. DOI: 10.1037/a0038200. Epub 2014 Nov 3. PMID: 25365778.

21. Jedel, S. et al. (2014). "A Randomized Controlled Trial of Mindfulness-based Stress Reduction to Prevent Flare-up in Patients with Inactive Ulcerative Colitis." *Digestion*. 89(2): 142–155. DOI: 10.1159/000356316. Epub 2014 Feb 14.

22. *Ibid.*

23. Brewer, J. A. et al. (2013). "Mindfulness Training for Smoking Cessation: Results from a Randomized Controlled Trial." *Drug and Alcohol Dependence* 130(1–3): 222–229. 2014;89(2):142– 55. DOI: 10.1016/j.drugalcdep.2011.05.027. Epub 2014 Feb 14.

24. Keng, S.-L., Smoski, M. J., and Robins, C. J. (2011). "Effects of Mindfulness on Psychological Health: A Review of Empirical Studies." *Clinical Psychology Review* 31(6): 1041–1056. DOI: 10.1016/j.cpr.2011.04.006. Epub 2011 May 13.

25. Kemeny, M. E. et al. (2012). "Contemplative/Emotion Training Reduces Negative Emotional Behavior and Promotes Prosocial Responses." *Emotion* 12(2): 338–350. DOI: http://dx.doi.org/10.1037/a0026118

26. Goldhagen, B. et al. (2015). "Stress and Burnout in Residents: Impact of Mindfulness-based Resilience Training." *Advances in Medical Education and Practice* 6: 525–532. DOI: 10.2147/AMEP.S88580. eCollection 2015.

27. Fjorback, L. O. et al. (2011). "Mindfulness-Based Stress Reduction and Mindfulness-Based Cognitive Therapy – A Systematic Review of Randomized Controlled Trials." *Acta Psychiatrica Scandinavica* 124(2): 102–119. DOI: 10.1111/j.1600-0447.2011.01704.x. Epub 2011 Apr 28.

28. Arch, J. J. et al. (2006). "Mechanisms of Mindfulness: Emotional Regulation Following Focused Breathing Induction." *Behaviour Research and Therapy* 44(12): 1849–1858.

29. Goldhagen, B. E. et al. (2015). "Stress and Burnout in Residents: Impact of Mindfulness-based Resilience Training." *Advances in Medical Education and Practice*. 6: 525–532. DOI: 10.2147/AMEP.S88580. eCollection 2015.

30. Greer, D. (2015). "An Online Mindfulness Intervention to Reduce Stress and Anxiety among College Students." University of Minnesota. ProQuest Dissertations Publishing 2015. 3718245. http://conservancy.umn.edu/handle/11299/175442.

31. Carmody, J., and Baer, R. A. (2008). "Relationships between Mindfulness Practice and Levels of Mindfulness, Medical and Psychological Symptoms, and Well-being in a Mindfulness-based Stress Reduction Program." *Journal of Behavioral Medicine* 31(1): 23–33. Epub 2007 Sep 25. DOI: 10.1007%2Fs10865-007-9130-7

32. Kenny, M. A., and Williams, J. M. G. (2007). Treatment-resistant Depressed Patients Show a Good Response to Mindfulness based Cognitive Therapy." *Behaviour Research and Therapy* 45(3): 617–625. Epub 2006 Jun 23. DOI: 10.1016/j.brat.2006.04.008

33. Creswell, J. D., Irwin, M. R., Burklund, L. J., Lieberman, M. D., Arevalo, J. M., et al. (2012). "Mindfulness-Based Stress Reduction Training Reduces Loneliness and Pro-inflammatory Gene Expression in Older Adults: A Small Randomized Controlled Trial." *Brain, Behavior, and Immunity* 26(7): 1095–1101. DOI: 10.1016/j.bbi.2012.07.006. Epub 2012 Jul 20.

34. Fjorback, L. O. et al. (2011). "Mindfulness-Based Stress Reduction and Mindfulness-Based Cognitive Therapy – A Systematic Review of Randomized Controlled Trials." *Acta Psychiatrica Scandinavica* 124(2): 102–119. DOI: 10.1111/j.1600-0447.2011.01704.x. Epub 2011 Apr 28.

35. Modesto-Lowe, V. et al. (2015). "Does Mindfulness Meditation Improve Attention in Attention Deficit Hyperactivity Disorder?" *World Journal of Psychiatry* 5(4): 397–403. DOI: 10.5498/wjp.v5.i4.397. eCollection 2015.

36. Gard, T. et al. (2014). "The Potential Effects of Meditation on Age-related Cognitive Decline: A Systematic Review." *Annals of the New York Academy of Sciences* 1307: 89–103. DOI: 10.1111/nyas.12348.

37. Khoury, B. et al. (2015). "Mindfulness-based Stress Reduction for Healthy Individuals: A Meta-analysis." *Journal of Psychosomatic Research* 78(6): 519–528. DOI:10.1016/j.jpsychores.2015.03.009. Epub 2015 Mar 20. Review. PMID: 25818837.

38. Sharma, M., and Rush, S. E. (2014). "Mindfulness-Based Stress Reduction as a Stress Management Intervention for Healthy Individuals: A Systematic Review." *Journal of Evidence-Based Complementary & Alternative Medicine* 19(4): 271–286. DOI: 10.1177/2156587214543143.

39. Howells, A., Ivtzan, I., & Eiroa-Orosa, F. J. (2016). "Putting the 'App' in Happiness: A Randomised Controlled Trial of a Smartphone-Based Mindfulness Intervention to Enhance Wellbeing." *Journal of Happiness Studies* 17(1): 163–185. DOI: 10.1007/s10902-014-9589-1

40. National Center for Complementary and Alternative Medicine. https://nccih.nih.gov/

41. Gillani, N. B., and Smith, J. C. (2001). "Zen Meditation and ABC Relaxation Theory: An Exploration of Relaxation States, Beliefs, Dispositions, and Motivations." *Journal of Clinical Psychology* 57(6): 839–846.

42. Monaghan, P., and Viereck, E. (1999). *Meditation: The Complete Guide.* Novato, CA: New World Library.

43. Sibinga, E. M. S. et al. (2016). "School-Based Mindfulness Instruction: An RCT." *Pediatrics* 137(1): 1–8. DOI: 10.1542/peds.2015-2532.

44. Goyal, M. et al. (2014). "Meditation Programs for Psychological Stress and Well-being: A Systematic Review and Meta-analysis." *JAMA Internal Medicine* 174(3): 357–368. DOI: 10.1001/jamainternmed.2013.13018.

45. Arias, A. J, Steinberg, Karen, Banga, Alok, and Trestman, Robert L. (2006). "Systematic Review of the Efficacy of Meditation Techniques as Treatments for Medical Illness." Journal of Alternative and Complementary Medicine 12(8): 817–832. DOI: 10.1089/acm.2006.12.817.

46. Brook, R. D., Appel, R. J., Rubenfire, M. et al. (2013). Beyond Medications and Diet: Alternative Approaches to Lowering Blood Pressure: A Scientific Statement From the American Heart Association. *Hypertension.* 61(6): 1360–1383. DOI: 10.1161/HYP.0b013e318293645f. Epub 2013 Apr 22.

47. Morgan, N., Irwin, M. R., Chung, M., et al. (2014). "The Effects of Mind-Body Therapies on the Immune System: Meta-analysis." *PLOS ONE* 9(7): e100903. DOI: 10.1371/journal.pone.0100903. eCollection 2014. Review.

48. Zeidan, F., Grant, J. A., Brown, C. A., et al. (2012). "Mindfulness Mediation-related Pain Relief: Evidence for Unique Brain Mechanisms in the Regulation of Pain." *Neuroscience Letters.* 520(2): 165–173. DOI: 10.1016/j.neulet.2012.03.082. Epub 2012 Apr 6.

49. Tang, Y.-Y., Tang, R., and Posner, M. I. (2013). "Brief Meditation Training Induces Smoking Reduction." *Proceedings of the National Academy of Sciences.* 110(34): 13971–13975. DOI: 10.1073/pnas.1311887110. Epub 2013 Aug 5.

50. Westbrook C, Creswell JD, Tabibnia G, et al. (2013). "Mindful Attention Reduces Neural and Self-Reported Cue-Induced Craving in Smokers." *Social Cognitive and Affective Neuroscience.* 2013 Jan;8(1):73-84. doi: 10.1093/scan/nsr076. Epub 2011 Nov 22.

51. Luders E. (2014). "Exploring Age-related Brain Degeneration in Meditation Practitioners." *Annals of the New York Academy of Sciences* 1307: 82–88. DOI: 10.1111/nyas.12217. Epub 2013 Aug 7.

52. Chen, K. W., Berger, C. C., Manheimer E, et al. "Meditative Therapies for Reducing Anxiety: A Systematic Review and Meta-analysis of Randomized Controlled Trials." *Depression and Anxiety.* 29(7): 545–562. DOI: 10.1002/da.21964. Epub 2012 Jun 14.

53. Rubia K. (2009). "The Neurobiology of Meditation and its Clinical Effectiveness in Psychiatric Disorders. *Biological Psychology* 82(1): 1–11. DOI: 10.1016/j.biopsycho.2009.04.003. Epub 2009 Apr 23.

54. Greer, D. "An Online Mindfulness Intervention to Reduce Stress and Anxiety among College Students." University of Minnesota. ProQuest Dissertations Publishing 2015. 3718245. http://conservancy.umn.edu/handle/11299/175442.

55. Gillani, N. B., and Smith, J. C. (2001). "Zen Meditation and ABC Relaxation Theory: An Exploration of Relaxation States, Beliefs, Dispositions, and Motivations." Journal of Clinical Psychology 57(6): 839–846. DOI: 10.1002/jclp.1053.

56. Desbordes Gaëlle et al. (2012). "Effects of Mindful-attention and Compassion Meditation Training on Amygdala Response to Emotional Stimuli in an Ordinary, Non-meditative State." *Frontiers in Human Neuroscience* 6: 292. DOI: 10.3389/fnhum.2012.00292. eCollection 2012.

57. Luders, E., Kurth, F., Mayer, E. A., et al. (2012). "The Unique Brain Anatomy of Meditation Practitioners: Alterations in Cortical Gyrification." *Frontiers in Human Neuroscience.* 6: 34. DOI: 10.3389/fnhum.2012.00034. eCollection 2012.

58. Chang, K. L. et al. (2015). "Chronic Pain Management: Nonpharmacological Therapies for Chronic Pain." *FP Essentials* 432:21–26. PMID:25970869.

59. Carpenter, Janet S., Gass, Margery LS, Maki, Pauline M., Newton, Katherine M., Pinkerton, Joann V., Taylor, Maida, Utian, Wulf H., et al. (2015). "Nonhormonal Management of Menopause-Associated Vasomotor Symptoms." *Menopause* 22(11): 1155–1174. DOI: 10.1097/GME.0000000000000546.

60. Leone, D. et al. (2014). "State of the Art: Psychotherapeutic Interventions Targeting the Psychological Factors Involved in IBD." *Curr Drug Targets* 15(11): 1020-9. Review.

61. Smith, B.L. "Hypnosis Today." Washington D.C.: *Monitor on Psychiatry* January 2011 50–52.

Chapter 14

1. Stetter, F., and Kupper, S. (2002). "Autogenic Training: A Meta-Analysis of Clinical Outcome Studies." *Applied Psychophysiology and Biofeedback* 27(1): 45.

2. Polak, A. Rosaura et al. (2015). "Breathing Biofeedback as an Adjunct to Exposure in Cognitive Behavioral Therapy Hastens the Reduction of PTSD Symptoms: A Pilot Study." *Applied Psychophysiology and Biofeedback* 40(1): 25–31. DOI: 10.1007/s10484-015-9268-y.

3. Dykema, R. (2006). *Yoga for Fitness and Wellness.* Belmont, CA:Thomson Learning.

4. Cramer, H. et al. (2016). "Prevalence, Patterns, and Predictors of Yoga Use: Results of a U.S. Nationally Representative Survey." *American Journal of Preventive Medicine* 50(2): 230–235. DOI: 10.1016/j.amepre.2015.07.037. Epub 2015 Oct 21.

5. Akhtar, P. et al. (2013). "Effects of Yoga on Functional Capacity and Well-being." *International Journal of Yoga* 6(1): 76–79. Available from: http://www.ijoy.org.in/text.asp?2013/6/1/76/105952.

6. Thirthali, J. et al. (2013). "Cortisol and Antidepressant Effects of Yoga." *Indian Journal of Psychiatry* 55(Suppl 3): S405–S408.

7. Pascoe, M. C. et al. (2015). "A Systematic Review of Randomised Control Trials on the Effects of Yoga on Stress Measures and Mood." *Journal of Psychiatric Research* 68: 270–282. DOI: 10.1016/j. jpsychires.2015.07.013. Epub 2015 Jul 13.

8. Shetty, P. et al. (2015). "Effect of Yoga on Autonomic Functions in Medical Students: A Pilot Study." *International Journal of Research in Medical Science* 3(5): 1046–1051.

9. Selvakumar, R. Effect of Selected Yogic Practices on Cardiovascular Endurance of College Students. http://tejas.tcarts.in/pdf/nov11_phyedu.pdf.

10. Kohn, M. et al. (2013). "Medical Yoga for Patients with Stress-related Symptoms and Diagnoses in Primary Health Care: A Randomized Controlled Trial." *Evidence-Based Complementary and Alternative Medicine* 2013: Article ID 215348. DOI: 10.1155/2013/215348. Epub 2013 Feb 26.

11. Monk-Turner, E. and Turner, C. (2010). "Does Yoga Shape Body, Mind and Spiritual Health and Happiness: Differences between Yoga Practitioners and College Students." *International Journal of Yoga* 3(2): 48–54. DOI: 10.4103/0973-6131.72630. PMID: 21170230.

12. Gong, H. et al. (2015). "Yoga for Prenatal Depression: a Systematic Review and Meta-analysis." *BMC Psychiatry* 15: 14. DOI: 10.1186/s12888-015-0393-1. Review. PMID: 25652267.

13. Kiecolt-Glaser, J. et al. (2010). "Stress, Inflammation, and Yoga Practice." *Psychosomatic Medicine* 72(2): 113–121. DOI: 10.1097/PSY.0b013e3181cb9377. Epub 2010 Jan 11.

14. Kumar, Shiv Basant et al. "Telomerase Activity and Cellular Aging Might Be Positively Modified by a Yoga-Based Lifestyle Intervention: A Case Report." *The Journal of Alternative and Complementary Medicine* 21(6): 370–372. DOI: 10.1089/acm.2014.0298. Epub 2015 May 12.

15. Kurwale, M. V., and Gadkari, J. V. (2014). "Effect of Yogic Training on Physiological Variables in Working Women." *Indian Journal of Physiology and Pharmacology* 58(3): 306–310.

16. Robert-McComb, J. J. et al. (2015). "The Effects of Mindfulness-Based Movement on Parameters of Stress." *International Journal of Yoga Therapy* 25(1): 79–88. DOI: 10.17761/1531-2054-25.1.79.

17. Jindani, Farah et al. (2015). "A Yoga Intervention for Posttraumatic Stress: A Preliminary Randomized Control Trial." *Evidence-Based Complementary and Alternative Medicine* 2015: Article ID 351746. DOI: 10.1155/2015/351746. Epub 2015 Aug 20.

18. Field, T. et al. (2013). "Tai chi/Yoga Reduces Prenatal Depression, Anxiety and Sleep Disturbances," *Complementary Therapies in Clinical Practice* 19(1): 6–10. DOI: 10.1016/j. ctcp.2012.10.001. Epub 2012 Nov 24.

19. Irwin, M. R., and Bower, J. E. (2016). "Mind- body Therapies and Control of Inflammatory Biology: A Descriptive Review." *Brain, Behavior, and Immunity* 51: 1–11. DOI: 10.1016/j. bbi.2015.06.012. Epub 2015 Jun 23.

20. Robins, J. L. et al. (2015) "The Effects of Tai Chi on Cardiovascular Risk in Women." *American Journal of Health Promotion.* DOI: 10.4278/ajhp.140618-QUAN-287. Epub 2015 August.

21. Wells, C. et al. (2012). "Defining Pilates Exercise: A Systematic Review." *Complementary Therapies in Medicine* 20(4): 253–262. DOI: 10.1016/j. ctim.2012.02.005. Epub 2012 Mar 13.

22. Wells, C. et al. (2014). "The Effectiveness of Pilates Exercise in People with Chronic Low Back Pain: A Systematic Review." PLOS ONE. 9(7): e100402. DOI: 10.1371/journal.pone.0100402. eCollection 2014.

23. Küçük, F., and Livanelioglu, A. (2015). "Impact of the Clinical Pilates Exercises and Verbal Education on Exercise Beliefs and Psychosocial Factors in Healthy Women." *Journal of Physical Therapy Science* 27(11): 3437–3443. DOI: 10.1589/jpts.27.3437. Epub 2015 Nov 30.

24. American Dance Therapy Association. http://www.adta.org/about_dmt.

25. Moore, C. (2006). "Dance/Movement Therapy in the Light of Trauma." In *Advances in Dance/Movement Therapy,* edited by S.C. Koch and I. Brauniger. Berlin: Logos Verlag. Pp. 104–115.

26. Leste, A., and Rust, J. (1990). "Effects of Dance on Anxiety." *American Journal of Dance Therapy* 12(1): 19–25.

Chapter 15

1. Clarke, T. C. et al. (2015). *Trends in the Use of Complementary Health Approaches among Adults.* National Health Statistics Report, no. 79 (February 10).

2. Navarro, V. J., et al. (2014). "Liver injury from herbals and dietary supplements in the U.S." *Drug-Induced Liver Injury Network Hepatology* 60(4): 1399–1408. DOI: 10.1002/hep.27317. Epub 2014 Aug 25.

3. Wang X. et al. (2015). "Creative Arts Program as an Intervention for PTSD: A Randomized Clinical Trial with Motor Vehicle Accident Survivors." *International Journal of Clinical and Experimental Medicine* 8(8): 13585–13591. eCollection 2015. PMCID: PMC4612983.

4. López-Teijón, M. et al. (2015). "Fetal Facial Expression in Response to Intravaginal Music Emission." *Ultrasound* 23(4): 216–223. DOI: 10.11771742271X15609367. Epub 2015 September 29.

5. Corrigall, Kathleen A., and Schellenberg, E.Glenn. (2015). "Music Cognition in Childhood." In *The Child as Musician: A Handbook of Musical Development, 2nd Edition*, edited by Gary E. McPherson. New York: Oxford University Press. 81.

6. Smith, J. C., and Joyce, C. A. (2004). "Mozart versus New Age Music: Relaxation States, Stress, and ABC Relaxation Therapy." *Journal of Music Therapy* 41(3): 215–224. DOI: 10.1093/jmt/41.3.192

7. Conrad, Claudius et al. (2007). "Overture for Growth Hormone: Requiem for Interleukin-6?" *Critical Care Medicine* 35(12): 2709-2713. DOI: 10.1097/01.CCM.0000291648.99043.B9.

8. Rahshenas, Nina et al. (2015). "Effect of Music Therapy on Stress: Is it Really Effective?" *International Journal of Emergency Mental Health and Human Resilience* 17: 192. DOI: 10.4172/1522-4821.1000192.

9. Salimpoor, Valorie N. et al. (2013). "Interactions between the Nucleus Accumbens and Auditory Cortices Predict Music Reward Value." *Science* 340(6129): 216-219. DOI: 10.1126/science.1231059.

10. Swaminathan, Swathi, and Schellenberg, E. Glenn. (2015). "Current Emotion Research in Music Psychology." *Emotion Review* 7(2): 189– 197. DOI: 10.1177/1754073914558282.

11. Bergland, C. (2012). "The Neuroscience of Music, Mindset, and Motivation: Simple Ways You Can Use Music to Create Changes in Mindset and Behavior." *Psychology Today*. https://www.psychologytoday.com/blog/the-athletes-way/201212/the-neuroscience-music-mindset-and-motivation

12. American Music Therapy Association. www.musictherapy.org

13. Chanda, Mona Lisa, and Levitin, Daniel J. (2013). "The Neurochemistry of Music." *Trends in Cognitive Sciences* 17(4): 179–193. DOI: 10.1016/j. tics.2013.02.007.

14. Gupta, Uma, and Gupta, B. S. (2014). "Psychophysiological Reactions to Music in Male Coronary Patients and Healthy Controls." *Psychology of Music* 43(5): 736–755. DOI: 10.1177/0305735614536754. Epub 2014 June 5.

15. Nilsson, Ulrica. (2009). "The Effect of Music Intervention in Stress Response to Cardiac Surgery in a Randomized Clinical Trial." *Heart & Lung: The Journal of Acute and Critical Care* 38(3): 201–207. DOI: http://dx.doi.org/10.1016/j. hrtlng.2008.07.008.

16. Särkämö, Teppo et al. (2014). "Cognitive, Emotional, and Social Benefits of Regular Musical Activities in Early Dementia: Randomized Controlled Study." *The Gerontologist* 54(4): 634–650. DOI: 10.1093/geront/gnt100. Epub 2013 Sep 5.

17. Longhi, Elena, Pickett, Nick, and Hargreaves, David J. (2015). "Wellbeing and Hospitalized Children: Can Music Help?." *Psychology of Music* 43(2): 188–196. DOI: 10.1177/0305735613499781. Epub 2013 August 22.

18. Onieva-Zafra, María Dolores et al. (2013). "Effect of Music as Nursing Intervention for People Diagnosed with Fibromyalgia." *Pain Management Nursing* 14(2): e39–e46. DOI: 10.1016/j.pmn.2010.09.004.

19. Conrad, Claudius.

20. Ludke, Karen M., Ferreira, Fernanda, and Overy, Katie. (2014). "Singing Can Facilitate Foreign Language Learning." *Memory & Cognition* 42(1): 41–52. DOI: 10.3758/s13421-013-0342-5.

21. Karageorghis, C. I., Mouzourides, D. A., Priest, D. L., Sasso, T. A., Morrish, D. J., & Walley, C. L. (2009). "Psychophysical and Ergogenic Effects of Synchronous Music During Treadmill Walking." *Journal of Sport & Exercise Psychology* 31(1): 18–36. http://bura.brunel.ac.uk/handle/2438/3117.

22. Beck, B. D. et al. (2015). "Coping with Work-Related Stress through Guided Imagery and Music (GIM): Randomized Controlled Trial." *Journal of Music Therapy* 52(3): 323–352. DOI: 10.1093/jmt/thv011

Index

A

ABC relaxation, 244–245
ABCDE approach, 47
Abdomen stage of autogenics, 267
Abdominal breathing, 233–235
Abusive relationships, 116–117
Academic entitlement, 69
Academic procrastination, 86
Academic stress
    introduction to, 68–69
    study styles, 69–71
    test stress, 71–73
Acculturation, 67
Acculturative stress, 67
Acetylcholine, 241
Acquaintance rape, 118–119
ACTH (adrenocorticotropic
        hormone), 24
Action stage, 131
Activating events, 47
Active listening, 105–106
Active meditation, 258
Active relaxation, 241
Acupressure, 284–285
Acupressure massage, 286
Acupuncture, 284–285, 286
Acute academic stressor, 69
Acute stress disorder, 53
Acute stressors, 6
    cardiovascular system, effects
        of on, 29
    gastrointestinal system, effects
        of on, 30
    immune system, effects of on, 28
    reproductive system, effects
        of on, 33
    skin, effects of on, 32
Adaptive behaviors, 140
Adjustment disorder, 52
Adrenal cortex, 23
Adrenal glands, 23, 24, 26
Adrenal medulla, 23
Adrenocorticotropic hormone
        (ACTH), 24
Aerobic exercise, 170, 171, 172
Affiliative humor, 208
Affirmations, 50
African Americans, 6
Aggressive communication, 107
Aggressive humor, 208

Aging, 34–35
Agreeable but assertive, 106–107
Alarm, 9–10
Alcohol, 74, 157–159, 173, 181
Alcohol audit, 158
All-or-nothing thinking, 47
Allostatic load, 26
Alpha waves, 255
Alternate-nostril breathing, 235–236
Alternative medical systems, 284–285
Alternative medicine, 283. See also
        Complementary and alternative
        medicine
Altruism, 104, 198, 199–200
Altruistic egotism, 104
Alveoli, 233, 234
AmEd, 181
American Art Therapy Association,
        290
American College Health Association
        (ACHA), 2, 63, 158, 168, 171
American Dance Therapy Association,
        278
American Music Therapy Association,
        291
American Psychological Association
        (APA), 5, 201
Amygdala, 23, 41, 42, 65
Anger, 155–156
Animal-assisted therapy, 289
Annual percentage rate (APR), 94
Anorexia nervosa, 187
Anticipatory academic stressor, 69
Anxiety, 51, 148
Apology letters, 196
Apple-shaped bodies, 183–184
Appreciation quotient, 153
Apps
    for biofeedback, 268
    financial management, 95
    for meditation, 254–255
    for price checking, 92
    social media, 109, 112
APR (annual percentage rate), 94
Aristotle, 195
Aromatherapy, 289
Art therapy, 285, 290–291
Asana, 269
Ashtanga yoga, 269
Assertive communication, 106–107

Assertiveness, 106–107
Attention, 245, 250
Attributions, 44–45
Autogenics, 265–267
Automatic stress responses, 10
Autonomic nervous system, 23
Autonomy, 151
Ayurveda, 285

B

Baby Boomers, 6
Backache, 31, 32
Balance, 200–201
Banking basics, 93–94
Bedtime breathing, 237
Behavior, 245
Behavior management, 140
Beliefs, 47
Belly breathing. See Diaphragmatic
        breathing
Belly fat, 30
Belongingness, 103
Benson, Herbert, 244
Big dreams, 133
Bills, 91
Binge drinking, 159
Binge eating, 186–187
Binge-eating disorder, 187
Biofeedback, 267–268, 285
Biologically-based therapies, 284,
        287–288
Biology of courage, 12
Biology of stress, 22–24
Biracial, 25
Body and stress
    aging, 34–35
    biology of stress, 22–24
    cancer, 33–34
    cardiovascular system, 28–29
    effects of stress on, 26
    excess stress, toll of, 26–27
    gastrointestinal system, 29–30
    immune system, 27–28
    introduction to, 21–22
    muscles, 30–32
    relaxing, 35
    reproductive system, 33
    skin, 32–33
    susceptibility and, 24–26
Body composition, 169

Body image, 181–183
Body language, 105, 218, 220
Bracing, 30
Brain, 41–43, 168–169
Breaking up, 119
Breathing
    alternate-nostril, 235–236
    controlled, 236
    counting or bedtime breathing, 237
    diaphragmatic breathing, 234–235
    diaphragmatic breathing with
        pelvic tilt, 236–237
    introduction to, 233
    introductory exercises, 235–238
    nasal switching, 235–236
    for pain relief, 237
    in tai chi, 277
    understanding, 233–234
    visualization, 238
    what you need to know, 235
    yogic, 237–238
Bruxism, 31
Buddhism, 255, 258
Budget, 91–92
Bulimia nervosa, 187
Bureau of Justice Statistics, 75
Burned-out workers, 219
Burnout
    causes of, 222
    early signs of, 223
    introduction to, 221–222
    stages of, 222–223
    vs. stress, 222

C

Caffeine, 180, 181
Caffeine intoxication, 180
Callousness, 222
Calm app, 254
CAM (complementary and alternative
    medicine)
    alternative medical systems,
        284–285
    biologically-based therapies,
        287–288
    categories of, 284
    creative or expressive therapies,
        289–292
    energy therapies, 284, 288
    manipulative and body-based
        methods, 284, 285–287
    mind-body medicine, 284, 285
    other techniques, 288–289
    for stress management, 284–289
    understanding, 283–284

Cancer, 33–34
Capillaries, 233
Carbohydrates, 177
Cardiorespiratory fitness, 169
Cardiovascular disease (CVD), 29
Cardiovascular health, 172
Cardiovascular system, 22, 26,
    28–29
Career selection, 216
Catastrophizing, 47
Cathartic writing, 207
CBT (cognitive behavioral therapy)
    cognitive restructuring or
        reframing, 46
    Rational Emotive Behavior Therapy
        (REBT), 46–47
    thinking traps, 47–48
    thought awareness, 45
    worrying, 48
Cell phones, 74, 228
Centering, 245
Chace, Marian, 279
Chair massage, 286
Challenge, 203
Challenge response model, 11
Change. See Personal change
Checking accounts, 91
Chest breathing, 233–234
Chi Kung, 288
Christianity, 255
Chronic insomnia, 174
Chronic loneliness, 108
Chronic procrastination, 86
Chronic stressors, 7
    cardiovascular system, effects
        of on, 29
    gastrointestinal system, effects
        of on, 30
    immune system, effects of on, 28
    mental health, effects of on, 50
    reproductive system, effects of
        on, 33
    skin, effects of on, 32
Climate change, 225
Codependency, 117
Co-Dependents Anonymous, 117
Cognition, 46, 245
Cognitive behavioral therapy (CBT)
    cognitive restructuring or
        reframing, 46
    Rational Emotive Behavior Therapy
        (REBT), 46–47
    thinking traps, 47–48
    thought awareness, 45
    worrying, 48

Cognitive Reappraisal Model. See
    Transactional or Cognitive-
    Reappraisal Model
Cognitive restructuring or reframing, 46
Cognitive therapy, 174
Cohabitation, 114
Collapse, as a stage of burnout, 222
Coming out, 111
Commitment, 203
Communication, 104–106
Commuting students, time
    management for, 88–89
Comparing and despairing, 47
Compassion, 198–199
Compensating, 47
Complementary and alternative
    medicine (CAM)
    alternative medical systems,
        284–285
    biologically-based therapies, 284,
        287–288
    categories of, 284
    creative or expressive therapies,
        289–292
    energy therapies, 284, 288
    manipulative and body-based
        methods, 284, 285–287
    mind-body medicine, 284, 285
    other techniques, 288–289
    for stress management, 284–289
    understanding, 283–284
Complementary medicine, 283
Compromise, 219
Compulsive overeating, 186
Computer-mediated communication,
    109–110
Concentration, 250, 257–258
Conditional tense, 136
Conflict resolution, 115–116
Confucianism, 255
Confucius, 195
Conscientiousness, 150
Consequences, 47
Consistency, 71
Contemplation stage, 130
Control, 203
Controlled breathing, 236
Coping muscles, 161
Coping stage, 13
Corticotropin-releasing hormone
    (CRH), 24
Cortisol, 23, 27, 29, 30, 34, 169
Coué, Émile, 50
Counting breathing, 237
Courage, biology of, 12

Creative or expressive therapies, 289–292
Credit cards, 94–95
Credit reporting agencies, 96
Credit score, 93
CRH (corticotropin-releasing hormone), 24
Crime, 75
Crisis, 222
Culture, 159
Curfews, 175
CVD (cardiovascular disease), 29
Cyberabuse, 110
Cyberbullying, 110
Cyberstalking, 110
Cynicism, 222
Czikszentmihalyi, Mihaly, 201

D
Daily hassles, 7
Dalai Lama, 195
Dance, 278–279
Date rape, 118–119
Day planning, 84
Debit cards, 94–95
Debt relief, 95–96
Decibels, 227
Deep breathing, 24
Deep muscle relaxation, 242–244
Deep tissue massage, 286
Defensive drinking, 159
Delegation, 219
Demeaning treatment, 220
Depression, 51–52, 55, 148
Description, 252
Destination goals, 133
Dharana Dhyana, 269
Diabetes, 27
Dialogue journaling, 207
Diaphragm, 233
Diaphragmatic breathing, 233–235
Diaphragmatic breathing with pelvic tilt, 236–237
Diathesis stress model, 24
Dietary Guidelines, 177–178
Digestive disorders, 30
Digital distress, 110
Digital financial management, 95
Digital natives, 63
Disability, 74–75
Discrimination, 67–68
Disorder, 82
Disordered eating, 186–187
Disputing irrational beliefs, 47
Distress, 4

Divorce, 119–120
Dopamine, 12, 43
Doubt, 222
Downward spiral, 148
Drugs, 74, 159–160
Dysfunctional relationships
  abusive relationships on campus, 117
  codependency and enabling, 117
  emotional and verbal abuse, 116–117
  intimate partner violence, 118
  recognizing, 116
  sexual victimization, 118–119
Dyspareunia, 33

E
Eating disorders, 187
Ecosystem, 224
Edison, Thomas, 204
Effects of challenging irrational beliefs, 47
Electroencephalogram (EEG), 267
Electromagnetic fields, 288
Electromyelogram (EMG), 267
Emerging adulthood, 65
Emotional abuse, 116–117
Emotional health, 146
Emotional intelligence, 146–148, 219–220
Emotional quotient (EQ), 146–147
Emotional reasoning, 47
Emotional spirals, 148–149
Emotion-based coping, 13
Empathy, 198
Enabling, 117
Endocrine system, 22
Endorphins, 169
Energy drinks, 180–181
Energy therapies, 284, 288
Engaged workers, 218
Engagement, 201
Entering freshman students, 64, 66
Enthusiastic workers, 218
Environmental health, 5
Environmental stress, 224
  cell phones, 228
  climate change, 225
  noise, 226–227
  pollution, 225–226
Epinephrine, 23, 24, 27
Episodic acute stressors, 6
  cardiovascular system, effects of on, 29

gastrointestinal system, effects of on, 30
  immune system, effects of on, 28
  mental health, effects of on, 50
  reproductive system, effects of on, 33
  skin, effects of on, 32
EQ (emotional quotient), 146–147
Escape routes, 204
Essential nutrients, 177
Essential oils, 289
Ethnicity, 25. *See also* Race and ethnicity
Eudaimonic happiness, 152
Eustress, 4, 109–110
Excess weight, 184
Exclusive, concentration, or focused meditation, 257–258
Excoriation Disorder, 32
Exercise
  and the brain, 168–169
  definition of, 169
  fitness fundamentals, 169–171
  F.I.T.T. Formula (for frequency, intensity, time, and type), 171
  guidelines for, 170–171
  health benefits of, 170
  options for, 172
  in stress-resistant lifestyle, 187
Exhaustion, 9, 10, 222
Expectations, 44
Expressive writing, 205–206
External locus of control, 43
Extraversion, 150
Eye contact, 105

F
Facebook, 109, 182, 215
Failure, 222
Family history, 25–26
Family stress, 107
Family ties, 107
Fast naps, 176
"Fat talk," 182–183
Fatigued workers, 219
Fats, 177
FCC (Federal Communications Commission), 228
FDA (Food and Drug Administration), 228
Fear, 154–155, 204
Federal Communications Commission (FCC), 228
Federal Trade Commission (FTC), 96
Fight or flight response, 10

Financial aid, 91
Financial goals, 92
Financial homeostasis, 90–92
Financial records, 90–91
First Generation Student Union, 66
First-generation college students, 64, 66
Fitness fundamentals, 169–171
F.I.T.T. Formula (frequency, intensity, time, and type), 171
Fixed interest rate, 94
Flexibility, 169, 172
Flow, 201
Focus, 70, 257–258
Food and Drug Administration (FDA), 228
Forehead stage of autogenics, 267
Forgiveness, 196–197
Freezing, 10
Freshman students, 64, 66
Friendship, 107–108, 116
Frugal living, 92–93
FTC (Federal Trade Commission), 96
FTC Identity Theft Affidavit, 96

G

Galvanic Skin Response (GSR), 267
Gambling, 157
GAS (general adaptation syndrome), 9–10
Gastroesophageal reflux disease (GERD), 30
Gastrointestinal system, 22, 26, 29–30
Gender, 24–25, 64, 106, 118
Gender identity
    coming out, 111
    emotional intelligence, 148
    homophobia, 111–112
    hooking up, 112–114
    online dating, 112
    partnerships, 112
General adaptation syndrome (GAS), 9–10
Genetics, 25
Gen-Xers, 6
GERD (gastroesophageal reflux disease), 30
Gestures, 105
Getting along with others, 104–107
"Gloomy glasses," 47
Gratitude, cultivating, 151–152
Greenhouse effect, 225
GSR (Galvanic Skin Response), 267
Guided imagery, 238, 285
    benefits of, 239–240
    introductory exercises, 240–241

understanding, 239
    what you need to know, 240
Gut feelings, 140

H

Habit reversal, 186–187
Happiness, pursuing, 152–153
Hardiness, 203
Hatha yoga, 269
Headaches, 31
Headspace app, 254
Health, 5
Health and performance, 13–14
Health habits. *See* Stress-resistant health habits
Healthy eating
    essential nutrients, 177
    guidelines for, 177–178
    liquid stress, 178–181
    mindful eating, 178
    nutrients, good sources of, 179
    nutrition and mood, 178
    in stress-resistant lifestyle, 188
Heart stage of autogenics, 267
Heaviness stage of autogenics, 266
Hedonic happiness, 152
Helper's high, 199
Helplessness, 222
Herbal medicine, 287
Heterosexual, 111
Hidden Minority Council, 66
Hinduism, 255
Hippocampus, 41, 42, 169
Hippocrates, 289
Hispanics, 6
Holistic methods, 283
Holistic perspective, 5
Holmes, Thomas, 7
Holmes-Rahe Stress Inventory, 7–8
Homeopathy, 285
Homeostasis, 9
Homophobia, 111–112
Homosexual, 111
Hooking up, 112–114
Hookup, 112–114
"Hookup culture," 113
Hopefulness, 153, 200–201
Hormonal stress response systems, 168
Human social genomics, 25
Humor, 207–209
Humor deniers, 208
Humor endorsers, 208
Humor enhancers, 208
Hunger signals, 185

Hydration, 178–181
Hydrotherapy, 288–289
Hyperventilation, 234
Hypnosis, 259
Hypnotic suggestion, 260, 266
Hypothalamic-pituitary-adrenal system, 276
Hypothalamus, 23, 24, 41, 42

I

"I" statements, 107
Identity formation, 25
Identity theft, 96
Illness and disability, 74–75
Immune system, 26, 27–28, 172, 208
Inactivity, 168, 171
Inclusive meditation, 258
Independence, 151
Inflammation, 168
Insomnia, 174
Inspirational quotations, 196
Insulin, 169
Insurance, 91
Integrative or integrated medicine, 284
Intellectual health, 5
Interest rates, 94–95
Internal locus of control, 43
Internet use, 74
Internships, 215
Intimacy, 114
Intimate partner violence, 118
Intimate relationships, 114–116
Introductory interest rate, 95
Intuitive eating, 185
Investments, 91
Islam, 255

J

Job insecurity, 223
Job interviews, 217–218
Job loss, 223–224
Jobsearch.about.com, 216
Journaling, 205–207
Judaism, 255

K

Karma, 197
King, Martin Luther, Jr., 195
Koans, 258
Kushner, Harold, 195

L

Laughter therapy, 207–209
Lazarus, Richard, 12
Learning and memory, 172

Learning disabilities, 75
Letters not sent, 207
LGBTQQI (lesbian, gay, bisexual, transgendered, queer/questioning, and intersex), 111
Life balance, 193, 200–201
Life change events, 7
"Lifestyle orientation," 151–152
LinkedIn, 215
Liver injury, 287–288
Loan and credit records, 91
Locus coeruleus, 42
Locus of control, 43
Loneliness, 108
Long work hours, 221
Long-term goals, 133, 134
Loophole language, 135
Lovingkindness Meditation, 258
Low-intensity workouts, 170
Lyubomirsky, Sonja, 152

M

Magnets, 288
Maintenance stage, 131
Mandala, 257
Manipulative and body-based methods, 284, 285–287
Mantra meditation, 257, 258
Mantras, 257
Marriage, 114–115
Maslow, Abraham, 151
Massage, 285–287
MBCT (Mindfulness-Based Cognitive Therapy), 252
MBSR (Mindfulness-Based Stress Reduction), 56, 252
McGonigal, Kelly, 14, 21
Meaning, tools for finding
    expressive writing and journaling, 205–207
    humor or laughter therapy, 207–209
Medical or sports massage, 286
Meditation
    active, 258
    apps and videos, 254–255
    benefits of, 255–256
    exclusive, concentration, or focused, 257–258
    exercise, 258–259
    introduction to, 255
    mind-body medicine, 285
    open or inclusive, 258
    practices of, 257–258
    religion and, 194, 195

understanding, 255
what you need to know, 256–257
Men
    body image, 182, 183
    communication, 106
    effects of stress on, 24–25
    emotional intelligence, 148
    stress on campus, 64
Mental focusing devices, 85
Mental health, 50
    acute stress disorder, 53
    adjustment disorder, 52
    anxiety, 51
    on campus, 51
    depression, 51–52
    intimate partner violence, 118
    post-traumatic stress disorder (PTSD), 53–54
    psychological approaches, 146
    suicide, 54–55
Mental rehearsal, 239–240
Meridians, 284–285
Metabolic fitness, 169
Metabolism, 172
Microaggressions, 68
Microassaults, 68
Microinsults, 68
Microinvalidations, 68
Micro-nap, 176
Millennials, 6
Mind and stress
    brain and, 41–43
    cognitive behavioral therapy (CBT), 45–48
    harnessing the powers of your mind, 55–56
    introduction to, 40–41
    mental health, 50–52
    perception-based theories of stress, 43–45
    psychological health, 41
    stress-related mental disorders, 52–54
    talking back to stress, 48–50
Mind-body medicine, 284, 285
Mindful breathing, 253
Mindful eating, 178
Mindful walking, 253
Mindfulness, 56
    apps and videos, 254–255
    benefits of, 251
    on the bus or subway, 253–254
    introduction to, 249–250
    mindful breathing, 253
    mindful walking, 253

practices of, 253–255
skills, 252
understanding, 250–251
what you need to know, 251–252
Mindfulness-Based Cognitive Therapy (MBCT), 252
Mindfulness-Based Stress Reduction (MBSR), 56, 252
Mindlessness, 252
Mind-reading, 47
Mindset, 15
Minerals, 177
Mini-nap, 176
Minority stress, 66–67
Minority students, 66–68
Molehills into mountains, 47
Money
    budget, 91–92
    financial goas, 92
    financial homeostasis, 90–92
    financial stress, 90
    frugal living, 92–93
    introduction to, 80–82
    management of, 89–93
    organizing basics, 90–91
    personal finances, 93–96
Mood, 151, 172, 178
Mood control, 156
Moses, Edwin, 132
Motivation for change, 133–134
Movement therapy, 278–279
Mozart, 291
Multiracial, 25
Multitasking, 87–88
Muscle dysmorphia, 182–183
Muscles, 26, 27, 30–32
Muscular strength, 169, 171
Musculoskeletal system, 22
Music therapy, 285, 291–292
The Myths of Happiness (Lyubomirsky), 152

N

Nadam, 258
Naikan, 197
Nano-nap, 176
Napping, 176. *See also* Sleep
Nasal switching breathing, 235–236
National Center for Complementary and Alternative Medicine (NCCAM), 255, 284
National College Health Assessment, 158
National Foundation for Credit Counseling, 96

National Institute of Alcohol Abuse and Alcoholism, 159
National Student Financial Wellness Study, 89
Nature, 195
Naturopathy, 285
NCCAM (National Center for Complementary and Alternative Medicine), 255, 284
Negative feelings, 154–156
Negatives, 49
Nervous system, 22
Networking, 217
Neuroplasticity, 43
Neustress, 4
Night life, 173
9-5 workers, 219
Niyama, 269
Noise, 226–227
Nonjudgmental attitude, 250, 252
Nontraditional-age students, 65–66
Nonverbal communication, 104–105
Norepinephrine, 23
Now imperative, 88
Nutrients, 177, 179
Nutrition and mood, 178

O

OA (Overeaters Anonymous), 186
Observation, 252
Occupational health, 5
Occupational stress
    burnout, 221–222
    career selection, 216
    causes of, 220–221
    coping with, 221
    definition of, 220
    emotional intelligence, 219–220
    finding a job, 216–218
    interview stress, 218
    introduction to, 214–215
    job interview, preparation for, 217–218
    job loss and unemployment, 223–224
    networking, 217
    preparing for the future, 215–216
    resume building, 215–216
    time and task management, 219
    types of workers, 218–219
    work and school balance, 215
    work life, 218–220
Occupational stressors, 9
Omvana app, 254
Online dating, 112

Online eustress, 109–110
Open meditation, 258
Optimism, 153
Order, establishing, 83–84
Ornish, Dean, 34, 195
Over-commitment, 219
Overeaters Anonymous (OA), 186
Overexertion, 169
Over-generalizing, 47
Oxytocin, 12, 24

P

Pain relief, breathing for, 237
Parasympathetic nervous system, 23, 24
Participation, 252
Partnerships, 112
Passive relaxation, 241
Passive voice, 136
Pear-shaped bodies, 184
Perception, 3
Perception-based theories of stress
    attributions, 44–45
    expectations, 44
    locus of control, 43
    self-efficacy, 43–44
Persistence, 70
Personal change
    action stage, 131
    behavior management, 140
    best time for, 131–132
    big dreams, 133
    boosting your power for, 136–139
    changing for good, 139–140
    choosing, 127–129
    contemplation stage, 130
    destination goal, 133
    getting in your own way, 138–139
    inevitability, 137–138
    introduction to, 126–127
    language of, 135–136
    long-term goals, 133, 134
    maintenance stage, 131
    motivation for, 133–134
    postponing, 131–132
    precontemplation stage, 129–130
    preparation stage, 130–131
    relapse, 131
    short-term goals, 134
    stages of, 129–133
    stressfulness of, 127
    visualization, 132–133
    what can be changed and what cannot, 128–129
    what you need to know, 127–128
Personal environment

establishing order, 83–84
    introduction to, 80–82
    management of, 82–84
    rules of order, 82
    study spaces, 82–83
Personal finances
    banking basics, 93–94
    credit score, 93
    debit and credit cards, 94–95
    debt relief, 95–96
    digital financial management, 95
    private information, protecting, 96
Personality traits, recognizing, 150
Personalizing, 47
Pet therapy, 289
Pets, 103–104
Pew Research Center, 109
Physical activity
    definition of, 169
    exercise and the brain, 168–169
    fitness fundamentals, 169–171
    F.I.T.T. Formula (for frequency, intensity, time, and type), 171
    guidelines for, 170–171
    health benefits of, 170
    options for, 172
    in stress-resistant lifestyle, 187
Physical Activity Guidelines for Americans, 170–171
Physical fitness, 169
Physical health, 5
Physical techniques, 264
    autogenics, 265–267
    biofeedback, 267–268, 285
    dance or movement therapy, 278–279
    Pilates, 278
    tai chi, 276–278, 285
    yoga, 268–276, 285
Physical violence, 118
Pilates, 278
Pilates, Joseph, 278
Pituitary gland, 23, 24, 42
PMR (progressive muscle relaxation), 234, 242–244
PMS (premenstrual syndrome), 33
Pollution, 225–226
Positive psychiatry, 148–153
Positive psychology, 148–153, 200
Positive spirals, 148
Positive traits, 200
Positivity
    boosting self-esteem, 149–150
    emotional spirals, 148–149
    gratitude, cultivating, 151–152

happiness, pursuing, 152–153
meeting needs, 151
optimistic and hopeful, becoming, 153
personality traits, recognizing, 150
self-compassion, 150–151
"undoing" stress, 149
Post-traumatic stress disorder (PTSD), 53–54, 268, 279
Posture, 105
Poverty, 9, 26
Power napping, 176
Powerlessness, sense of, 220
Practice, 85, 140
Pranayama, 237–238, 269
Pratyhara, 269
Prayer, 194, 195
Precontemplation stage, 129–130
Prefrontal cortex, 41, 42
Prejudice, 66–68
Premenstrual syndrome (PMS), 33
Preparation stage, 130–131
Primary appraisal, 12
Priorities, 140, 219
Privacy, 110
Private information, protecting, 96
Problem-based coping, 13
Prochaska, James, 129
Procrastination, 86
Progressive muscle relaxation (PMR), 234, 242–244
Protein, 177
Protestantism, 255
Psoriasis, 32
Psychological approaches, 144
coping muscles, 161
emotional health and, 146
emotional intelligence, 146–148
introduction to, 145
negative feelings, detoxifying, 154–156
positivity, 148–153
risky behaviors, 157–161
Psychological Balance Inventory, 40
Psychological health, 5, 41
Psychological violence, 118
Psychoneuroimmunology, 27
Psychosocial stressors, 9

Q
Qigong, 288

R
Race and ethnicity, 25, 66–68, 111–112
Racism, 67–68

Rahe, Richard, 7
Rape, 118–119
Rational Emotive Behavior Therapy (REBT), 46–47
Raynaud's disease, 267, 268
Real talk, 135–136
Real time, 86–87
Reappraisal, 13
REBT (Rational Emotive Behavior Therapy), 46–47
Receipts, 91
Reciprocal golden rule, 76
Reflective journaling, 207
Reflective listening, 105–106
Refocus, 6
Rehearsal, 85
Reiki, 288
Rejection, 119
Relapse, 131
Relapse rehearsals, 205
"Relationship addiction," 117
Relationship management, 220
Relationships
dysfunctional, 116–119
ending, 119–120
forming, 107–109
friendship, 107–108, 116
improving, 120
intimate, 114–116
introduction to, 102–103
life balance, 200
loneliness, 108
sexual and romantic, 110–114
shyness, 108
social anxiety, 108–109
Relaxation
ABC relaxation, 244–245
benefits of, 241–242
progressive muscle relaxation, 242–244
understanding, 241
what you need to know, 242–244
Relaxation response, 244
Relaxation therapy, 174
Relaxed workers, 219
Relaxing, 35
Religion, 194, 195
Religiosity, 194
Religiousness, 194
Repetition, 71
Reproductive system, 22, 26, 33
Resilience, 201
alternate plans, 204–205
blocking your escape routes, 204
characteristics of, 202

coping with ups and downs, 209
dealing with setbacks, 203–204
introduction to, 193
lessons from resilient people, 202–203
no failure to fear, 204
relapse rehearsals, 205
Resistance, 9, 10
Resistance exercise, 171, 172
Respiration stage of autogenics, 267
Respiratory system, 22
Resume building, 215–216
ResumeHelp.Com, 216
Resumes, 216
Reverse anorexia, 182–183
Risky behaviors, 74
alcohol use, 74, 157–159, 173, 181
drugs, 74, 159–160
gambling, 157
tobacco, 160–161
Romantic relationships, 110–114
Rotter, Julian, 43
Routines, 85
Rules of order, 82
Rumination, 29, 48
Rutgers University, 109

S
Samadhi, 269
Same-sex marriages, 115
SAR (specific absorption rate), 228
Sarno, John, 31
Savings, 91
Schedule of Recent Experiences (SRE), 7–8
Schultz, Johannes, 266
Secondary appraisal, 12
Sedentary living, 168
Self-actualization, 151
Self-awareness, 220
Self-compassion, 150–151
Self-defeating humor, 208
Self-disclosure, 110
Self-efficacy, 43–44, 90
Self-enhancing humor, 208
Self-esteem, 149–150
Self-hypnosis, 259–260
Self-knowledge, 206
Self-management, 220
Self-reflection, 197
Self-soothing, 32
Self-talk, 49
Selye, Hans, 3, 4, 9–10
Serotonin, 12
Sexting, 110

Sexual and romantic relationships, 110–114
Sexual coercion, 118
Sexual orientation, 111
Sexual relationships, 110–114
Sexual response, 33
Sexual risk taking, 118
Sexual victimization, 118–119
Sexual violence, 118
Shame, 222
Shiatsu massage, 284, 286
Short-term goals, 134
Shoulds, 47
Shyness, 108
Single-mindedness, 252
Skeletal muscles, 30
Skin, 26, 32–33
Skin Picking Disorder (SPD), 32
Sleep. *See also* Napping
    amount needed, 173–174
    curfews, 175
    habits for getting enough, 174–176
    sleep environment, 175
    sleep ritual, 176
    sleeplessness on campus, 173
    stress, toll of, 171–173
    stress and, 171–176
    stress-induced insomnia, 174
    in stress-resistant lifestyle, 187–188
    student night life, 173
    worrying, 175–176
Sleep disturbances, 173
Sleep environment, 175
Sleep restriction therapy, 174
Sleep ritual, 176
Smart phone use, 74
Social anxiety, 108–109
Social anxiety disorder, 108–109
Social distractions, 70
Social health, 5
    definition of, 103
    getting along with others, 104–107
    introduction to, 102–103
    modern technology, 109–110
    support and, 103–104
Social intelligence, 104
Social isolation, 108
Social media, 109
Social physique anxiety, 182–183
Social Readjustment Rating Scale, 8
Social support, 9, 103–104
Socioeconomic status, 9
Soft drinks, 179–180
Soft language, 135
Soto Zen meditation, 257

SPD (Skin Picking Disorder), 32
Specific absorption rate (SAR), 228
Spiritual health, 5, 194
Spiritual intelligence, 194
Spirituality
    enriching your spiritual life, 194–195
    forgiveness, 196–197
    introduction to, 193
    karma, 197
    Naikan, 197
    prayer, 195
    spiritual health, 194
    spiritual intelligence, 194
    values, 197–200
SRE (Schedule of Recent Experiences), 7–8
Stand and defend reaction, 12
Stereotypes, 67–68
Stimulus control therapy, 174
Stranger rape, 119
Stream-of-consciousness journaling, 206
Strength training, 171, 172
Stress
    in America, 5–6
    biology of, 22–24
    bodily responses to, 10–13
    vs. burnout, 222
    common stressors, 7–9
    definition of, 3–4
    dimensions of health and, 5
    general adaptation syndrome, 9–10
    good, bad and neutral, 4
    health and performance, 13–14
    introduction to, 2–3
    optimal level of, 13–14
    rethinking, 14–16
    stressors, types of, 6–7
    toll of, 171–173
    "undoing," 149
Stress eating, 186
Stress fat, 183–184
Stress in America survey, 5
Stress mindsets, 15
Stress on campus, 61
    academic stress, 68–73
    common stressors, 73–75
    coping with, 76
    introduction to, 62–63
    students under stress, 63–68
"Stress overload," 220–221
Stress paradox, 14
Stress response, 22–24
Stress signals, 105

Stressors
    common, 7–9
    definition of, 3
    types of, 4, 6–7
Stress-related mental disorders
    acute stress disorder, 53
    adjustment disorder, 52
    post-traumatic stress disorder (PTSD), 53–54, 268, 279
    suicide, 54–55
Stress-resistant health habits
    body image and stress, 181–183
    disordered eating, 186–187
    healthy eating, 177–181
    introduction to, 167
    naps, 176
    physical activity and exercise, 168–171
    sleep, 171–176
    stress-resistant lifestyle, 187–188
    weight and stress, 183–185
Stress-resistant lifestyle, 187–188
Student loans, 90
Student night life, 173
Student Stress Scale, 62
Students under stress
    under age 25, 65
    entering freshman and first-generation students, 66
    gender differences, 64
    minority students, 66–68
    nontraditional-age students, 65–66
    statistical profile, 63
    stress levels, 64
Study skills, 70–71
Study spaces, 82–83
Study styles, 69–71
Submission, 10–11
Substance use and abuse, 118
Suicide, 54–55
Sun salutations, 275
Susceptibility, 24–26
Swedish massage, 285–286
Sympathetic nervous system, 23, 276
Synapses, 42–43

T

Tai chi, 276–278, 285
Taoism, 255, 277
Task management, 219
Taxes, 91
Technostress, 5
Telomeres, 34–35

Temperature, 267
Temporomandibular disorder (TMD), 30, 31
Tend-and-befriend, 12
Tension myositis syndrome (TMS), 31
Test anxiety, 69
Test preparation strategies, 72
Test taking strategies, 72–73
Therapeutic humor, 208
Thinking traps, 47–48
Third-person writing, 207
Thoracic breathing, 233–234
Thought awareness, 45
3-day time diary, 81
Thriving, 15–16
Tibetan Buddhism, 56, 250
Time
  introduction to, 80–82
  living in real time, 86–87
  management of, 84–89
  management of for commuting and working students, 88–89
  multitasking, 87–88
  now imperative, 88
  procrastination, 86
  taking time for yourself, 85–86
  visualization of, 84–85
Time diary, 81
Time management, 219
Time off from work, 219
Tinnitus, 227
TM (transcendental meditation), 244, 257
TMD (temporomandibular disorder), 30, 31
TMS (tension myositis syndrome), 31
Tobacco, 160–161
To-do lists, 219
Total body massage, 285–286
Traditional Chinese medicine, 284, 288

Transactional or Cognitive-Reappraisal Model, 12–13
Transcendental meditation (TM), 244, 257
Transferable skills, 216
Transgender, 111
"Transtheoretical" model, 129
Trauma, 9
Trichotillomania, 32
Triggering events, 140
Twitter, 215
Type 2 diabetes, 27

U
Ulcers, 30
Underexertion, 169
Unemployment, 223–224
The Upside of Stress (McGonigal), 14, 21
U.S. Department of Agriculture (USDA), 177
U.S. Department of Health and Human Services, 170–171

V
Vaginismus, 33
Values, 151, 197
  altruism, 199–200
  clarifying, 198
  compassion, 198–199
Variable interest rate, 94–95
Verbal abuse, 116–117
Violence and crime, 75
Visceral fat, 30
Visual mantras, 257
Visualization, 132–133, 196–197, 238–241, 266
Visualization breathing, 238
Vitamins, 177
Vogt, Oskar, 266
Volunteering, 215

W
Waist shape, 183
Walking meditation, 258–259
Warmth stage of autogenics, 267
Warranties, 91
Water, 177. See also Hydration
Weight, 183–185
Weight gain, 30
Willpower, 137
Women
  body image, 181–183
  communication, 106
  effects of stress on, 24–25
  emotional intelligence, 148
  experience of stress, 6
  stress on campus, 64
Workaholics, 219, 220
Working students, time management for, 88–89
Workspace, 82–83
Worry trees, 48
Worrying, 48, 175–176
Worst-case scenario, considering, 140

Y
Yama, 269
Yawn, 33
Yerkes-Dodson Principle, 13
Yoga, 285
  benefits of, 276
  common poses, 269–274
  introduction to, 268
  sun salutations, 275
  understanding, 269
  what you need to know, 276
Yogic breathing, 237–238

Z
Zazen meditation, 258
Zen meditation, 258